Theos Bernard, the White Lama

THEOS BERNARD, THE WHITE LAMA

Tibet, Yoga, and American Religious Life

PAUL G. HACKETT

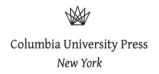

Columbia University Press
New York

Columbia University Press
Publishers Since 1893
New York   Chichester, West Sussex
cup.columbia.edu
Copyright © 2012 Columbia University Press
All rights reserved
Library of Congress Cataloging-in-Publication Data
Hackett, Paul G.
Theos Bernard, the White Lama : Tibet, yoga, and American religious life /
Paul G. Hackett.
p. cm.
Includes bibliographical references and index.

ISBN 978-0-231-15886-2 (cloth : alk. paper) — ISBN 978-0-231-53037-8 (electronic)
1. Bernard, Theos, b. 1908. 2. Yogis—United States—Biography. 3. Scholars—United
States—Biography. 4. United States—Religion—1901-1945. I. Bernard, Theos, b. 1908.
II. Title.
B132.Y6H24   2012
294.3′923092—dc22
[B]
2011011638
♾

Columbia University Press books are printed on permanent and durable acid-free
paper.
This book was printed on paper with recycled content.
Printed in the United States of America
c 10 9 8 7 6 5 4 3 2 1
References to Internet Web sites (URLs) were accurate at the time of writing.
Neither the author nor Columbia University Press is responsible for URLs that may
have expired or changed since the manuscript was prepared.

To Theos Bernard

. . . and all those whose religious vision exceeded their grasp

CONTENTS

ILLUSTRATIONS

PREFACE

How few ever think that there will be one around to check up on them.

— THEOS BERNARD[1]

BEFORE HE HAD EVEN SET FOOT on his home soil in the fall of 1937, Theos Bernard declared to a reporter for London's *Daily Mail*, "I am the first White Lama—the first Westerner ever to live as priest in a Tibetan monastery, the first man from the outside world to be initiated into Buddhists' mysteries hidden even from many native lamas themselves."[2]

Over the weeks and months that followed, Theos's account of his life and the events that befell him in Tibet would grow greater and greater in proportion, coming to nearly obliterate any trace of his actual activities. By March of the following year, having called in a few favors back home, he arranged an alumnus lecture at the University of Arizona, and arriving in Tucson, he pulled out all the stops.

When the curtains parted before a packed house, all in attendance saw Theos Bernard, religion scholar, explorer, and mystic, seated in a chair on a dais in the middle of the stage, next to a movie projector and surrounded by ritual artifacts and Tibetan robes. "Come with me," he invited the audience, "in a flight in the Clipper Ship of the imagination from San Francisco across the vast Pacific . . . into the heart of Asia, the Land of the Lama— Tibet!" and with a carefully practiced grandiose style, Theos Bernard, "the White Lama," unfolded his story, explaining how he had fulfilled an ancient Tibetan prophecy and become "the first white man ever to live in the lamaseries and cities of Tibet . . . initiated into the age-old religious rites of Tibetan Buddhism [and] . . . accepted by the Tibetans as one of them"—or so he claimed.

As the evening progressed, Theos provided even more details of his "recognition" by the Tibetans as a reincarnation of the eighth-century master Padmasambhava. He told of his dark retreat "in the dungeons of the Potala Palace" where midway through his internment, Buddhist monks descending into the black depths of those catacombs were astonished to find him bathed in a "white light" where none could possibly exist, thereby confirming his fulfillment of the prophecy of the coming of the "white lama," a man who would herald and bring about the spread of the truths of Buddhism to the Western world.

With each of Theos's descriptions, the assembled audience was held rapt with attention to every detail. His old grade school principal, Mary Price—who had made the journey from Tombstone to Tucson to hear him speak—recounted that throughout his lecture, Theos walked in his robes through the aisles of the auditorium that was "absolutely quiet except for Theos talking and the sound of your neighbor breathing." It was "the most emotionally packed thing and best talk" she had ever heard in her life—so emotional, she recalled, that Theos was a long time coming down from the stage, surrounded by many people, including four or five of his old law school professors.

After the evening had wound to a close, Theos joined his mother, brothers, and Mary Price for the long drive back to his old home of Tombstone. As the car traveled along the dusty road south toward the Mexican border, Mary asked Theos, privately, if what he had said on stage was actually true. "Every word," was his response.

While Theos Bernard *had* gone to Tibet, *had* met various lamas, and *had* participated in rituals there, beyond those simple facts, little more of what he said on that spring evening, or afterward, had the slightest ring of truth to it. Nonetheless, from the practical standpoint of what he was attempting to accomplish, that lecture in Arizona was a success. Theos received endorsements sufficient enough to secure a contract for a major lecture tour from a public relations firm in New York, and while the details were being arranged, returned to California to spend time with his father, Glen. There, with Glen's help, he began to refine a public persona that would capitalize on the prevailing moods and interests in 1930s America and to no small degree, establish a personal mythology that would serve as a foundation for his life in the years to come.

What actually happened to Theos Bernard over his forty years can only be pieced together from the fragments left in his wake when he disappeared in the fall of 1947. Over the months and years that followed, his friends and family would struggle to make sense of his life as well as their own role in it, some with greater or lesser success—even passing on this obligation to others. The end result would be a scattering of primary and secondary source documents across North America, from Arizona to New York and California to Florida, as well as in parts of India and Tibet, each locale holding different pieces of a puzzle offering glimpses into his life. This book is the result of my attempts to collect those pieces and put together that puzzle. This is the story of Theos Bernard.

In talking about Theos Bernard, there are a number of different ways of approaching him. It is possible to speak of Bernard in terms of his accomplishments in his role as a pioneer. As a first-generation American explorer in Tibet, he was only the third American to successfully reach Lhasa,[3] the capital, and the first "Westerner" (American or European) to do so as a religious pilgrim. While there, Bernard amassed what would be the largest collection of Tibetan texts, art, and artifacts in the Western Hemisphere for more than thirty years[4] and documented, in both still photography and 16-mm film, an age-old civilization on the eve of its destruction. Bernard presented the first dissertation in religion at Columbia University in 1943 and in doing so was the catalyst for the founding of the religion department there. Bernard was the first Westerner to recognize the uniqueness of the scholar Gedun Chöpel (*dge 'dun chos phel*, 1903–51) when they met in 1936, and attempted to bring him to America in 1941. Bernard was also the first American student of Geshe Ngawang Wangyal (*ngag dbang dbang rgyal*, 1901–83), who would later teach at Columbia University before establishing himself as a teacher in New Jersey and, like Dezhung Rinpoche in Seattle,[5] would become the *guru* and *paramguru* to a large contingent of today's American scholars of Tibet. Bernard's list of "firsts" could be continued.[6]

Alternately, it is possible to speak about his role in and influence on subsequent academic and popular interest in Indo-Tibetan religion and culture. Guided by his father over his last two decades, Bernard was groomed as both a scholar and a new religious leader for America in the traditions of Indian yoga and Buddhist tantra. In the late 1930s, he embarked upon a journey to India and Tibet that would set the tone for a whole generation of religious seekers from Europe and America in the 1960s. Within only a few years of his death, Bernard's book on haṭha yoga would be translated into French, German, and Spanish. Slightly more than a decade later, his semiautobiographical works would also become standard reading for a whole generation interested in "Eastern" religions and traveling to India.

Much as 1960s American culture cast its shadow over the latter part of the twentieth century, so too the early twentieth century inhabited a world strongly defined by the nineteenth. The cultural landscape of late nineteenth-century America—which, in many ways, set the stage for Bernard's life—was host to an explosion of alternative religious movements that ran the gamut from modification and innovation to complete repudiation, from Spiritualism and Universalism to Mormonism, Christian Science, and Theosophy. While key figures were producing or revealing new scriptures and pseudepigrapha, others, dubiously credentialed, were importing ideas from India and China wholesale and utilizing them to reformulate normative Protestant Christian ideals.[7] So vibrant were these enterprises that the twentieth-century alternative religious movements that would directly result from them seem little more than their cultural stepchildren by comparison. More significantly, however, the subsequent manifestations of these traditions in American society would retain the marks of that first generation of religious innovators, instantiating the nineteenth-century Protestant ideals of pietism and affective religiosity, anticlericalism, personal unmediated access to knowledge of the divine, and populist and egalitarian notions of participatory religion—all of which were effectively missing in the source traditions of Asia that were being drawn upon. With these movements taking on a life of their own, their putative origin seems to have been less a source of new ideas than a source of new symbols, words, and images divorced from their actual meaning— a *tabla rasa* for the projection of religious fantasies. It was a realm whose pinnacle was Tibet.

Indeed, throughout the late nineteenth and early twentieth centuries there remained, occasionally peeking above the surface, this mythic image of Tibet—a physically esoteric land concealing an even more esoteric body of mystical knowledge. Reports of "high lamas" and ornate temples filled with all varieties of gods and golden riches were standard in newspapers of the day, from references to the "Deliah Lama" to the adventures of Marmaduke M. Mizzle in the "lamasery" of Shigatse.[8] A land "bounded on the south by the highest mountains in the world . . . Tibet could be imagined as a domain of lost wisdom,"[9] and by the 1930s this myth was being projected across America with full force.

James Hilton, in his wildly popular[10] novel *Lost Horizon*—and later the film by the same name—gave these ideas a palatable expression in American mainstream culture. Although the literary trope of "hidden kingdoms" and "lost worlds" was standard for many a writer, from Jules Verne to Arthur Conan Doyle, with the exploration and mapping of most of the known world by the early twentieth century, such tales were the expression, and eventually the last gasp, of nineteenth-century adventurism. By well into the early twentieth century, few spots in the world remained "unexplored" and suitable as a home for "the unknown." While Merian C. Cooper and Edgar Wallace set their "home" on a mist-shrouded island in unnavigable waters in the South Seas, Hilton set his in Tibet, and in 1933, as the icon of just such a lost world, King Kong, was scaling the heights of the Empire State Building before the eyes of moviegoers across the nation, Hilton's *Lost Horizon* was beginning to climb the sales charts in William Morrow's New York publishing offices only a dozen blocks away.

What both visions offered the American public was the hope that another world existed somewhere—a world not ravaged by economic depression, threatened with war, or simply beaten down by the oppressiveness of the mundane. Without even the solace of a cold beer,[11] many Americans found comfort instead in the myth of such "other" worlds, outside of their own and untouched by time. What differentiated Hilton's book from the many that had gone before, however, was its theme. While other authors penned tales filled with pulse-pounding dangers or titillated their readers with descriptions of exotic princesses, Hilton's narrative instead capitalized on the public's enthusiasm for mystical truth, offering the promise of a hidden sanctuary where the knowledge and values of mankind were being preserved and sheltered from the chaos of the everyday world. It was a sanctuary that could only exist in the last such unconquered refuge: Tibet.

Like the otherwise run-of-the-mill conspiracy novel of recent years, *The Da Vinci Code*, Hilton's otherwise run-of-the-mill "lost world" adventure story was distinctive for its religious—specifically, Christian—overtones. Despite the fact that Tibet was and remained the greatest Buddhist kingdom the world had seen in over two thousand years,[12] the sacred "truths" being preserved in Hilton's "hidden valley" of Shangri-La were European truths guarded by a Capuchin friar who had discovered the secret of eternal life. To the "High Lama" of Shangri-La, it was clear that there would be "a time when men, exultant in the technique of homicide, would rage so hotly over the world that every precious thing would be in danger, every book and picture and harmony, every treasure garnered through two millenniums, the small, the delicate, the defenseless—all would be lost." More than just physical artifacts, it was also the "universal truths," endangered and forgotten in the world outside of Shangri-La, that concerned the monks of that "lamasery." As one lama in Hilton's novel asked, "Must we hold that because one religion is true, all others are bound to be false?" implying a deeper truth that they had found underlying the various religious "truths."

Tibet was—for Hilton and so many other writers who tried to capitalize on the book's success (Bernard included)—the natural sanctuary for all knowledge and the place to which those who sought it would have to journey. It was a destination that only a few—privileged by wealth, power, or mysterious good fortune—could reach. In an era when a well-funded explorer could circulate among the highest echelons of society, Bernard did precisely that. In his brief lifetime, Bernard met, associated, and corresponded with the social, political, and cultural icons of his day, from the Regent and leading politicians of Tibet to saints, scholars, and diplomats in British India, and such notables as Sir Francis Younghusband, Charles Lindbergh, Mohandas Gandhi, Jawaharlal Nehru, and Franklin Delano Roosevelt.

Bernard himself first came into the public eye in 1937, when his exploits in Tibet landed him on the front page of *The New York Times.* It was the same year that Frank Capra released his film version of *Lost Horizon.* When Theos Bernard returned to New York that fall, he brought with him precisely the images and stories he needed to play into the popular mythic identity of Tibet as Shangri-La. Of Shangri-La itself, the film concluded with the declaration, "I believe it because I want to believe it." Of the many who flocked to see and hear Bernard regale audiences with his adventures, they too believed him because they wanted to believe. Although not so imaginative (though at times almost as fictitious) as Hilton's story, Bernard's own account was just as romantic, for unlike those who had gone before, he was seeking something different. Alexandra David-Neel, William McGovern, and others had all told what there was to find, he declared, "but no one has revealed what lies behind that which exists, and here is my task." For Bernard as well, it was a foregone conclusion that there was special knowledge to be found in Tibet. Indeed, by the 1930s, this fascination with Tibet as a locus of esoteric knowledge was by no means novel. If anything, it was merely the latest round in a series of ongoing exercises in the counter-cultural circles that he was participating in. It was yet another episode in the search for a new, undiscovered level of reality within the realm of human grasping—knowledge of which the right person could bring back to the West.

Thus, in telling the story of Theos Bernard, this book also recounts the story of one "America"—a counterculture America that was irresistibly drawn eastward toward the spiritual landscape of India and Tibet. From the earliest murmurings of vague and ill-conceived fascinations in the late nineteenth century down to the cottage industries of the present, this mythic image of the East—and of Tibet in particular—has been and remains a compelling icon in the American psyche. What inspired such journeys of both mind and body for many, and where it led for one, is what this book hopes to tell.

ACKNOWLEDGMENTS

SEVERAL FRIENDS HAVE BOTH HELPED and encouraged the writing of this book over the years. First and foremost in that list is Craig Schenck, who has been both a sounding board and source of insights into the mind and life of Theos Bernard. Like Theos Bernard, having attended the University of Arizona as an undergraduate and pursued my Ph.D. at Columbia University in New York, I owe a certain debt of gratitude to Bill Magee, who continually counseled me against following too closely in Theos's steps. I owe an equally unrepayable debt of gratitude and love to Rabia Magee, who, from my earliest days in graduate school, housed me, fed me, clothed me, and cared for me in more ways than can be listed.

To my close friends and fellow graduate students at Columbia, David Kittay, John Campbell, and Erika Dyson, who have helped, supported, entertained, tolerated, and occasionally (when necessary) berated me, I give my deepest, heartfelt thanks and affection. Similarly, to Bryan Cuevas, whom I have been fortunate enough to call a friend from my earliest days in graduate school up through the present, deepest thanks for his counsel and continued camaraderie from Charlottesville to Berkeley, to Lhasa, New York, and many points in between. Likewise, to Chris Kelley and Stephanie Syman, Tom Creamer, Michael Horlick, Pema Gutman, Odette Worrell, Peggy Shannon, and many others, who freely offered their friendship, encouragement, and support, and other countless friends and acquaintances as well, who have endured being subjected to the "tales of Theos Bernard" over the years (not to mention my irritability as my research neared its conclusion)—I cannot express my thanks enough.

Numerous other people have contributed both directly and indirectly to this research. I would like to thank Gen Lozang Jamspal for his assistance with deciphering some of the more obscure references in Tharchin's written Tibetan and his help with numerous Tibetan cultural cues and historical anecdotes. Thanks also to Bob Love, who shared early versions of his research on Pierre Bernard with me, and to Cathy Albanese, whose helpful discussions provided me with additional perspectives and insights on American religious culture. Thanks to Kathleen Taylor, who provided her copies of correspondence between Glen Bernard and Atal Behari Ghosh, and to June Calendar for sharing some of her reminiscences of Viola Bernard.

Special thanks are also due to Barbara Graham of the Helen Graham Park Foundation, who not only saved numerous primary source materials from certain destruction but also generously made them available for research and study, as well as offering her kind company. Though I never had the chance to meet her, Viola Bernard herself contributed to the telling of Theos's story, by saving and archiving every letter and cablegram he wrote as well as his diaries and copies of all personal papers and interviews, compiled from the early 1980s until her death in 1997.

I wish to convey my deepest thanks and gratitude, as well, to the family of the house of Tsarong, including Mr. Dundul Namgyal ("George") Tsarong, Mrs. Yangchen Dolkar Tsarong, Mr. Jigme Tsarong, Mr. Paljor Tsarong, Mrs. Namlha Takla, and their families, who continue to uphold the great name of Tsarong through their generosity and kindness. Thanks also to the many individuals in Kalimpong and Darjeeling who graciously shared their time, stories, historical documents, and photos with me, including Nilam Macdonald at the Himalayan Hotel (Kalimpong); Mr. Sherab Tenduf La at the Windamere Hotel (Darjeeling); Mr. Hlawang Pulger at the Bellevue Hotel (Darjeeling); Swami Prabuddhananda of the Ramakrishna Vedanta Ashram (Darjeeling); Mr. David Tharchin, who made the contents of his grandfather's office available to me for research during my stays in Kalimpong; and Rai Sahib Sonam Kazi, first minister of Sikkim and his family; in Dharamsala, the venerable Geshe Lhakdor, director of the Library of Tibetan Works and Archives, and the members of his staff; Daniel Entin, director of the Nicholas Roerich Museum, and Dr. Alena Adamkova, director of the International Roerich Memorial Trust, each of whom took time from their busy schedules to answer my questions about the Roerich family; and finally, to the many people throughout the Kulu Valley, in Lahoul and in Spiti, who kindly took me into their confidence and provided much information—only portions of which, at their request, are related here—all of whom must remain anonymous.

Similarly, I remain indebted for the assistance and encouragement that I received from Amy Heinrich, director of the Starr East Asian Library at Columbia University, and from the staff of the Columbia University Health Sciences Archives, Stephen Novak, Bob Vietrogoski, and Henry Blanco, and for their help and friendly company during the many weeks and months I spent in their offices. Thanks to the staff of the British Library as well for assistance in accessing the Oriental and India Office Collections, in particular, Tim Thomas, David Blake, and Penny Brook.

Thanks to the faculty and staff of the University of California at Berkeley; at the Bancroft Library: Anthony Bliss, David DeLorenzo, Jane Rosario, and Lauren Lassleben; at the Hearst Museum: Victoria Bradshaw, Joan Knudsen, Manda Maples, and Malu Beltran; and the faculty and staff of the Center for Buddhist Studies: Robert Sharf and Liz Greigg. Thanks also to the staff of the Smithsonian Institution (Suitland, MD), New Mexico Palace of the Governors (Santa Fe, NM), the University of New Mexico Center for Southwestern Research (Albuquerque, NM), the National Postal Museum Library (Washington, DC), the Jacques Marchais Museum of Tibetan Art, and the National Archives and Records Administration.

Many thanks to Tsewang C. Tethong of the University of British Columbia and Elizabeth Napper of the Tibetan Nuns' Project, who kindly gave their time and assistance in identifying and locating references and sources.

Special thanks go to Isrun Engelhardt, Heather Stoddard, Elliot Sperling, and my many other friends and colleagues in the field of Tibetan studies who have assisted and encouraged me in the pursuit of this subject over the years. I would be remiss, however, not to mention the influence on my life of my teacher for the many years I lived in Charlottesville, Virginia, the very venerable Geshe Jampel Thardo. Without his patience, guidance, and presence in my life as a true *kalyanamitra*—then and since—I would never have survived those first few years of my education, let alone reached this point. No less so, I remain eternally indebted to my advisor, Jey Tsong Khapa Professor of Indo-Tibetan Buddhism here at Columbia University, Professor Robert Thurman, who years ago provided the opportunity to continue my studies when I had given up trying and has never failed to be a source of encouragement, support, guidance, and friendship throughout this entire experience.

Finally, special thanks are due to Wendy Lochner, Christine Mortlock, Leslie Kriesel, and Peggy Garry at Columbia University Press, who helped make the publication of this book a reality, guiding me through the final days leading to its publication.

Theos Bernard, the White Lama

ONE

Life in the Desert

The vibrations . . . of many spiritually seeking souls come floodlike to me
[and] I perceive potential saints in America and Europe, waiting to be
awakened.

—ŚRĪ YUKTEŚWAR[1]

TO BE BORN IN AMERICA just after the turn of the twentieth century
meant coming of age in a land on the verge of a new cross-cultural renaissance. For several decades, many religious figures, like the more famous
Swami Vivekananda and others, toured the cities of America, introducing
people to "the wisdom of the East." When examined in detail, many of the
themes that resonate throughout the American religious subcultures of
today had their roots in this first generation of Indian mystics and their
Anglo disciples and religious seekers.

"I am not a believer in miracles," Vivekananda declared to a *Washington
Post* reporter in 1894, "they are repugnant to me in matters of religion."
"Mr. Kananda," the correspondent went on to report, presented "the, to
orthodox sects, rather original proposition that there is good in the foundation of every religion, that all religions, like languages, are descended
from a common stock, and that each is good in its corporal and spiritual
aspects so long as it is kept free from dogma and fossilism." Nonetheless,
Vivekananda reaffirmed the basic tenets of his Indian religious roots while
couching them in modern terms:

> I claim no affiliation with any religious sect, but occupy the position of
> an observer, and so far as I may, of a teacher to mankind. All religion to
> me is good. About the higher mysteries of life and existence I can do

no more than speculate, as others do. Reincarnation seems to me to be the nearest to a logical explanation for many things with which we are confronted in the realm of religion. But I do not advance it as a doctrine. It is no more than a theory at best, and is not susceptible of proof except by personal experience, and that proof is good only for the man who has it. Your experience is nothing to me, nor mine to you. I am not a believer in miracles—they are repugnant to me in matters of religion. You might bring the world tumbling down about my ears, but that would be no proof to me that there was a God, or that you worked by his agency, if there was one.[2]

Vivekananda's statements easily could have been issued fifty or a hundred years later by an American adopting a decidedly Protestant Christian form of Indian spirituality. Yet it is hard to tell whether Vivekananda simply expressed Vedic ideas in a manner palatable to American audiences or was promoting a now commonplace, nascent Indian worldview—the result of British colonialism.[3] Either way, such comments were common in the alternative religious circles of the late nineteenth and early twentieth centuries in America as Indian religious culture began to make its mark on the cultural landscape. Indeed, not long after the arrival of such figures as Vivekananda, Paramahansa Yogananda, and others, someone remarked,

In the imagination of the great majority of Americans, foreign missions has been an altogether one-sided affair. Taking for granted the superiority of Christianity, they have pictured the Christian movement as going out to over spread the world.

To thoughtful minds, it has long been obvious that there would soon come a time when the great Eastern religions, sure of the superiority of their spiritual life over the mechanized living of the Western world, would come to us with the deep conviction that they were the heralds of the world's true gospel. . . .

Christianity is at work in India and Hinduism is at work in the United States . . . and there is no possibility of American religion escaping the influence of the great Indian faiths.[4]

It was in the midst of just such a fervor arising from that intermingling of cultures that Theos Bernard was born, on Thursday, December 10, 1908, to two "students of the East," Glen Agassiz Bernard and Aura Georgina Crable.[5]

Although born in Pasadena, California, Theos was raised by his mother in Tombstone, Arizona, having been abandoned by his father before the age of two. Returning to her childhood home, Aura Crable was very discreet about the father of her child and the circumstances of their meeting. When asked, she would only say that he had been a fellow student at a divinity school in New York City, and that he had left her to follow his religious calling.

Although some of the details of Aura's story may have raised the eyebrows of her neighbors—such as her son's rather un-Christian name, Theos Casimir Hamati Bernard, or the volumes of books on Indian philosophy crowding the shelves of her home—the polite discretion of the times afforded her a cushion of safety and anonymity. Working as a postmistress in the town and filling in as pastor in the local Episcopal church, Aura formally divorced Glen and seven years later (according to strict Episcopalian rule) remarried, to a local mining engineer from Scotland. With Jon Gordon, Aura had three more sons, Ian, Dugald, and Marvene, and together they raised the four boys in the deserts of southern Arizona.

Although it may not have been the wide Mississippi of Tom Sawyer or Jim Hawkins's pirate-infested islands of the Caribbean, the hills and canyons of southern Arizona were a fit adventure land for teenage boys. Where a scant fifty years earlier, Cochise and his Apache warriors had fought the U.S. cavalry, by the 1920s the Dragoon Mountains were dotted with makeshift mining camps and filled with families of prospectors. The Gordons' own camp lay a short distance from Tombstone, just over the hills from their house behind Sheepshead Mountain.

Growing up in that small town, the Gordon boys spent their summers in the hills, playing poker with the miners, swimming in riverbeds filled by the summer monsoons, chasing each other through the desert scrub nestled between granite cliffs, and occasionally blowing up parts of that landscape with sticks of dynamite stolen from local mines. Theos and his brothers joined the newly founded Boy Scouts, Theos and Dugald both becoming Eagle Scouts. Theos also participated in the "Lone Scouts" program, a regimen of studies designed for boys living in isolated parts of the country. As a Lone Scout, he learned skills outside mainstream scouting in a program that stressed independent activities and self-reliance, as well as proficiency in written and radio correspondence and survival skills.

In addition to these influences, his stepfather tried to instill in Theos and his brothers an appreciation for a scientific, though not a rigid, approach to life. Dugald recalled an incident when his father was hired by a local property owner to assay his land for its mining potential. When Jon Gordon and Dugald arrived to perform the task at hand, they found a second man, a dowser, had been hired for the same purpose. Gordon was given a map to the mine and a compass and instructed to go underground to map the locations where he thought the ore would be, while the man with a dousing rod was set up above ground to do the same. When both had finished, the property owner compared their results and showed the two men that their assessments agreed. "Do you believe this?" Dug asked his father. "Well, son," Gordon replied, "these are the kinds of things you will be having to make decisions about in your life . . . don't reject something that you don't understand until you have a basis for doing so." It was this sort of attitude on the part of his stepfather, combined with his mother's strong religious influence, that Theos later acknowledged as having shaped many of his preconceptions about the world.

Among the Gordon boys, Theos, being the oldest, was the leader his younger brothers looked up to. He played football in high school as captain of the team, together with his two close friends, Billy Fowler and Dan Hughes. He was the favored son everyone thought would make the family proud, and he was receiving a good education as well. Despite its remoteness, the Tombstone school system was good for its day. When high school graduation came, there was no doubt in the minds of all three friends that they would go to college. Billy chose to study engineering, while Dan and Theos chose law.

The decision to pursue a legal career was not difficult for Theos. His grandfather, William Harwood, had been the first mayor of Tombstone, had played an instrumental role in the Arizona Territorial Assembly's bid for statehood, and was involved in the founding of the University of Arizona, while his uncle Francis was a lawyer in Prescott to the north. Times were changing for Tombstone, and even though Theos, Dan, and Billy would be the only graduating students from Tombstone High School in 1926 to go on to college, he and Dan wouldn't even be the first local kids to go to law school.[6]

While Dan's father had made some money early on as a cattle buyer in northern Mexico[7] and Billy's family had seen good fortune in the mines, the Gordon household was not well off, and the costs of a college education

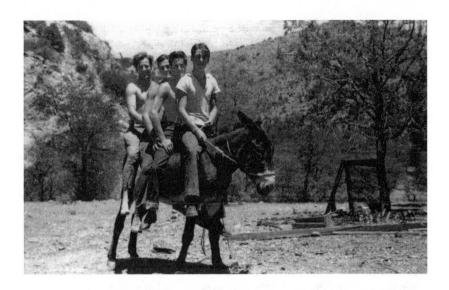

Figure 1.1 The Gordon brothers in the Dragoon Mountains: Theos, Ian, Dugald, and Marvene (AZHS)

were not small. Although Jon Gordon had been educated as a geologist and had a good grasp of geological theory, he had poor practical mining skills and an even poorer business sense. As a result, while many of the families around them grew wealthy from the mines, the Gordons failed to prosper. Nonetheless, with a bright future in front of him, Theos got a paper delivery route in Tombstone, while the rest of the family contributed what they could to his college fund. Jon Gordon didn't show Theos any special favors, though. Even when he would stay out late—at a high school dance one town over in Saint David, or just carousing with his friends—Gordon would roust him out of bed at 5 a.m. to do chores, hoping to instill in him a sense of duty and the value of hard work.

Entering college in Tucson at the newly founded University of Arizona, Dan and Theos were accepted to the College of Arts and Sciences, and Billy to the College of Engineering; they all lived together in the college dormitories and spent their time like typical college boys, drinking and chasing girls. Unlike Billy and Dan, however, Theos was more reckless and worse yet, couldn't hold his alcohol. "A couple of drinks," Dan remarked, "and Theos would start raising Cain." On one occasion after coming home from a movie, the boys had gotten a bottle of liquor and carried on drinking in the parking lot behind Cochise Hall dormitory. After a few drinks, Theos was once again out of control. Deciding to go to his room, he jumped up and started climbing the fire escape up the back wall of the building. Convinced he would fall to his death, Billy and Dan started yelling at him to come down. "You think I'll fall?" he said, and laughing, let go of the fourth-floor railing and leaned backward, dangling by his knees for several minutes.

As a young man, Theos was both athletically fit and academically well grounded, and entered college well prepared for the experience on all fronts. A rugged, yet handsome football player, he attracted the young women of Tucson with ease, and—as his friend Dan observed—when it came to such things, Theos was "a red-blooded American boy"; on more than one occasion, his boss noted, Theos would be seen standing on the street, saying good-bye to a girl in the morning before coming in to work at the part-time job he'd taken to support himself in school.

Near the close of his first year of college, Theos underwent the same ritual hazing all freshmen traditionally experienced at U of A—being thrown in the fountain in front of the first building on campus, "Old Main." On a cold, rainy spring day, however, the chill from a simple prank developed into first a chest cold, and then rheumatoid pneumonia. Getting worse day by day, Theos was hospitalized and eventually withdrew from school early, a scant two weeks from the end of the academic year. A victim of medical incompetence on the part of the school's resident doctor, Theos probably would have died had his mother not intervened, insisting on taking him home to Tombstone and the doctor of her choice.

Theos was now under the care of a family friend and osteopathic doctor who believed in the mind's ability to influence and heal the body, but Aura still had reasons for concern. By the time Dr. Agnew saw him, Theos was so stiff and weak from his illness that he was completely unable to move and had to drink fluids through a tube. Put on a special regimen with constant medical supervision and spending the summer as an invalid, he only gradually recovered.[8]

Regaining his strength enough to return to school in Tucson a few months later, Theos spent the next year completing his core curriculum classes and by the spring of 1928 was ready to progress in his studies. When he returned to Tucson for his third year of college in the fall, he officially switched from the College of Liberal Arts and Sciences to the College of Law. With the stock market crash of 1929, however, life became much more difficult for everyone in Tucson, especially Theos. Struggling under increased hardship, he continued his studies and with the help of a scholarship in his final year,[9] managed to graduate in June 1931 with his Bachelor of Law (L.L.B.) degree.

Theos stayed on in Tucson while his friends Billy and Dan left to look for work. It was a difficult year for Theos. His childhood friends had gone, and he was "on the streets" looking for work as America sank deeper into economic depression. As the weeks passed, the life he had chosen for himself was looking less and less appealing. Just after graduation he was lucky enough to find a summer job clerking for a local judge and working part-time in a law office, but it didn't provide much of a life. His friend Dan, however, had gotten a job as a court interpreter for a judge back in Tombstone, Judge Sames. Through his new contacts, Dan managed to get Theos a job with the *Tucson Daily Citizen*, a newspaper owned and operated by a friend of Judge Sames, General Frank Hitchcock. As the months passed while he worked at his different part-time jobs, Theos became more and more convinced that a law career was not for him.

By January 1932 he had decided to return to school, and began taking classes at the university again while he tried to sort out his life.[10] Working his professional connections in Tucson, he managed to get a job for the summer as a court clerk in Los Angeles, where two fellow alumni from the Arizona law school were then living. Determined to make a career move, Theos took the opportunity to attend summer classes at USC as well. It was then and there, in Los Angeles, that he reconnected with his estranged father, Glen, after a twenty-year separation.

In the course of his studies and travels over the years, Glen Bernard had been a student of several different teachers. Born in 1884 in Humeston, Iowa, he was the second oldest in a family of all boys. Before Glen had turned ten, however, his father began to have severe mental difficulties; eventually he was institutionalized. Taxed with the strain of raising five boys under these circumstances, their mother, Kittie, sent the oldest, Perry, to Lincoln, Nebraska, to an uncle who could offer a stable environment and provide a strong male role model.

Before the Golden Spike was struck in 1869 completing the transcontinental railway, Nebraska had marked "the end of the line"—the farthest destination easily attained of an ever westward-moving "gateway" to untamed lands. By the time Perry Bernard arrived twenty-five years later, the cities of Nebraska had grown much more cosmopolitan, so much so that in his new home of Lincoln, Perry chanced to meet a strange resident, a Hindu yogi who went by the name of Sylvais Hamati.[11]

With or without anyone's consent—no one is sure—Perry became a student of Hamati, learning yoga and the fundamentals of Indian philosophy, eventually becoming the titular head of Hamati's organization, The Tāntrik Order in America, for which he adopted the name of (Dr.) Pierre Arnold Bernard—some say, to capitalize on the notoriety of a famous French physician—and to which he would eventually (and unilaterally) append a long list of credentials.[12] Over the next twenty years, Pierre, with the occasional assistance of Glen[13] and their brothers and friends, established and ran a series of sanitariums and "clinics" in the Pacific Northwest, from San Francisco to Seattle, St. Louis, and Chicago, before eventually moving to New York.[14]

By 1907, the Tāntrik Order seemed to be on solid footing, so much so that Hamati decided to return to India, turning over the operation and direct oversight of the organization to the Bernard brothers and their inner circle of followers. Within three years, however, the organization was in trouble. Pierre—by then branded in the tabloid newspapers as "The Omnipotent Oom"—found himself on the wrong side of the law, facing multiple charges of fraud and morals violations for his dalliances with young students at his yoga studio after being unfairly tied in with the "white slave trade" scare. Meanwhile, Glen had run off with a young orphaned girl who had come to New York to study for the lay ministry,[15] Aura Crable—whom Glen affectionately, if somewhat pretentiously, referred to as "L'Aura."

Although Pierre recovered from these setbacks—though without losing his tabloid moniker—Glen disavowed his brother for what he considered a debasement of the teachings through capitalization on yoga for material and personal gain. By 1910, within a few years of being married, Glen, maintaining his sincerity in the study and practice of yoga, told Aura that he could not live the life of an ordinary man—a "householder," in Indian religious parlance—but had to follow the religious life. The "Yogic Sciences" to which Glen claimed to be devoted required careful study and commitment; "spurious occultists"—as he later came to characterize his brother—were merely "prostituting a science of which they know not so much as the first principles."

With this justification, Glen abandoned Aura with a one-year-old baby, sending her back to her childhood home of Tombstone, but their relationship remained amicable—even affectionate—belying a more than sympathetic attitude on Aura's part for Glen's aspirations. Even in the midst of discussing their divorce proceedings, Aura declared to him, "I can never cease to desire to keep you and how I hope my opportunity will come . . . for I always want to know you have love for me, for your life is dear, very dear to me."

Despite her affections and understanding, Glen went through with the divorce, and it seems that he and Aura never saw each other again. Following a brief return to New York in 1911, Glen spent ten years working as a common laborer for the railroads and in the mines of California, and as a part-time electrician. All the while, however, he continued studying with various Indian scholars and yogis, most notably the early companion of Paramahansa Yogananda in America, Swami Dhirananda, a disciple of two famous yogis in India: Swami Kebalananda and Śrī Yukteśwar.

By the time Theos arrived in Southern California, Glen was living in Los Angeles in the spiritual shadow of Yogananda's ashram nearby in Mount Washington—the Self Realization Fellowship. Although Yogananda and Dhirananda had had a falling out, there is nothing to indicate that Glen had a strained relationship with Yogananda himself, who, it is said, visited him on more than one occasion.[16]

Glen took the opportunity of his son's presence that summer to bridge the distance in their relationship, and to introduce him to Indian philosophy and the practices of yoga as a long-term treatment for his physical condition. Even though to all outward appearances Theos had recovered from his undergraduate illness, in actuality he had not, for it had been quite severe, leaving him chronically physically weak with an enlarged heart.

Over the course of the summer, Theos learned the basics of yoga, from the preliminary practices to simple postures, his favorite being the headstand. Glen also took the time to teach his son some of the fundamentals of Hindu philosophy. When he returned to Tucson in the fall, Theos had a new direction and purpose in life, and he knew what he needed to do to fulfill it.

Returning to the University of Arizona, Theos got a job at the Law Library and rematriculated for a full course load, this time concentrating on philosophy and religion, taking courses on classical literature, philosophy, and classical Greek to complement his earlier study of Latin. He also began to do yoga in his spare time and eagerly showed off what he had learned to his brothers.[17] About his rationale for this time of his life Theos later wrote:

> I had been told that I should find some way to become economically independent. It seemed to me that if I ever became enmeshed in the practice of law, there would never be any time left for my other studies; so I decided that I would follow the direction of philosophy. . . . If I was ever to give instruction in these Eastern teachings in America, it would first be necessary that I fully acquaint myself with our own philosophical heritage. In the end, I hoped I would be in a position to interpret the East in light of the West.[18]

Though his purpose seemed clear, Theos had little in the way of resources to finance such an ambitious goal. Although he claimed he had secured a connection to Columbia University by having met a "Dr. Culp,"[19] a Columbia professor who was lecturing while on vacation in New Mexico and Arizona in the summer of 1933, Theos knew well that an Ivy League school was beyond his financial means.

By the early 1930s, the streets of Tucson were filled with thousands of unemployed men, and many people had debts from the corrupt "Morris Plan" banks that had offered poor and low-income workers unsecured loans. Theos had debt collectors after him, and was anxious to earn as much money as he could in the hope of leaving Tucson. In a bold move, he went to one of the collection agencies that was pursuing him and rather than paying his debt, offered instead to work for the firm as a collections agent for a percentage of the returns. Thomas Tormey, the head of the agency, took him up on the offer, and although Theos never paid his own bill, he did work for the agency and managed to earn some cash.

The opportunity that Theos needed appeared in early spring 1934. Dan Hughes remembered that it was a warm spring afternoon in Tucson when he and Theos were sitting in the Law Library, working. Dan, in need of distraction, picked up a back issue of *Fortune* Magazine, and leafing through the pages, came across a story of a man in New York with his own elephant.[20] He pointed out that the man in question was also named Bernard, and Theos immediately identified him as his uncle, someone his father had undoubtedly told him about.

A far cry from the press accounts of his past—or anything else that Glen might have told him about his uncle—the profile of Pierre Bernard in *Fortune* depicted a successful businessman and financial pillar of the community of Nyack, New York. Though there was mention of "teaching Yoga and Sanskrit around the country," the adventures of "the Omnipotent Oom" were little more than an anecdotal backdrop. Long forgotten as the fraudulent proprietor of "the Temple of Mystery" sanitarium, Pierre was described as having "a flourishing practice in treating brain and nervous diseases in New York City." Moreover, he was now a bank president; the head of construction, real estate, and mortgage companies; and the owner of his own stable of elephants and a fleet of vintage Stanley Steamers. In the depths of the Great Depression he was, in a phrase, stinking rich.

Without any hesitation, Theos took pen to paper and wrote a letter to his long-lost uncle introducing himself, speaking of his love of yoga, his hopes for the future, and his aspirations of attending school in New York. A few weeks later, a small envelope appeared in the mail for Theos, postmarked Nyack, New York. It was his uncle's reply, in the form of an invitation to attend the annual Easter Party at the Clarkstown Country Club.

TWO

New York and New Mexico

I have . . . goals, ends, purposes for this life—it may not appear that I ever accomplish a great [deal], but as long as I make a certain development, this span of life's eternal circle has been complete. I feel that I have brought something [that is] a little out of the ordinary and that it must have its chance to express itself and continue on in its growth. This is a feel[ing] that has been with me for many years and something that is far more than an idea—it is a feeling—perhaps from the unconscious, but it has manifested itself many times in the conscious when I have been with myself in silence.

—THEOS BERNARD[1]

OVER THE COURSE of the previous fifteen years, Pierre Arnold Bernard—known simply as "P.A." to the members of his country club—had carved out a private social and religious empire for himself. To the club's patrons he provided a combination of *de facto* marriage brokering among the like-minded offspring of New York socialite circles and a socially liberal atmosphere of education and entertainment (mostly the latter). To the younger crowd, he provided a protected enclave and constructive outlet for a post-Victorian generation seeking a spiritual redefinition of themselves and the world around them, as well as a shelter—for those whose families could afford it—from the harsh realities that most people faced during the depths of the depression.

Although punctuated by visits from American and European notables—from New York Governor Franklin Delano Roosevelt and Leopold Stokowski to Queen Elizabeth—the atmosphere at the country club remained very insular. Early in his career in Nyack, New York, just twenty miles north of Manhattan across the Hudson River, Pierre Bernard established his own real estate company; shrewdly buying up most of the property adjacent to the country club, he then sold it off to the membership at a considerable profit. P.A. maintained his solid base of support by encouraging—if not arranging—marriages between members and between their children. Perhaps in a lapse of judgment, he hadn't tried to stop his friend Winfield Nichols when he announced his betrothal to one of P.A.'s patron's daughters, the psychologically troubled Barbara Vanderbilt. It was an inaction that Pierre would regret, for when the marriage turned sour, he soon lost the favor of the Vanderbilt family despite having disavowed his friendship with Nichols from that point on. Putting up with such foolish con men was the price the intelligent ones had to pay for their success. Pierre survived, and so did his country club—with new patrons—and for most the scandals only added a little more spice to life in an environment where everyone knew everyone, if not as neighbors, then by reputation.

In April 1934, a newcomer arrived at the club whom Pierre soon realized he would have to contend with as well: his nephew Theos. Muscular, tan, and handsome, Theos made an impression on the partygoers at the club—including his uncle's wife, Blanche DeVries, who later claimed she "swooned" at the sight of him—as a handsome new face among a well-known closed community. Although to his family and friends in Arizona he was known as Theos Gordon (using his stepfather's surname), when Theos arrived in Nyack, he introduced himself as Theos Bernard, using his legal name to emphasize his relationship with his uncle. As she later recalled, "it was a beautiful Easter day," and to a young Viola Wertheim, a day made more special by meeting Theos. "We met and we were drawn to each other." For Theos, the day would prove special as well, for, any other considerations aside, Viola was one of the principal patrons of the Clarkstown Country Club, and marriage to her would provide precisely the sort of financial backing that he needed in order to attend Columbia University.

Viola Wertheim had grown up in New York City in the early 1900s, born to a family of wealth.[2] Her parents having divorced at an early age, she and her sister, Diana, lived with their mother, spending their days under the care and supervision of various tutors. It was their music instructor who got them interested in Eastern philosophy, and by extension, in yoga and Pierre Bernard's country club—a teenage interest fed by "the secretiveness . . . excitement . . . and cult-like nature of it all." Enraptured by the novelty, "Vi" and "Di" (as they were called) began staying at the country club for

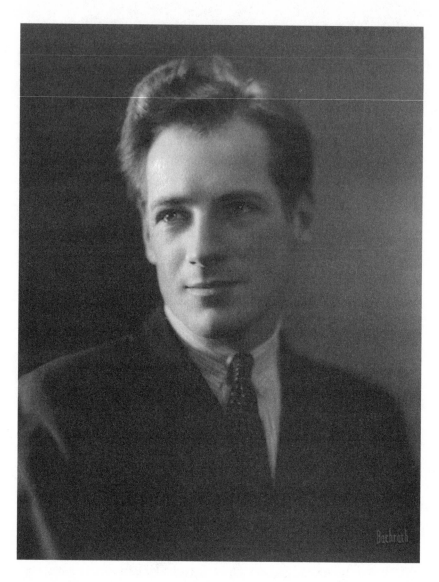

Figure 2.1 Theos Bernard, ca. 1930 (CUHS)

extended periods of time. Fearing her daughters were being drawn into a cult, their mother, Emma, went so far as to purchase land and build a house directly adjacent to the club so she could keep an eye on them.[3]

While Diana seems to have viewed her life at the CCC (Clarkstown Country Club) as a social adventure, Viola took a more serious interest in Indian religion and philosophy. At the age of sixteen she went so far as to study

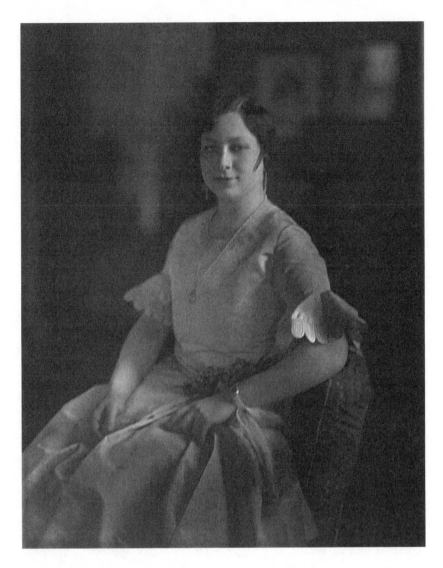

Figure 2.2 Viola Wertheim, ca. 1930 (CUHS)

Sanskrit with the noted linguist A. V. Williams-Jackson, then a professor at Columbia University. As the years passed and the more sordid aspects of the club's "cult-like nature" became increasingly apparent to her, she slowly distanced herself. She still attended social functions from time to time and remained very close to Pierre's wife, Blanche (or simply "De-Vries" to her friends and associates).[4]

By the end of that spring day in 1934, Theos and Viola had struck up a close friendship, and although Theos had to go back to Arizona, he vowed to return to New York immediately after graduation. True to his word, he graduated from the University of Arizona on May 30, and four days later, hitching a ride with the father of a friend, left Tombstone for New York.

Within a matter of weeks, Theos and Viola were deep in a romantic relationship. "Theos and I decided that we were so completely sure of ourselves and of each other that to waste this leisure of the summer together by waiting any longer would be very wrong as it means all our first adjustments in marriage would have to be made while we were working," she wrote, explaining herself to her brother, Maurice. She continued,

> We decided we'd get married on the third of August, and then take a six weeks trip out west to meet his family. Theos wants to get his Ph.D. in Philosophy—he was enrolled for the fall at Harvard, but is now going to go to Columbia, and we'll live in New York and study together and make a grand go of things, I know.

But there were many more concerns for Viola than the simple adjustment to married life, the most important being her fiancé's surname. Although the sensationalistic reports about Theos's uncle Pierre had faded from the front pages of the tabloids, the telephone and telegraph operators in Nyack, it was rumored, were on the payroll of the local papers, and "Oom the Omnipotent" was still a household name in New York City.[5] Few journalists of the day would have allowed the name of Bernard to pass unnoticed—as Viola's sister, Diana, had learned when she married Pierre's personal secretary, Percival Whittlesey, some years earlier.

Reassuring her brother that it would be a mistake to think that "a quick marriage was necessary, and that the family didn't approve," she spoke glowingly of Theos's acceptance by the whole family. As she had had to do with her mother, Viola pleaded with Maurice not to hire a private detective to investigate Theos's background: "since father's death we've used detectives against each other, always with good intentions, and always with unpleasant results as far as our family relationships were concerned. I assure you in this case there is not the slightest necessity and there would be the strongest hurt."

Reassuring him repeatedly that Theos was not simply pursuing her for her money, she told him:

Theos, himself, has considerable zinc holdings in Arizona, which tho less lucrative right now than in the past (obviously) are still adequate to make him financially independent. . . . I wrote this to answer questions you might hesitate to ask. I am entering this new phase of existence with eyes and heart wide open—my decision was reached through the assistance of every ounce of judgment, analysis and maturity at my command. . . . If the future proves I had made a mistake, mine will have been the responsibility and mine the price to pay, and no one else's.

More than a statement of mere mutual financial accountability—a lie on her part, she well knew—her letter to her brother was a heartfelt personal plea to not ruin a relationship she felt deeply about.

We seem to share interests, hobbies, opinions and point of view, in addition to loving each other which all add strength to the foundation. For me he fulfills more aspects of myself than I ever hoped from anyone— and I seem to for him. The key fits the lock if you know what I mean—I'm sure you do. His kinship to Dr. Bernard is an asset in the sense that my contact with the club and Dr. Bernard has been so close and of such long standing that it would be harder for me to work out an utterly complete understanding with a man who couldn't appreciate my point of view towards the Nyack situation. . . . Theos is a strong, definite and independent person and our life together is something quite completely our own and only ours in every sense.

Ironically, as the news of their impending marriage filtered through their social circle, the strongest objections came not from Viola's family but from Theos's. When they heard the news, both his father and his uncle were opposed to the marriage: Glen because he thought Viola was merely a tool being used by Pierre to get his hooks into his son, and Pierre because he feared Theos was stealing one of his principal funders—a fear that was quite justified.

Theos managed to persuade his father that his fears were ungrounded, or at least, not unseen by Theos himself and marginal given the potential benefits. "It is a little after 4am," he wrote,

but I must give you the latest developments. I have just finished a long conference with P.A. who has been on his high horse. We did not give into anything—but did get him quieted down. . . . At present—& has been of this opinion for some time—she feels that P.A. is doing everything to keep her around for her money (you know the answer) however she is still feeding him—but it is not going to cut in on *our* lives to cause us any unhappiness. He is trying to school us both for going to school—wants us to live here—and also is trying to persuade us not to take our trip West—damn him—he is crazy—he is cutting his own throat—for she is suspicious of all—I am beginning to drop hints—eventually I will tell her some facts—not until she is ready, however. She just turned over $25,000 to him—so you see her loyalty even tho she is suspicious—she hates to believe it. . . . Anyway—Dad—I see much trouble ahead marrying this girl with all her dough—if I was not so far into it—I would tell her no— unless we severed all—it would start us out on a different basis. The way it is—I am going to have to do a certain amount of "playing the game"— however—it is probably worth it—I am getting ahead & she is with me 100%—he had better never get too funny. If he plays his cards right & we support him—he (*might*) will the place to me—god knows who he could leave it to—& it is a beautiful place—make us a luxurious country estate with our other one next door. I wonder if P.A. could be that decent—to even think of me—my wife has virtually made him.

Theos's hopes on all counts were naïve, for Pierre had no intention of giving up so easily, let alone of submitting to his nephew's control over Viola, even in the context of their new relationship. Lulled into a false sense of security, Theos believed that P.A. had been convinced, but it was not so:

P.A.—as you said—he cannot keep his hands off. Until yesterday, a day before—we were going fine—not a word from him—but it couldn't last. He got wind of the fact that we had just leased an apt. & that I had registered at Columbia and did he get hot and bothered—the 1st excuse—he came out with it all. Today he is trying his darndest to knock a Ph.D. and talk me out of going thru with it—trying to get Vi to give up her work. Here is what he has done to her—She has been here 10 years—has never got anywhere with yoga & says she has never seen anyone here who has—But he tells her that he is *now* ready to give up *his secrets* of yoga to *her* and let her get somewhere; so she doesn't know whether she is missing the opportunity of a life time by refusing his hand or not. She has faith in him—feels he has something—doesn't know what—so she is up in the air. . . . He makes me sick.

As Viola did with her family, Theos assured his father that he was serious about his relationship with Viola:

She is in favor of me & feels we should go ahead and get something *definite* that we understand—following an academic training. . . . Vi and I want to grow together and we feel that by working together at school will be the best way. . . .

I do like this girl—and do not want P.A. causing us any trouble—she will be one with whom I can always work—broke or rich—so she is a treasure. Her money helps—but her character means more.

The only remaining concern for Theos, his father pointed out, was breaking the news of his engagement to his mother back in Arizona.

The Ariz. girl is a question—knowing her temperament—I am going to give her the story all at once—then try to smooth it down. I would rather tell her than have another tell her—and all my friends will soon know. If she will be halfway decent—I will go 95% of the way—but she will have to obey. I know her will and what she can and will do—however—I will do my best with good intentions.

Theos succeeded in dealing with the situation and in the end, Pierre was forced to see the futility of his objections, for ultimately neither he nor Glen had any say in the matter. Viola too prevailed over the voiced and unvoiced concerns of her friends and family and on Wednesday, August 1, 1934, she and Theos were married in a private ceremony in New York City.[6] Initially thinking to take their honeymoon in New Mexico and Arizona, they eventually decided on a train trip through Chicago up into the Canadian Rockies, from where they drove down to Los Angeles to board a ship bound for New York via Central America.

By mid-September they were back in New York, in their apartment on the east side of Midtown Manhattan near Cornell Medical School, where Viola was studying, and settled into married life. For Viola, medical school coursework was a major focus of her life, while for Theos, though likewise enrolled in a full load of courses at Columbia, the preoccupations were the same, with one exception: all but two of his classes were for "residence credit," that is, credit only for attendance, with no grade given. He was auditing nearly all his courses.

At least part of Theos's rationale for taking this approach to his education at Columbia seems to have been a certain disdain for what constituted the academic discipline of "philosophy." When Theos passed through its doors in 1934, the department at Columbia still bore the mark of the recently retired yet still highly esteemed philosopher of pragmatism, John Dewey. Theos's own advisor and chair of the department, Herbert Schneider, had been one of Dewey's students, and like Dewey took a pragmatic approach to philosophy. It was not the sort of approach Theos was interested in, and it left him feeling "very discouraged."

Despite their coursework and the constraints it placed on their lives, Theos and Viola found the time to take occasional vacations together, whether upstate at the country club on the weekends or skiing in Canada and swimming in Cuba. By the beginning of the spring of his first year at Columbia, however, having had his fill of Greco-Roman and continental philosophy, Theos had decided to try his luck in the anthropology department, in the subfield of comparative religion. Looking for summer employment along those lines, Theos worked his contacts in the philosophy department.

Early that spring, Theos was put in touch with Morris Cohen, a philosopher at City College of New York. Cohen's son, Felix, had been employed as a lawyer for the U.S. Department of the Interior's Bureau of Indian Affairs (BIA), where opportunities for lawyers with experience in the American Southwest were just becoming available. Following the Meriam Report of 1928 exposing the extreme levels of poverty and illness in Native American communities, Felix Cohen and the Commissioner of Indian Affairs, John Collier, had drafted a new set of guidelines to restructure the tribal governments, guidelines that eventually became the Indian Reorganization Act of 1934. By 1935, the Department of the Interior was prepared to implement the provisions of the act across the country. Hearing that the BIA was seeking lawyers with anthropological experience, Theos would have considered himself a perfect candidate for one of the posts—were it not for his health.

Concerned about the lasting effects of Theos's early illness, Viola insisted that he visit a cardiac specialist. The doctor's findings were not good.

Theos's chest x-rays revealed an enlarged and weakened heart with potentially life-threatening valve lesions. Understandably upset at the prospect of her husband suddenly dying or being reduced to the state of an invalid, Viola worried all the more given Theos's penchant for reckless behavior, especially in her absence.

Moving forward with his plans just the same, Theos drew the assignment for the New Mexico Pueblos, and Viola began to plan the summer in northern New Mexico with him so she could avoid being separated from her husband, monitor his condition, and exercise some restraint over his activities. But by the end of the spring it became clear that Viola would have to remain in New York well into July to finish her internship in obstetrics at an outpatient clinic in the Bronx, so, resigned to spending several months apart, just before Theos left for New Mexico they took a short trip to Haiti and Jamaica.

Although a year earlier Viola's mother had bought them a new car—a 1934 Cadillac Club Sedan—as a wedding present, Emma Wertheim allowed Theos to take her own car, an old convertible Roadster, for his trip out west. From the day he left, Theos phoned, wrote, or cabled Viola nearly every day throughout the summer, despite being occupied with work from the moment he arrived. Nonetheless, he and Viola missed each other dearly, being separated at length for the first time since their marriage. Viola wrote of the emptiness she felt in her heart, feelings made more painful by the realization that her commitments would most likely prevent her from visiting Theos at all and they would have to spend the entire summer apart.

Suggesting that they plan their eventual reunion in Guatemala, Theos tried to console her, saying, "Remember we are philosophers at heart if not in name and the ever changing panorama of life only tends to deepen our insight into the futilities of the objective world and worth of the feelings of souls together [and] my one purpose is to have a perfect expression of love between us." Promising to write her every day with the details of even the most mundane events of his life, Theos did precisely that, and unlike Theos, Viola saved every letter and scrap of paper he sent her.[7]

While Viola was forced to focus on the physiological aspects of the human condition, the summer afforded Theos the opportunity to reflect on the grandeur of life in the desert—as well as practice his skills at representing it on paper.[8] Accompanying Commissioner John Collier, Theos spent his first week attending conferences and traveling around the Southwest, visiting the pueblos and reservations of New Mexico and Arizona. No less striking in 1935 than it had been hundreds of years earlier to so many others who saw it then or hence, the town of Taos, New Mexico and the journey to reach it were both inspiring and captivating to Theos:

> The drive up is an excellent example of beauty out of nothing, for the road is nothing but a ruff, bumpy, dirty, dusty road winding its way along the thick and muddy Rio Grande under a dry and scorching desert sun hedged in on both sides by barren rocky hills which rise abruptly from the river, forming sheer cliffs at the top with rock slides beneath, which only need a huff and poof to dislodge them. From this description you may begin to wonder where one is going to find something that can be called beautiful. It is the barrenness itself that reflects the beauty, and your uncertainty of getting through that stimulates you to a point of appreciation. At the end of this canyon which extends for many miles, you rise up on a mesa which continues up to the base of Mt. Taos whose peaks are covered with snow and where few white men tred, for it is the sacred possession of the Indians and they patrol it very closely; so I will have to climb it this summer.[9]

Although he was unaware of it, Theos had drawn the most difficult assignment among the bureau's locales. Of all the Native American communities in the area, Theos chose to focus on the Taos Pueblo, one of the most stable and strong in the Southwest—a position it held by maintaining a strict isolationist policy toward outsiders. Even knowledge of the Taoan language was forbidden to non-natives. Worse yet, the strength of the Taos community meant that Theos would have little leverage in getting the BIA's constitution adopted by the tribal elders. The Governor of the Pueblo explained that the social organization of the community and their religion were intertwined in a manner that had been passed down "from mouth to mouth" for centuries and they had no intention of relating its details to Theos, much less allowing representatives of the U.S. government—or any other white men, for that matter—to dictate changes to it.

While his prospects for successfully completing his official job were small, Theos held out hope that he would still be able to negotiate some sort of agreement between the Pueblo council and the BIA or, at the very least, be able to compile a report suitable to submit to the anthropology department at Columbia. While he waited for the situation to improve,

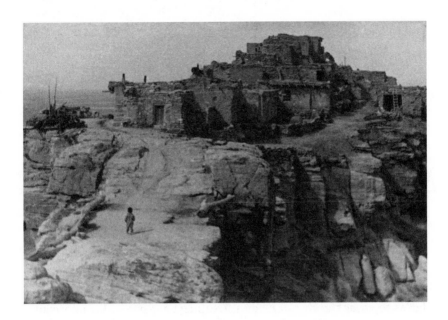

Figure 2.3 Walpi (Hopi) Pueblo, Arizona, July 1935. Photo by Theos Bernard (NAA)

Theos took the opportunity to practice his photographic skills with the new Leica camera he had brought with him, experimenting with different lenses and settings. Try as he might, the camera was difficult to master, and he lamented his inability to steal the occasional forbidden photograph of a Native American ceremony or even take a suitable portrait of the Pueblo governor.[10] It was a simple enough problem, but for Theos it, like so many others, led to deeper reflections, which he shared with Viola:

> the present governor who is also the medicine man for the pueblo—he has a beautiful face filled with a million wrinkles of kindness, I would like to get a good picture of it—before the end of the summer if I may—if I keep trying and can win their friendship—all I can do is be sincere, and this I want to develop, for it is something that we tend to lose in our own culture because of the many faces that we have to put on in order that we may gain certain ends—it is difficult to be simple, plain, and sincere—but I am looking forward to the day when this will be the only side of my life I will have to live—for to me it is through that that we are able to grow spiritually—even if you do not think that we have a spirit.

This is one of the reasons that makes me love you so dearly . . . with you I can be as I truly want to be . . . you are my anchor and rudder in life, no matter what I do, I find that I need you more and more—each day you become more a part of me.

Despite his sincerity, and even with the assistance of one of Collier's local contacts, Theos was unable to gain the kind of inroads into Pueblo society he had hoped for, much less instigate institutional change. Even after he secured an invitation to meet with the tribal council, though he was allowed to ask many pointed questions about the structure of the Pueblo government, it was rather *pro forma* and only later, on camping trips with his Pueblo informants, Tony and Adolph, was he able to glean meaningful information. Although he would complain and berate them about their lack of enthusiasm for what they saw as taking dangerous risks,[11] nonetheless Theos felt a certain degree of responsibility for his contacts, going so far as to cover the cost of medical treatment for one of his informants' family members suffering from trachoma.

Having read his accounts of it all, Viola expressed concern over Theos's fast-paced schedule, even reiterating the warning given to him by his physician not to overexert himself, but he simply would not listen. Theos continued his activities—both professional and recreational—with abandon, from racing around the countryside at 70 miles an hour in his mother-in-law's Cadillac to climbing to the peak of Mount Wheeler at 13,000 feet. One evening, however, after a 36-hour, 600-mile round-trip, Theos returned to Santa Fe fatigued, with his heart pounding and short of breath—effects that recurred off and on for a week.

Despite such setbacks, by July Theos was feeling far more confident of the knowledge he was acquiring—on a personal level, if less so in the context of his job—and even wrote to one of his professors at Columbia, Ruth Benedict, chair of the anthropology department, suggesting that she let him teach her "Southwest Indians" course upon his return, if not teach a course of his own, and requesting copies of her notes on the "Papago"[12] Native American community. But despite his declarations of expertise, his professors remained far from enthusiastic about the idea of turning over their courses to a master's student with merely a year of rudimentary courses under his belt. Such a lackluster response prompted a certain degree of resentment toward academia in general, which he expressed to Viola as ambivalence about me being an anthropologist . . . that in the last analysis that the decision is up to me—true if it is of any importance but I hardly think so here. You know what my one desire is and anything else is only one which will work in the best with the world of affairs—and I hardly give a dam [sic] what it is. If you like to have an anthropologist around—O.K., if you prefer philosophy—maybe O.K. then too, if you prefer a business man, well, we will see. I want something that is worthwhile and not too confining as philosophy is likely to be and that will lend itself to my one purpose which you are familiar with.

For Theos, whatever career path he chose would be merely a social formality, and a temporary one at that, compared to his deeper interest in yoga and Indian religion. For the present, he felt, the mundane activities of employment were "perfectly all right, for we both have work that has to be done, but later one of us will have to give up their job so that we can be together." The same would hold true, he told her, even in the following year when they would go to India, after which they could "steer their paths together," including having children.

As time passed, Theos was feeling more and more comfortable about his choice of locations for the summer, for the lands of Taos—the area that had inspired Ansel Adams to abandon his previous photographic habits for a more modern realistic style[13]—was one of the most beautiful locales in North America, even if the town proper was populated by a predominantly artist community and an assortment of spiritual seekers, for whom Theos had a certain degree of disdain:

The people were a very nice group of useless souls trying to find a way in life, but never enough internal stimulus to hold them to the path of true understanding. They were all artists. . . . They are intensely interested in something which they call occultism—well I gave myself away by showing an interest which I can not help once I see the reflection of a desire. They have gone the usual course—through Theosophy, Rosicrucian, Baha'i-ism, and then into eastern philosophy. They are acquainted with a great deal of literature and all such intellectual things, and as they have shown to me, the intellectual side has been too heavy and they have fallen by the wayside. . . . They have never been able to find a way of applying what lies behind the mental to the problem of everyday living. . . . They seem to sense that I know something and continue to pound away, but I always find a way out, but of course I can't very well leave them unless I point to some path. It is all rather amusing, but I seem to always run on to this sort of thing and if fate does not bring it to me, I dig it up. From them I can learn nothing, except as I am able to understand their problem and will be better able later on in life to lay a way for those of this type to follow. . . . It is always a little distasteful for me to talk with people of this type, for they are so filled with words and their actions are so poverty stricken. They have contacted such shallow depths that their understanding or ability for receiving is warped, and you can only talk to them through their own language. But there are ways of making them follow when you find that there is a desire to follow but not the courage of heart to go alone.

Nonetheless, Theos remained enamored of the area surrounding Taos Mountain. "The country is perfect," he told Viola, "and I know that you would like it . . . so I could see no reason for not choosing it." Of course such considerations and ruminations were not what he was being paid for, and by early July when he filed his first report to the Bureau of Indian Affairs after weeks of silence, their response was not a happy one. "I caught hell today from the main office," he told Viola—especially from Collier, since he had ignored the recommendation that he study the San Juan Pueblo rather than the one at Taos, given the known difficulties of working there.

Having to bite his tongue in the face of their anger and plead his case to the bureau, he got members of the committee overseeing the operations to admit that he "seemed to be doing unusually well." But the hardest part for Theos wasn't conducting the research or reporting his findings, it was having to deal with criticism and submitting to bureaucratic authority. "If they would leave me alone here I could get most anything out of them [the Taos Pueblo]," he wrote to Viola. The BIA administrators, other than his immediate supervisor, "are just about to get under my skin, but no—I can fool them, too—I will continue to smile and let them think that everything is all right. . . . I want to learn all that I can, and so I will try to please until I have what I want . . . dam them—I will see to it that this experience proves invaluable to me."

Indeed, his experiences with members of the Pueblo were proving to be of exceptional value to Theos, offering insight into yet another culture, for their way of life, upon reflection, *did* seem superior to the troubled and confusing approach of the average American, even if it didn't quite live up to the level of esteem he accorded to Indian philosophy.

We had a long talk about the world, its beginning and how life continues on it—etc. all along metaphysical and ethical lines which was rather interesting. They are true natural philosophers. One is almost inclined to think that there is something in that more or less naïve viewpoint of life. At least it does not seem to tie up their insides in knots as is the tendency of many of our complex viewpoints—except the viewpoint you and I have—that is the one and only true outlook and nothing but good will come of it if just a little understanding is used with it. One cannot proceed with anything by mere blind faith. Faith will lead you into a blind drift every time if some reason is not applied—but there is a right and wrong way of applying reason, and there is a place for faith.

However, Theos was under orders to leave Taos and conduct a survey of all the other pueblos, which he agreed to, grudgingly.

Just the same, when Duncan Strong, his traveling companion from the BIA, arrived, he encouraged Theos to continue his activities and negotiations at the Taos Pueblo:

Dunc thinks that I am doing all right. He says that I can expect all the old foggies [sic] to think that I am doing everything wrong, but not to be bothered about it for I am the first person in this country to ever try such an experiment and that I have everything to gain and nothing to lose and therefore stay with it. They have been at their old ways for sometime and have produced very little and now if I can find a new way of securing information that I will have made a really very encouraging contribution to the field. . . . This will be the first time that anthropology has been used for a practical purpose and it is [his] feeling and that of several others that if it is going to stand up as a science that it will have to reproduce something that can be used and that I am making the first effort.

With a renewed sense of the value of his insights and a certain degree of vindication from a colleague, Theos thought again of Columbia:

Many more trips like this and there will [be] little left for me to cover in this neck of the woods. Gee, if I could only give Benedict's course on the South West Indian it would put everything in fine shape. It seems to me that one who has studie[d] the country and the ways of the Indians and then traveled over the entire area should have some qualifications for teach[ing] such a course.

It was a conviction concerning his qualifications that would increase in the weeks that followed as he met archeologists on the payroll of the BIA and visited more and more reservations. But all these activities were put on hold when Theos received word that having successfully passed her latest medical exams, Viola was flying out for a visit.

Although Viola managed to come for a week at the end of July, she was unable to stay any longer, and as a result they had to spend their first wedding anniversary apart. Returning to Taos, Theos promised that it would never happen again, and wrote to her:

> This summer has wiped out all questions and melted us together once and for all. There is no more adjustment for us to [do]. The only adjustments that are left are the ones that we as one have to make to the ever changing circumstances. The [separation] of the summer has been really worth while and told us a great deal, and the week we were together showed us how right we were.

Convinced of the strength of his relationship with Viola, Theos was equally convinced of his ever growing knowledge of the Pueblo communities, knowledge that outstripped that of his boss, Collier, whom he felt "only has the outside facts to talk about," but—unlike Theos—no real insight. So assured of himself, he concluded that he would undoubtedly be put in charge of Ruth Benedict's course on Southwestern Indians at Columbia, if not hailed as the foremost authority on them; after his experiences during the summer, Benedict was "just going to have to start teaching on some other section of the country."

Not everyone was as confident of Theos's abilities as he was, from Collier in his assessment of his reports to his colleagues' lack of faith in his ability to safely drive a car. One rainy evening in particular, "with the rain all day, the road home was like a sheet of ice; so even the return was unusually frustrating. Molly drove. They would not trust me. It seems they think that I drive a little fast."

Putting the best face on things, Theos decided to return to New York in time for the start of classes, although he had originally planned otherwise. Even before meeting with Collier, Theos resigned himself to the inevitable.

I am very much inclined to believe that I am not stay[ing] on here, of course I can give him [Collier] a big song and dance and perhaps persuade, but I do not feel that I should. . . . I do want to finish up something here; so if he does not want me to stay, I will try to figure out something that will be of some use and try to do it before the year is over.

Indeed, as he feared, Collier insisted that Theos study a second pueblo, for comparison purposes if nothing else. Making a small concession, Collier agreed to allow Theos to continue interacting with representatives of the Pueblo in Taos so long as he agreed to move his base of operations to the Acoma Pueblo, some sixty miles west of Albuquerque and almost two hundred miles from Taos.

Theos's hopes having been slightly deflated, he wrote to Viola reminding her—and himself—of their true, primary interest: India.

There are definite plans for next year which mean a great deal more to me than it would mean to me if I rose to be the greatest anthropologist of this country and any ten other countries. . . .

I should keep the fact in mind that we have a friend in India and that it will behoove me to be there with him and after all that is what I am after in this lifetime and it is the only thing that makes me feel that I am doing something that justifies my existence. These other many things tend to only create a feeling that they are only an excuse to be waiting. . . . From the looks of things, it will be best for me to go there and make the next small step in my development, or at least, gather that which is to be used for that end and a little while later.

Although voiced in mundane terms of logistical concerns, far more central to Theos were the metaphysical implications for his own life, reflections he could not keep to himself:

I am aware of the necessity of my completing something of this nature in this world to which I have been born—it too is a part of my own understanding. . . . I have . . . goals, ends, purposes for this life—it may not appear that I ever accomplish a great [deal], but as long as I make a certain development, this span of life's eternal circle has been complete. I feel that I have brought something [that is] a little out of the ordinary and that it must have its chance to express itself and continue on in its growth. This is a feel[ing] that has been with me for many years and something that is far more than an idea—it is a feeling—perhaps from the unconscious, but it has manifested itself many times in the conscious when I have been with myself in silence.

Although he had given voice to such thoughts in Viola's presence before, when he set them down in writing this time they disturbed her. It was true that Theos and Viola shared a certain appreciation for Indian philosophy and the larger issues surrounding yoga and the like, but Viola was training in medicine, which included psychiatry. An interest in a religious system was one thing; deep-seated convictions of spiritual purposes in life were another thing altogether. Upon receiving her response, Theos found himself trying to recover from his earlier, hastily written words:

> For some reason or other, I got talking to you tonight. This I have done very seldom on paper, but it all started coming and before I could call a hault [sic], I had said enough that it was best to finish or at least, continue for a while. I much prefer having you near when I do this, for I have such screwy inward feelings that you may not quite understand what I am talking about sometimes. . . . I am not saying that I am sorry—I am saying that I love you and love you dearly—I doubt if even you understand even tho you profess to know all about it.

Still concerned about a misunderstanding, before even mailing his letter, Theos placed a phone call to Viola.

> There did I talk to you tonight—I enjoy talking to you more than anything else that I do. That is what we are for—as you have said—and I want us to learn to talk to each other and so bring our lives closer together—as you say that we may have the same roots. . . . I am glad that we can always talk these things over and then decide together and so stick with one another—this is the way we want our lives to always go—hand in hand.

Having reassured her to a certain degree, Theos continued to write for the rest of the summer, but restrained himself from expressing such thoughts beyond their association with his career and his decision to commit to either philosophy or anthropology, at least until he could do so in person again:

> I want to see what each department is offering this year and what possibilities I have, because a final decision has to be reached this fall—and I have been driving toward philosophy for a good many years now and it is going to take a great deal to pull me away, from the academic standpoint. As far as my life is concerned—it is impossible. I have my inner ambitions and plans for activity in my later life and want to make sure that the direction that I go today will not take me to [sic] far afield. You have a very screwy individual around—and the problem is to make sure that too much screwy-ness is not stirred up for the time being. This [is] enough for the present—we will go into it later.

Try as he might, however, the subject of his own purpose in life was something that Theos kept returning to, mostly instigated by Viola's feedback on his career decisions:

> I do not think you have the right attitude, for regardless which direction I go—anthro or phil—I will always feel that they are both so unnecessary and inconsequential that it will be difficult for me to hold on to the end. There is only [one thing] for me and you well know what that is and until that is my entire life, I will never be satisfied. I finished up satisfying people and attaining what others consider to be of some significance when I was admitted to the bar [to] which I can always return. If it is ever necessary, I will be admitted to the N.Y. bar, but as far as something worthwhile is concerned this to me is far more honored than any other degree or profession bar none, at least, it is the only [thing] that I have any tolerance for. This other training that I am doing now is just doing two things—marking time and giving me information about the West that may be a little helpful in selling certain Eastern Teaching if it should ever become necessary that I have to sell the thing that means so much to me and that nobody else seems to understand. As far as the degree is concerned—it makes no difference whats so ever [sic], however it would be nice to tack onto the name if needs be, but I will probably never have any direct use for it.

Finally, he concluded, "it will be a great deal easier for me to get my Ph.D. in anth at Col. [Columbia] than it will be in phil. because of the backing and interest that I am receiving; so it might be well for me to take advantage of it." And so, planning his return east, Theos plotted a circuitous route through the Southwest and California, touring the country—accompanied by DeVries, his uncle's wife and his wife's best friend—before heading to Washington to submit his final report and returning to New York, Columbia, and Viola.

THREE

Two Parallel Paths (I)

What is needed most today is for someone having an intellectual understanding of these scriptures to actually go through the various ritual stages,
thus gaining by experience an estimate of the truth of the teachings.

—THEOS BERNARD[1]

AS JOHN COLLIER sat in the offices of the Bureau of Indian Affairs (BIA)
reading Theos's report on his time spent among the pueblos of New Mexico, he grew more and more annoyed; it was far from anything he had expected or asked for. Along with his own letter, he sent the report to William
Duncan Strong, the staff anthropologist for the Smithsonian Institution's
Bureau of American Ethnology, who had been "loaned" to the BIA as a consultant and had worked with Theos in New Mexico, asking for his opinion.
When he received Strong's response a few weeks later, it was not what Collier had hoped for either. In addition to using the opportunity to present his
own assessment of the problems faced by (and some times exacerbated by)
the BIA, Strong defended Theos and argued further that rather than con-
demning his approach, it should be taken as a model for future fieldwork:

> The investigator to whose report these remarks are appended was a
> beginner at ethnographic research and this, paradoxically enough, was
> why he was chosen to inaugurate the new program. Unpleasant historic
> contacts, combined with a naturally esoteric political and religious or-
> ganization, have led the majority of pueblo peoples to develop a mas-
> terly protective mechanism of silence or evasion against all scientists
> seeking factual information on such subjects. The ethnologist has per-
> force met guile with guile and as a result the great mass of fragmentary

ethnological information extant has been secured and published in the face of native opposition.

Unfortunately many of the leading ethnologists that have worked in the Rio Grande area have either become so imbued with evasive patterns learned from the Indians or so besmirched in native eyes through revelatory publications that their usefulness in the present crisis seemed doubtful. Hence a student whose methods were unconditioned by past usage was chosen for the direct approach. Bernard's ethnographic results are thin, due primarily to lack of time but also to lack of experience. *However, he demonstrated quite clearly that the direct approach through the pueblo political bodies at Taos and Acoma was not only possible but enthusiastically received by the Indians themselves.* With adequate time to approach the inner values and sanctions behind their formal and, in some cases, evasive expressions he would undoubtedly have been able to present for either Taos or Acoma a living picture of a functioning pueblo. He, or others, can still do this, and *until it is done* the idea of preserving pueblo life by constitutional means must remain an absurdity.

Beside his definite recommendations regarding organization with which, in the main, we agree, Bernard demonstrated that the tactful, sincere and objective student of their affairs will be welcomed by almost any of the functional pueblos. His failure to secure adequate factual material, aside from his inexperience, *lay primarily in the shortness of his stay and secondarily to the fact that he was shifted from one place to another through administrative action.* Now is the time to place at least two young but thoroughly trained anthropologists among the Hopi and the Rio Grande pueblos, respectively, to begin this new type of work. Within six months we venture to say that the Bureau of Indian Affairs would receive invaluable information regarding many of their most acute problems. With the passage of some years of this intensive observation such direct values would be increased tremendously. No administrator, inevitably swamped in routine economic and legal matters, can get this information. Only a student thoroughly trained in ethnology and social science and working with *but independently* of the administrative forces can do this.[2]

That Collier had viewed the Taos Pueblo as a subject of investigation he wished to preserve for himself seems clear from his negative response to Bernard's initial assignment there as well as Strong's clear personal critique in the closing remarks of the letter.[3] More difficult for Collier was how he would represent the results of the program he was overseeing. In presenting his *Annual Report to the Secretary of the Interior* months later, Collier omitted all mention of such issues, stating simply that Dr. Duncan Strong had returned to the Bureau of American Ethnology and that during the previous summer "a number of anthropological collaborators were sent out to various tribes . . . to gather facts that will help insure that the constitutions being drawn are based on the actual social organization and institutions of the particular tribe or group, thus giving reasonable assurance that such constitutions will become an integral part of tribal life."[4]

Theos, for his own part, had left such concerns behind. He knew what he had needed to do that summer and in his own mind had just done it: the successful completion in New Mexico of a dry run for India. It mattered little what Collier and others thought—his research was not for their consumption, nor something that they should even know about. Indeed, by now one thing that Theos had learned from both his father and his uncle was never to state publicly what he privately thought and felt. America, in their opinion, was not a friendly place for nondevotional religious practitioners; moreover, it was downright hostile to the sort of yogic religious activity that all the Bernards were actively pursuing.

"God made me the messenger of the new heaven and the new earth of which he spoke in the Apocalypse of St. John," Christopher Columbus wrote in 1500, "and he showed me the spot where to find it."[5] For many at the time, this "New World" was not merely a fortuitous discovery by a faulty cartographer. It was a find that, in the wake of the fall of Constantinople, would lend to the nascent Protestant movement in Europe a feeling of validation and historical predestination, seeing the American continent as a land ripe for conquest and reformulation along the lines of the utopian ideals espoused for a "Christian" (i.e., Protestant) country.

Three hundred and fifty years later, the United States had not turned out as Columbus or anyone else following him had hoped. By the mid-nineteenth century, social tensions between the northern and southern halves of the country were on the verge of tearing the nation apart, and when the dust of the brutal and bloody Civil War had settled, the scars it left on the American populace and landscape were just as much psychological as they were physical. The states of the old Southern Confederacy lay in smoldering ruin, waves of non-Protestant and non-Christian immigrants were landing on both the eastern and western coasts of the country, the rapidly industrializing cities in the North were becoming increasingly secular, and rural areas were rife with alcoholism and promiscuity. If anyone had thought that America would evolve into a Christian utopia—a "Millennial Kingdom"—before, by the late nineteenth century it was a myth that few could sincerely espouse.

Beyond its obvious social dimensions, this clear failure to build a perfect Christian kingdom in America had far more disturbing implications: it seemed nothing more than a testament to the ineffectualness of human agency in the world. Over the decades that followed, many Americans would struggle to come to terms with this realization in their religious lives. It would take close to fifty years in Christian circles for a new mythology to reform, around a literalist interpretation of scripture advocating an adherence to certain "fundamentals."[6] Others in the country still committed to earlier Protestant ideals—in spirit if not in word—would explore many different avenues of religious identity for themselves and the country as a whole. Some would look to science for guidance.

Harkening back to the idea of "natural theology," which had given rise to the scientific disciplines a century earlier, members of the growing "Spiritualist" movement began to consciously frame themselves against detractors as advocates of a "science" of higher-order phenomena. In the words of one defender of the movement:

> If he [the scientist] has not time to leave his fossils and insects, to cease his delving into the earth for dead stones, or to relinquish his fine-spun theories of philosophy, let him not carp at those who have had time to listen to the intelligences who come with word of mouth and can give positive testimony to the world—who can prove as the result of their investigations that it is true our friends live.[7]

Repeatable "investigations" (seances) with properly trained investigators (spirit mediums), it was claimed, could demonstrate the existence of an otherwise invisible psychophysical reality (a metaphysical hidden world). In adopting the language of science, the Spiritualist movement attempted to claim legitimacy for its findings. Despite being flawed in many popular applications, by the end of the nineteenth century such appeals to empirical methodologies had high stature, serving as a motivation for others with more Indic fascinations, such as the Theosophical Society, as well as scholars in nonscientific academic circles to do likewise.

Indeed, just as the scientific community of the nineteenth century had cut its theological roots and moved away from the ideal of validating the Christian religious worldview toward a more descriptive approach to reality, many notable scholars of religion and society were finding such an approach equally appealing. Individuals like William James and Rudolph Otto, for whom the validity of religious experiences in general was personally affirmed, concluded that the lack of apparent validation for any one religious tradition through scientific methods should be taken to imply the superficial relativism of all religions. What they all concealed, it seemed, was an ultimate religious "Truth" accessible only through induction. These men presumed that a "numinous" reality—a realm of "the divine"—existed and was the object of both experience and worship in religious traditions. While this view may have drawn criticism as some attempted to derive a typology of religions and religious experience, the existence of a universal and commonly accessed realm of "the sacred" or "divine" was a palatable premise easily accepted by the more liberal segments of the general populace.

In the spring of 1936, as Theos sat at his desk to compose his master's thesis for Columbia University on the state of research into Indian tantric ritual, such an idea was not just a theory but rather an obvious truth. For Theos and others, insofar as all religions could be said to partake in a common religious Truth, it seemed only reasonable that some might be more accurate representations of this Truth than others. To Theos, the religions of India (and soon, he would add, Tibet) were just such traditions. But such ideas were dangerous ones to express in an academic environment. In negotiating his way through the university system, he knew he would have to make his choices and tread with caution.

Indeed, at the end of the previous summer, Theos had summarized his thoughts on academia for Viola in light of their pending trip to India, while at the same time agonizing over his best course of action at Columbia University:

> I do feel that it will be best to arrange things so that we go over there next year even if it necessitates putting off the degree for a couple of years longer, I can always use the extra years of academic training as much as I despise it. The only thing that will ever satisfy me is philosophy for that is the creative field which is for me. There is nothing creative in anthro as far as I am concerned—it is only restoration[8] and this

does not please me very much. However there is nothing that is being taught in the schools of phil today that means a great deal to me, for I am positive that they are all off on the wrong foot and therefore it is difficult for me to work with them. The thing that I want to do for the rest of my life is to develop myself and thereby set an example that is worthwhile for others to follow. This is the one thought that I have held to for so many years and it has directed my actions in many cases. If a thing is not good enough for me to live twenty four hours of the days, I do not want to waste my time talking about it—I do not see this putting ones beliefs off for an armchair discussion and then living exactly the opposite to his beliefs and teachings. They must all be one for me and this is what I propose to do and I think that my life so far will exemplify the fact that I have at all times held to this principle. In a few years I am going to want to spend all of my time in talking, writing, and practicing my own philosophical beliefs which are of Eastern origin so there will be no room for the training that I have received in anthrop. So the questions boils itself down to this—which is the easiest way to get a Ph.D. and which will give me the best excuse to go to India and study that which I am interested in, and which will permit me to carry on as I wish in the teaching of what I have been able to learn both through reading and through practice. In every case the answer is just about phil., but I do hate to bother with what I have to go through in getting the degree. It will be a great deal more interesting working in the other department. . . . True enough I will get more cooperation and recognition from the anth department than the other so it might be best to choose it from this standpoint and I am sure that it will be a lot easier to get the degree. I will do like many others have done—waste their lives until they are forty getting ready to do what they think is best because they first wanted to satisfy everyone else—to hell with the rest of the world—they do not know what is right— if they did our civilization would be a lot different today. The individual has to decide what is best and then go out and get it for them and the first few generations usually have to be martyrs before the mob catches on that they were trying to help them.

Far from expressing these thoughts to his academic advisor, Theos had to put his best face forward when he returned to Columbia. Deciding to take what he saw as the quickest path to a Ph.D., he matriculated for a full course load in anthropology. Theos was anxious that he and Viola not

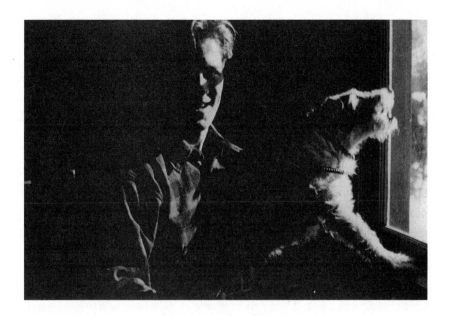

Figure 3.1 Theos Bernard with Jumbo, ca. 1935 (CUHS)

waste any more time than necessary in academia so that they could "be off to work on that which has so subtly welded our paths together—when we come back—you can have babies or practice and anything of the many trivial trails of life that catch your fancy and I can do likewise."

But Theos's first priority when he returned to Columbia was making a good impression in the anthropology department, although it would prove to be a challenging environment. Franz Boas—first professor in anthropology at Columbia, who had just retired in 1935—had turned over leadership of the department to one of his two main students, Ruth Benedict, Theos's new advisor. Both Boas and Benedict were instrumental in shaping the nascent field of anthropology. Boas had argued for a rigorous methodology focusing on a "four-field approach" of human evolution, archeology, language, and culture, while Benedict emphasized the importance of the concept of culture while attacking what she saw as racism and ethnocentrism in the field. Although Theos made a good effort in telling his would-be professors of his activities over the summer, even giving a talk at Columbia on his research among the pueblos of northern New Mexico, his work was far from methodologically rigorous. The talk was well received, but not surprisingly, insufficient to convince the department to give him a lectureship. Instead, Theos was forced to carry a full courseload for the fall. By the following spring, it was clear to him that he would not be able to submit a master's thesis on yoga to the anthropology department, and instead Theos registered for thesis research in the philosophy department, choosing the chair, Herbert Schneider, as his advisor.

At the time, Schneider was the only professor of religion in the department—indeed, he held the only academic position in religion at Columbia, the Schermerhorn Chair of Religion and Social Works—and although he agreed to supervise the thesis, he did not share many of Theos's personal or professional attitudes toward religious matters. Schneider was, for the most part, still very much a follower of John Dewey, his own advisor, and his pragmatic approach to philosophy. Dewey himself felt that what could be called "Truth" was something evolutionary in nature and, in opposition to more romantic portrayals, was not constituted by or related to some transcendental or eternal reality. It was merely something based on experience that could be tested and hence, shared by all who would investigate it.

Schneider himself, asserted what could be seen as a complementary approach to this worldview, taking an ethnographic perspective. "Philosophy," he wrote,

> shows traits which distinguish it from science or from whatever one may choose to name the cooperative and systematic search for experimental evidence. Any historian of philosophy knows that philosophers have usually imagined themselves as seekers or finders of one or more objective truths. A philosophy is usually cast by its author into the form of a systematic demonstration of propositions that purport to be true.[9]

In arguing for his approach to research, Theos was aiming at a metaphysical version of Dewey's pragmatism, which was nearly the precise opposite of Schneider's conception of the discipline, putting him squarely into Schneider's pejorative characterization of a "romantic" philosopher. Observable in a nascent form in his master's thesis, Theos's basic suppositions about Indian yoga in theory and practice would eventually be fleshed out:

> [The Indian approach is] not unlike those employed in teaching geometry. First the student is given the proposition that the sum of the angles of a triangle is equal to two right angles. This must be accepted as

axiomatic, until it is finally demonstrated through reason to be an actual fact. Still it is only a rational conviction which does not necessarily carry certainty. The truth of this proposition can be verified only by actually cutting out from a piece of paper a triangle and measuring the angles, thereby actually experiencing beyond any measure of doubt that the sum total of the three angles is *180* degrees or the equivalent of two right angles. This last procedure of obtaining direct knowledge or realization of a geometrical truth might be said to correspond to the realization of transcendental truth through Yoga.[10]

In his mind, not only was he pursuing "one or more objective truths," he was proposing something far more radical: that he himself could and would validate them for all to see. To this extent, his thesis was far more a personal manifesto than an academic study. Expressing sentiments that would be echoed some forty years later by many Americans with regard to the Tibetan tradition, Theos observed the precarious state of research in Indian tantric yoga in 1936:[11]

The men in India who have such training are rapidly dying and with them goes this knowledge, for the younger people who are rapidly becoming Europeanized no longer see its value. One of the first tasks of the student in this field today must be to gather together those manuscripts which are left so that the future may have them if for no other reason than for the possibility of preserving one of the strands that has gone to make up the ball of the cultural heritage of the world. . . .

Since Sir John Woodroffe, who uses the name of Arthur Avalon in many of his writings, has recently passed away, as have two of the pundits who worked with him, it is rather doubtful whether this work will be continued at the present time, or must wait until a new impetus from some other source takes it up again. However, what is much needed at this time is someone willing to work with one of those Eastern teachers, so rapidly dying off, who will first familiarize himself with the existent Tantrik literature, and then devote several years of his life to the practice of its method, thereby enabling himself to gain a conscious insight into its many problems.

Further characterizing the imperative incumbent upon "a student"— a thinly veiled reference to himself—Theos continued: "What is needed most today is for someone having an intellectual understanding of these scriptures to actually go through the various ritual stages, thus gaining by experience an estimate of the truth of the teachings." For, as he observed,

> There seem to be no records in the literature of any occidental student of this subject having run the gamut of its training and endeavoured to understand in this manner its praised latent potentialities. It is hardly conceivable that men of intelligence could hold to a body of truth so tenaciously for centuries if there was not a scintilla of value in it. One of the difficulties that it has had to contend with these many years in the Western world is that no one here is willing to experience for himself that which it embodies.

Theos thus envisioned his master's thesis as a first step in this process, that is, "to present systematically the various steps in the rituals which are given for the Shakti Tantra and relate them to the metaphysical reasoning which is the basis for this form of Tantra."

The first challenge Theos faced was unraveling the "confused state" of literature on tantra as it existed in the 1930s. From a survey of that literature, he concluded that there were only two reputable scholars of Indian tantra in the world: "Arthur Avalon"[12] and Benoytosh Bhattacharyya. Relying almost exclusively on the works of these two men, Theos composed his thesis as a summary of the "state of the art" of research into Hindu and Buddhist tantra, noting Bhattacharyya's frequent references to the Tibetan Kangyur and Tengyur—the two halves of the Tibetan Buddhist canon.

In his thesis, Theos reported the then standard chronology of the history of tantra, beginning with "the aborigines of India [who] were supposed to have had a highly developed practice of magic when the Aryan invasion took place." As a result, Tantrism was theorized to have "originated in primitive magic, but took definite form under the stimulus of Buddhism." It was the Buddha, Theos argued, who could be credited with the real systemization of tantra. Born in the mid-sixth century B.C.E. amid the intermingling of Āryan Vedic culture and indigenous prototantric beliefs, the Buddha "could not fail to take account of these beliefs of the masses and in order to satisfy this second class of the laity, he had to incorporate some sort of mantras, Dhâraṇîs, Mudrâs and Maṇḍalas." It was a theory argued by Bhattacharyya in his *Introduction to Buddhist Esoterism* just a few years earlier:

In the Manjusrîmûlakalpa, which formed part of the extensive Vaipu-lyasûtra literature of the Buddhists and was probably composed in the first century of the Christian era, we find quite an astonishing number of mantras, Mudrâs, Maṇḍalas, and Dhâraṇîs, which must have taken their origin in the early centuries B.C., and probably from the time of Bud-dha himself. Later on, in the Guhyasamāja, which is considered as the first systematic Tantrik work of the Buddhists, and which was probably written in the third or fourth century A.D., we find Buddha saying to the congregation of the faithful, that as the people were not sufficiently enlightened he did not preach the Tântrik system when he was born as the Dîpankara and Kasyapa Buddha.[13]

From reading Bhattacharyya, Theos claimed that the purpose of the Buddha's systemization of these materials was "to introduce the Shakti element into Buddhist Tantra particularly for obtaining emancipation through Yoga and Samādhi."

More significantly, he pointed out, "Yoga is the process by which the Jiva is brought to unite with the paramâtma [and] it is not a separate sys-tem of eastern philosophy, a frequent misconception, but rather a tech-nique common to them all in variously modified forms." Hence, the basis of understanding tantra was understanding yoga. To do this would require an exploration of the legacy of Indian Buddhist tantra for, after this initial systemization by the Buddha—represented by the Guhyasamāja Tantra—"the Buddhists put out a great deal of literature on the Tantras, and during the Tântric Age (8th and 9th Centuries), it is said that thousands of works were written which later filtered through the Himalayan passes to Tibet and Mongolia, and thence to China and Japan, leaving their effect on large sections of the populations of these countries." The significance of this, he noted, was that "a great many of those original works which were in Sanskrit are now preserved in the Tibetan Tangyur."

As for the non-Buddhist forms of tantra, Theos repeated Bhattacha-ryya's observation that "the bulk of literature which goes by the name of the Hindu Tantras arose almost immediately after the Buddhist ideas had established themselves, though after the Tāntric age, [and] even up to the last century, Tântric works continued to be written by the Hindus."[14] Since the validity of this hypothesis was corroborated by Woodroffe,[15] the avail-able evidence suggested that the truly authentic tantric tradition was not only Buddhist but also only to be found in Tibet.

Nonetheless, Theos felt that discussions of the attainments of "magic powers"—*siddhis*—in both Buddhist and Hindu tantric traditions pointed to and were causally related to "the interrelation between Buddhist and Hindu Tantra and the confusion which is to be found in the literature." Given the state of the field, it was difficult to separate Buddhist from Hindu tantric materials, and "no less difficult to distinguish the authentic from the spurious." And although he lamented that this was "an almost endless task," headway was being made by the man Theos felt to be the only reliable researcher in Buddhist tantric studies at the time, W. Y. Evans-Wentz, who had just published his *Tibetan Yoga and Secret Doctrines*.

Following Woodroffe's lead, Theos set forth the basic outline of his research in his master's thesis, presenting the tantric literature as

> above all a practical scripture primarily concerned with action and ritual which the undiscerning may think has, in any case been prescribed to an excessive extreme. It is so concerned because, though action cannot alone and directly secure liberating knowledge, the attainment of the latter must necessarily be preceded by right action. For how otherwise can such spiritual knowledge be gained? In order to secure the development of the Jîva's body, certain physical exercises are necessary. Similarly both these and other mental and spiritual exercises are required if liberating knowledge (brahmanjnâna) is to be attained. Such exercises are generically termed "sâdhana," and include both worship (pûjâ) and all its ritual.[16]

While moving his narrative into a consideration of the subject of tantric *sādhanas*, Theos had to dance around a touchy subject. Ghosh and others who had written on the subject had clear disdain for Western presumptiveness regarding ritual:

> Sâdhana has historically varied with race and creed. The Hindu has his own in the Tantra which is called Sâdhana Shâstra. The provision of such a definite training is the strength to a greater or lesser degree of all ancient orthodoxies, just as its absence may prove to be the rock on which the more modern forms of religion may split. Doubtless to newer "Protestant" spirit, whether issuing from Europe, Arabia, or elsewhere, all ritual is liable to be regarded as "mummery," except possibly the particular and perhaps jejune variety which it calls its own. For even the

most desiccated "Protestantism" has not been able altogether to dispense with it.[17]

Theos chose instead to draw upon Woodroffe's book of essays on the *Śākta Tantra-śāstra—Shakti and Shakta*—and to a lesser extent, its sequel—the treatise on *kuṇḍalinī* yoga by Ghosh and Woodroffe, *The Serpent Power*, both of which presented the subject far more theoretically, without sociological commentary.

Despite having based his earlier statements on Bhattacharyya's claims of a Buddhist origin of tantra, Theos presented Indian ritual practice as Woodroffe had, as fundamentally linked to the cosmogonic principles of "Hindu" Saṃkhya philosophy. Viewed from that perspective, tantric practice hinged on the primordial, substantive, and creative force known as *prakṛti* and its three qualitative forms (*guṇa*), characterized as "presentation" (*sattva*), "movement" (*rajas*), and "veiling" (*tamas*). Their three functions, Theos explained, were complementary: "That of the Sattvaguna is to reveal consciousness, while the Tamasguna has the opposite function of suppressing or veiling consciousness. Rajasguna is to 'make active' and as such it works on Tamas to suppress Sattva, or on Sattva to suppress Tamas."

Quoting Woodroffe, Theos explained that "sādhana" came from the Sanskrit root √*sādh*, meaning to exert or to strive, and that therefore a *sādhana* was "the striving, practice, discipline and worship in order to obtain success or Siddhi which may be of many kinds." Hence, he declared, "the ultimate object of all Sādhanā is to develop Sattvaguna, but the means by which this goal is attempted will differ according to one's capacity. . . . The order he will go through will vary according to his intellectual and spiritual development. All ritual is aimed at the control of the mind, for this is the tool by which one is able to gain control over the Spirit."

Throughout his explication of the fundamental features of tantric ritual (*pūja*), Theos returned again and again to one common feature as emphasized by Woodroffe: the importance of conscious understanding by the participant (*sādhaka*) in his or her actions during the process. For example, with regard to self-consecration (*nyāsa*), he declared,

> The principle involved here is that by associating every part of the body with the Divine, the mind and body are made divine to the consciousness of the Sādhaka. Many people have given this ritual a great deal of undue criticism, saying that its gestures were a lot of nonsense. This would be

very true if they were carried out without any intelligence behind them: The originators knew however, that "thought is everything, molding our bodily features, moral and intellectual character and disposition, leading to and appearing in our actions." Therefore the aim is to follow this ritual with will, attention, faith and devotion.

In such terms, Theos took great pains to counter the notion of "degenerate practices" and antinomianism, usually attributed to tantra.

If it will be remembered that one of the objects of Tantrik ritual is to "forward the morality of the sense by converting mere animal function into acts of worship," many of the misconceptions that are likely to result from studying parts of this ritual would never occur. In the many instances that it has received severe condemnation, it is because those who were advocating it in one form or another were using a religious ritual for their own immoral license. If the ritual is strictly adhered to, there is nothing in it that can be thought of as immoral. Its principles are based on the theory that one of the surest ways of gaining control over the intangible is by first gaining absolute control of the tangible which is so closely linked. It has taken the three strongest appetites of man and endeavoured to lift them from the carnal and attach them to the Brahma by the power of suggestion.

Moreover, he argued, the view of human functions was even less dualistic than it might appear, and—again quoting Woodroffe—although one could speak of lifting "appetites of man . . . from the carnal," in reality,

The attitude which is taken toward all desires and functions of man are not that they are in and of themselves evil. "Man is, in his essence or spirit, divine and one with the universal Spirit. His mind and body and all their functions are divine, for they are not merely a manifestation of the power (shakti) of God but that power itself. . . . Nothing in natural function is low or impure to the mind which recognizes it as Shakti and the working of Shakti. It is the ignorant and, in a true sense, vulgar mind which regards any natural function as low or coarse."

Theos was careful to point out that although the *pañcamākara* ritual—or "ritual of the five 'M' aspects (*pañca-ma-akara*: madya, māngasa, matsya, mudra, & maithuna)—conveys the notion of complete engagement in transgressive behavior, only the highest class of practitioner, a Vīra, would be qualified to engage in the rituals on a literal level, while the Divya and Paśu classes would engage in symbolic versions of the rite."

A quotation will convey the symbolic meanings used by the Divya. "Wine" (Madya) according to Kaula Tantra is not any liquid but that intoxicating knowledge acquired by Yoga of the Parabrahman which renders the worshipper senseless as regards the external world. "Meat" (Mangasa) is that Sattvik knowledge by which through the sense of "Mineness" (a play upon the word Matsya) the worshipper sympathizes with the pleasure and pain of all beings. Mudrā is the act of relinquishing all association with evil which results in bondage. Coition (Maithuna) is the union of the Shakti Kuṇḍalinī, the "inner woman" and World-force in the lowest centre (Mūlādhāra Chakra) of the Sādhaka's body with the Supreme Shiva in the highest centre (Sahasrāra) in the upper Brain.

Only viewed in this light, he explained, should the role of yoga—specifically *kuṇḍalinī* yoga "since it is the distinctive Tantrik form," rather than Dhyāna/ Bhāvanā yoga, which was "purely a mental process"—be understood.

In *kuṇḍalinī* yoga, Theos continued, the *kuṇḍalī* creative force (*śakti*) "sleeps" in the lowest or root *cakra* (*mūlādhāra-cakra*) of the subtle body, and hence liberation (*mukti*) is only obtained

when it is aroused and brought up to unite with the consciousness of the Supreme Shiva. The process or means by which the Jiva is united with the Paramātmā is called Yoga. This union which is attained by the Sādhakas is one only of imagination, while in Yoga, it actually takes place.

Following Woodroffe's lead, Theos proceeded to similarly describe the four formal implementations of yogic practice (*mantra-, haṭha-, laya-* and *rāja-yoga*):

Even though the aim of all Yoga is the same, there are said to be four common forms which are: Mantrayoga, Haṭhayoga, Layayoga and Rājayoga. It is possible to find other divisions which are made, but these mentioned are the basic ones and all others are just the many ways of saying the same thing. After all, it is not the division that is of importance, for it is only for the purpose of classification. It will soon appear that in fact, they all use the same basic methods and only differ in the manner in which they place the emphasis, however, it might be mentioned here that all are agreed that perfect liberation can only be attained through Rājayoga, and these others are only steps in preparation for this highest form of Yoga. The stress is as follows: In Mantrayoga, it is on worship and devotion; in Hathayoga, it is on the physical (its power and function to affect the subtle body), in Layayoga, it is placed on the supersensible Pīthas (seats or centres) and supersensible forces and functions of the inner world of the body, and Rājayoga, it is on the intellective processes.

From this Theos proceeded to summarize the aspects of the yogic subtle body as they related to kuṇḍalinī yoga, according to Woodroffe, along with eight-branched (aṣṭaṅga) yoga and the preliminary practices and purifications discussed in the Gheranda Saṃhitā and Haṭha Yoga Pradīpikā of Svātmāramasvāmin.

Although his presentation was a fairly accurate condensation of Woodroffe's research, peppered throughout with Sanskrit technical terms, beyond verifying his citations, it is highly unlikely that anyone on Theos's thesis committee had any basis for assessing the accuracy of its content.[18]

While Theos was actively engaged in studying the works of Woodroffe, Ghosh, and Alexandra David-Neel, Viola was completing her coursework in medical school and preparing herself for their journey to India, before her anticipated internship the following spring at the Jersey City Medical Center. Their academic obligations under control, Theos and Viola attempted to maintain their focus on their trip and the importance of their "friend in India"—none other than Theos's father, Glen.

FOUR

Two Parallel Paths (II)

I don't believe there is a more lonely individual living than the well-trained yogi. Yet just as he is capable of the greatest loneliness, he is also capable of the greatest happiness. So to put it in a few words a companion in yoga is a blessing rare to be found.

—GLEN BERNARD[1]

IN THE FALL of 1912, a young Brahmin named Sukumar Chatterji stood on a dock in San Francisco. Having made the journey from India, he had plans to study journalism in America, but this was not to be his fate. Like so many newcomers to the American shores, his naïveté would prove to be a critical weakness; falling victim to the schemes of fradulent "friends," before he knew it, Chatterji had lost all his money and was penniless on a foreign shore. Left to his own resources, he began working at odd jobs here and there in the Bay area—the state fair in Sacramento, a potato farm in Stockton, any work wherever he could find it. By the spring of 1914, Chatterji had stabilized his life and was modestly employed in San Francisco's Chinatown district as a musician for the Theosophical Society, presenting himself to inquirers as a snake-charmer from Bengal.[2]

In early 1915, Chatterji's fortunes appeared to be improving when he met a man named Heramba Lal Gupta, who invited him to participate in a growing Indian expatriate movement. The members of the Gadar Party, as they called themselves, were putting into motion plans to incite a revolution in India and overthrow British rule. Introduced to other members of the group, Chatterji was told that "men were already in Afghanistan, Persia, Africa, China, Siam, Burma, Nepal, and Java, and were to start for India, collecting as many men, arms, and ammunition as possible" along the way.

Signing on to the cause, Chatterji was given $700 in gold and on May 23, boarded a ship bound for the South Seas, traveling in disguise as Prince Morali Murarilael Sharma, along with a compatriot, Jodh Singh (traveling as Prince Hassan Zada). Several weeks later, they arrived in Manila, where they were met by two men who claimed to be representatives of the German government. Chatterji and Singh were given instructions by these "German officials" to act as couriers, relaying coded messages and funds between various German consulates in Asia and agents in the field. For the better part of a year, Chatterji traveled from country to country, ferrying messages between his contacts and even writing an article for an Indian nationalist newspaper published in San Francisco associated with the Gadar Party. In his article, Chatterji asserted that India's true ally was Germany, going so far as to claim that the only reason Germany had gone to war was to free India from the British. This likely proved to be his undoing: in April 1917 U.S. federal agents in San Francisco began arresting members of the Gadar Party, adding Chatterji's name to their list of "wanted men." At almost the same time, during one of his trips, Chatterji—now a known "subversive"—was apprehended by British agents in Bangkok. Charged with treason and thrown into solitary confinement, he remained there for the better part of six months.

Chatterji's story—and his life—might have ended then and there, were it not that more of his fellow conspirators were being arrested across the United States. In addition to the activities of the Gadar Party, for several years German agents, it was alleged, had been supporting unions and encouraging strikes in an attempt to prevent the United States from entering the war in Europe by economically destabilizing the country from within. Fortunately for Chatterji, several of the men arrested were also charged with espionage against the British Empire, that is, "against the territory or dominions of any foreign prince or state, or of any colony, district, or people, with whom the United States are at peace,"[3] since part of the Indian revolution plot—the Jacobsen Plot, as it came to be known—involved the assassination of an American team in India.

In 1917, "Capt. Cook, the arctic explorer" was preparing another expedition, this time to the Himalayan mountains. Led by one of their German contacts, Paul Boehm, Chatterji and others had planned to waylay Cook's party, seize their papers, and impersonating them, proceed to India in order to incite revolution. Boehm, however, was arrested by the British in

Singapore, and along with three other men, was indicted in Chicago. Chatterji confessed his part in the plot, and although he still faced charges of treason in India, he was extradited to the United States, where he and Jodh Singh agreed to testify for the prosecution.

When the court trial of Paul Boehm, Albert Wehde, and Gustav Jacobsen was finally decided in 1920, all three men were sentenced to three years' imprisonment at Leavenworth Penitentiary.[4] Although he denied any bargaining took place in exchange for his testimony, Sukumar Chatterji did express his desire to remain in America, which appears to have been fulfilled. Following his testimony, Chatterji disappeared from public view for several years, only to reappear in 1922 in San Francisco once again, this time teaching yoga in and around San Francisco's Haight-Ashbury district, having reinvented himself as an "East Indian Philosopher and Scientist."[5] It was then and there that Glen Bernard met him and became one of his students.

Thus, in the early 1920s, while young Theos was still a teenager in southern Arizona, Glen Bernard was hard at work studying breathing meditation (*prāṇāyāma*) in San Francisco with Chatterji, transcribing his lectures, and researching the literature of the Bengali tantric tradition. Over the course of several months, Chatterji lectured on both the traditional presentation of breathing exercises and its parallels with contemporary scientific knowledge concerning respiratory functions. As the classes progressed, Chatterji's lectures expanded into a broader discussion of ayurvedic medicine and its relationship to Hindu philosophy.

Chatterji taught every week under the auspices of the Fiat Lux Society of San Francisco, and Glen took copious notes on the lectures—covering both theory and practice—over the course of two years, from 1922 through 1924, a portion of which were published as a small book on Saṃkhya philosophy entitled *Cosmic Creation*. Glen, continuing to study and practice yoga as well as the rudiments of Sanskrit, focused on the fundamental principles of ayurvedic medicine, diet, and chemical compounds, studying the recently published translations of the Indian medical treatises, the *Caraka Saṃhita* and *Suśruta Saṃhita*.

Following his studies with Chatterji, in the fall of 1924 Glen began preparing for his own journey to India, while continuing to study haṭha yoga and philosophy with Wassan Singh (a.k.a. Haṭha Yogi Wassan) and Swami Yogananda in Los Angeles. Working and saving his money, by the end of 1925 Glen was ready to go. He applied for a new passport, and upon its

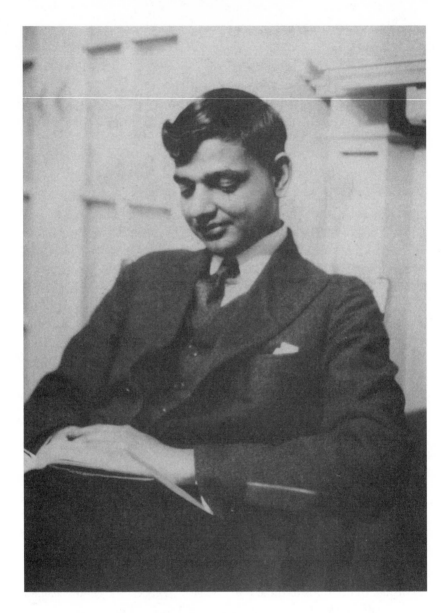

Figure 4.1 Sukumar Chatterji (BANC)

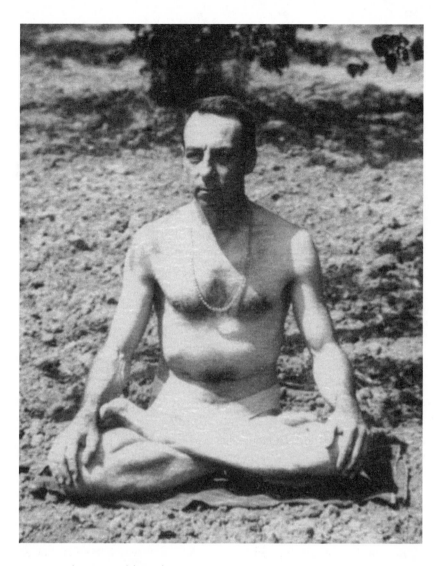

Figure 4.2 Glen Bernard (BANC)

receipt in early December, obtained the necessary visas from the British consulate in Los Angeles and quickly boarded a ship bound for India.

After passing through Hong Kong and Singapore, on February 16, 1926, Glen arrived in Calcutta, home to the Bengali yoga tradition and his former teacher, Sukumar Chatterji, who had returned to India and was living in Cawnpore on the outskirts of the city. Chatterji put Glen in touch with fellow students of *his* teacher, who then took Glen to meet Swami Kebalananda.[6] Over the course of the following months, Glen developed close friendships with Kebalananda and several of the other disciples of Śrī Yukteśwar, as well as with other teachers in the area, including the students of Swami Vivekananda, Atal Behari Ghosh, and the family of Swami Vimalānanda—the latter accepting Glen as his student and giving him meditation (*dhyāna*) and mantra recitation (*japa*) teachings.

While he continued to study and practice yoga, far more significantly than anything else he did, Glen became good friends with Atal Behari Ghosh—the Sanskritist then working with a fellow disciple of Sivacandra Vidyarnava, Sir John Woodroffe, on the editing and translation of the *Kularnava Tantra* and other texts. Atal Behari Ghosh—who was only ever attested as the secretary of the Āgamānusandhānasamiti (The Agamas Research Society), an organization funded by the Mahārāja of Darbhanga, Maheshwar Singh—was a rigorous scholar and in fact, the man to whom the pseudonym "Arthur Avalon" actually referred.[7] Through Ghosh, Glen would also befriend another young man studying in the area, Walter Yeeling Evans-Wentz.

Although Glen spent only a few months in India, he remained in close correspondence over the subsequent ten years with Ghosh, who considered him "a friend who sympathizes with my labours." Glen, for his own part, considered Ghosh very much in the role of a teacher and saw himself as his pupil.[8] Ghosh thought Glen a man of unusual temperament for his respect and earnest interest in the tantric tradition, particularly when compared to many of Ghosh's Indian associates—"the men who are looked upon as 'educated' in this country—you know the type I mean . . . Woodroffe said nothing truer when he spoke of these intellectual hermaphrodites as 'mind-born sons of the British.'"[9]

In America, Glen informed him, the situation was not much better. Americans were infatuated with science and its marvels for their own sake. Ghosh remarked, in reply,

> The postcards you sent are highly interesting; they show how the modern mind is functioning to its own detriment. "Looking at the Moon" is another picture showing how the minds of the young are being perverted. What use is it to anybody to know what the surface of the moon is like? They are all for the organization of useful knowledge—Do they intend having an American Colony in the Moon?

No less a bane to Glen than the blindly scientific minded were their opposites, fake religious leaders. Ghosh was able to offer some consolation regarding fraudulent "swamis" and those who would capitalize on American interest in yoga for personal gain, reassuring him that the problem was universal and merely a sign of the degenerate era they lived in, "not confined to any particular country." Offering his insights, Ghosh stressed to Glen the significance of his work on the *Kularnava Tantra*, and more importantly, how he could help him.

My interpretation of the Kularnava is going to be one of which I shall be proud to the end of my days. The trouble is that I am interrupted so frequently here that I lose my thread and lose a lot of time having to pick them up again. As I read these passages, now I see things there which are anything but what I myself saw in them fifteen years ago. I see a wonderful way of putting the gross to illustrate the subtle workings of the mind and the way it rises to higher and yet higher spheres. There is not a single man here with whom I could discuss it. Even my Pandit who has been working with me for eighteen years is of no help. If I could get the next door house in Chaibassa and transplant myself permanently there and if I had a congenial co-worker, I could make better progress and better work, too.

I am handicapped other ways also, the President is not responsive in his financial support—and I am ordered about as to what I should do. To relieve me of all this I often times wish that you would succeed in your intentions and settle in this country for some time at least—or at any rate, remain here longer than you did last time—which you will be able comfortably to do if there be two houses in Chaibassa, but no use dreaming.

Over the years that followed Ghosh maintained a congenial working relationship with Glen, asking him to assist with his projects and solicit help. To this end, Ghosh asked if Glen "could get at any newspaper man willing to notice my society and give a laudatory notice of my President [the Mahārāja of Darbhanga] . . . also let me know if you have circulated the appeal and if there is any response or likely to be." The financial aspect of his endeavors was a great source of worry for Ghosh, for "the President (Mahārājādhirāja of Darbhanga) is keen as ever regarding the publications; it is true so long as he is alive he will keep it going but what after that?"

But Glen had no luck in that regard; in fact, he was often lucky to keep himself housed and fed. Despite his failure to return quickly to India or secure funding, Ghosh continued to encourage him in his endeavors and was very much a friend in his self-imposed solitude in America. It was Ghosh as well, a mere month after Glen's return to the States, who broke the news of the death of his guru:

> You will be pained to know that your Guru passed away on the 5th of this month. I came to know of it on this 9th. His end was most peaceful—he simply crossed the borderline. I feel the loss very much—for though I seldom met him, he was always uniformly kind to me and was really a good man. . . .
>
> I hope you will make good progress in your Sadhana at the place you are returning to. Your Guru was full of hope as to your ultimate success. He died at a most wonderful moment in a most wonderful manner. People like him do not die—they simply pass out of our ken.

Glen had written to Swami Vimalānanda often in the months following his return, up until the swami's death, and he remained in contact with his late guru's family and the man's eldest son, Kalikacharan Roy Chaudhuri, who took over running his father's temple, the Bairabananda Kalikāshram in Belur Math. Chaudhuri assured Glen,

> It is consoling to remember that Father gave you enough to lead you to self-realization. He gave you one of the most powerful of the siddha mantras. If you follow the directions, I have not the least doubt that new vistas of spiritual progress will open up before you automatically. Give it as much practice as your circumstances and energy permit and you are sure to forge rapidly ahead. I am strengthened further in this conviction by the fact that Father made a good prognosis of your spiritual progress from certain signs which he read in your physiognomy.

In closing, he offered that "whenever you think that we may assist you in any way—answering any question or giving any information, we will do it most gladly for your asking . . . [and] when and if you come to India, always remember that you are most cordially welcome to our home." Although Ghosh had warned Glen that the sons of Swami Vimalānanda were "not quite up to the mark," Kalikacharan Roy Chaudhuri did his best to help Glen gain an understanding of the practices and instructions given by his father. Chaudhuri, as promised, described in detail in his letters the many individual elements of the meditational devices (*yantra*) and their signification in the context of tantric practice.

Between Ghosh and Roy Chaudhuri, Glen had a wealth of information at his disposal. Ghosh kept him apprised of his own progress and the cutting-edge work being done by Evans-Wentz, as well as his own opinion of the place of Tibetan Buddhism in the Indian religious tradition.

> The book by Dr. Wentz which will first come out is "The Tibetan Book of the Dead." It is in the press as I was told by him. The other book is "Life of Melarepa" which will be taken up almost immediately. These are both Buddhistic books but what he has sought to establish is that Buddhism in its essential character is not opposed to Vedanta—which is the correct interpretation.

When Evans-Wentz's *Tibetan Book of the Dead* finally did come out, Glen conveyed his enthusiasm to Ghosh, who admitted, "I had something to do with Dr. Wentz's book."

> It requires elaboration I admit, but so far as it goes it is all right. His next book *Melarepa* [*sic*] will I hope also [be] useful. He has two other books in contemplation and asked me to look through them when typed and I promised to do so. I also called his attention to a Sanskrit book on Buddhist Yoga. I have so far seen fragments of it and have not yet been able to get the entire manuscript.

Leaving aside the work of literary research, Ghosh offered Glen assistance with all of his personal practices as well, from mantra recitation to breathing and diet:

> I gather that you are finding some difficulty with your mantra. Am I right? . . . When you are practicing concentrate on what you have in mind. Do not let your mind be detracted by the opinions of persons and societies. I realize it is difficult in a country like yours where everyone seems to be boiling over—but it is necessary that your mind should be

directed towards what you have chosen to attain. The opinions of societies and individuals divert the mind imperceptibly. I am sure you can succeed against these, but it is best not to run any risks. You are perfectly right that you will experience what is now beyond your "conscious" understanding. I have added the adjective for what seems to be beyond your understanding is not really so.

As to having everything on a rational basis your desire is quite consistent but you will have to take certain things on trust to start with. This reasonableness will dawn before you as you progress. . . . You are not to, and [I] am sure you will, despair. To control the mind you may try one of two things—fix your gaze on the tip of your nose when repeating your mantra in japa. If you find this tiresome, you may fix your gaze on a speck of light when doing japa. You will soon find yourself dissolved in the light and the outer world will fall away from you. I am glad you have got the Asana in control. It is an important step forward. As for Pranayama—never exert yourself more than you can do with ease and comfort. This is not to be done in a way that is easy for the sadhaka. . . .

The all important thing—the regulation of your food—is what troubles me—I cannot say what is needed as particular things. You may in the early stages confine yourself to milk and fresh vegetables—If you understand the workings of the Doshas you can easily see the directions where danger is apprehended and take precautions. The quantity of opium needed for a days use is a pill about three times the size of a mustard seed. It does not have any deleterious effect. I am taking this dose now and am all the better for it. Europe is afraid of opium for the stuff is misused there in the same way as alcohol also is. But you can control Vayu by using milk or milk sauce in your food. . . . But you must bear this in mind always that anything which does not agree with you is to be relinquished. This applies to inhalation and everything. You might keep a note of this and let me know so that I could be of help. . . . As to short cuts, do not think of them just yet; for this you have to be with an adept for some time.

Although all the issues that Glen raised with Ghosh were indeed central to his religious practice, there were additional reasons for his interest in diet. While in Calcutta, Glen had taken the time to establish contacts with a number of people working in the field of ayurvedic medicine and the chemical import-export industries, partly in the hope of establishing international commercial ventures—none of which appears to have been successful—and to secure a source for ayurvedic medicines.

Glen remained in contact throughout those years with another friend of Ghosh's in Calcutta: his personal physician and fellow seeker of religious truths, Kaviraj Narendranath Bidyanidhi, a chemist and pharmacist. Upon his return to the United States, Glen found work as a metallurgical engineer and deployed his skills to both professional and personal ends. By 1928 he was shipping samples of cinnabar regularly from California to Bidhyanidhi in Calcutta, where mercury would be extracted for use in medicinal preparations, samples of which Bidhyanidhi found to be "of much benefit."

Querying Bidhyanidhi on the specifics of the different formularies, Glen returned to his study of the translated Indian medical treatises, the *Caraka Saṃhita* and *Suśruta Saṃhita*. With Bidhyanidhi's help, he researched mercury and arsenic compounds as potential treatments for cancer (including Hodgkin's disease), typhoid, smallpox, gonorrhea, and syphilis—medications that Bidhyanidhi shipped and Glen began selling up and down the coast of Southern California.[10] He also began ingesting some himself, having been assured by Bidhyanidhi that "mercury so used in the treatment of Syphilis is prepared in strict accordance with Shastraic rules and the result is that there is no apprehension of its having any baneful effect on system of the patient."

Over the course of their communications, Glen asked for Bidhyanidhi's insights into diagnostic techniques. As his friend pointed out, though, "it is very very difficult to teach these ideas through correspondence" and he instead invited Glen to return to India in 1929, when Woodroffe was expected to return as well. Little more than two weeks later, in October 1928, Atal Ghosh similarly wrote to Glen informing him that to raise more funds,

> I may have to ask you to come out, if you are so inclined, to India to help the project. . . . Nothing is yet certain, but as I always dream dreams, I write to ascertain if I may rely on your help if the occasion arises. The people are so mad with publicity that they scarce think of their Dharma. It must be worse in Europe and the rest and India is affected by contact— a sort of calcification.

Although he remained hopeful that Glen would be able to return to India, he remarked, "I suppose your efforts have not led to anything like success for I would have heard from you if it did." Nonetheless, he still asked Glen to do what he could remotely.

I am waiting for your opinion of the Mahanirvana (Great Liberation). If a third edition comes out, your opinion may help to improve it. I have finished reviewing the text and commentary and it is a decided improvement over all previous publications. For I had the advantage of consulting Mss. which are practically flawless.

But Glen was still unable to return, and as time passed, Ghosh repeatedly found reasons to invite him back to India. Still thinking about the Kumbha Mela to be held in Allahabad later that year, Glen wrote to Ghosh inquiring about it. Ghosh, naturally, encouraged him to attend, as there was a chance that Woodroffe would be attending too, staying until March 1930. By the following September, Ghosh had obtained more information:

The Kumbha Mela will be somewhere about the middle of January. If you could come you may have a chance of seeing our new President. Sir John [Woodroffe] is not coming out this year. He wishes to stay back for his daughter's examination who will be sitting for her B.A. degree next year. He indicated coming out October 1930.

But the implications of this were far more than social for Ghosh:

I am beginning to feel that it may not be possible for me to work with him [Woodroffe] for very long. He is growing too learned for me, and as you noted sometime back, he is getting too oxonised.[11] The books in the Power series written in collaboration with Mr. Kerji[12] are nonsense and to me unintelligible. They are likely to have a mischievous effect on some minds. The last book which has just come out is to my mind worse yet. I am not going to take any immediate action and you keep it to yourself. The best thing for you is what you have decided upon—namely to have a rigid training and then come out.

Glen did wish to collaborate with Ghosh, even if by long-distance correspondence. But September 1929 also brought troubling financial news. Ghosh wrote to Glen, "I was away at Simla to see the Maharaja who is our new President for you will be sorry to know that the Maharaja of Darbhanga is dead." A short time later, Ghosh expressed his disappointment: "The interest of the new President of our Society in its work seems to be rather weak. My letters are not attended to. I wrote to Woodroffe about it for it was he who proposed his name and I merely seconded it—these men want to be advertised. In the meantime I am going on with my work." And so, in the interest of bringing in Glen as his collaborator to replace Woodroffe, Ghosh suggested,

> If you can get any of your backers interested, let me know in time—so that I may send you the papers by installments. If you send any of the papers you have with you—I should like to see what they have done with these and then follow them up. What I intend is to present the Tantra in as many of its aspects as I possibly can and show where they harmonize.

By the spring of 1930, after a brief illness, Ghosh was hard at work editing the *Sarada Tilaka*, a tantric presentation of Samkhya philosophy.[13] He also began to think of collaborative projects that he and Glen could work on. With the third edition of *The Serpent Power* about to come out, with "some alterations and an addition here or there," and Ghosh was enthusiastic about having found another assistant in his research:

> I am glad however to tell you that I got offer of help from a learned recluse from Kathiawar in Gujarat who is willing to come and stay with me if necessary and I can arrange to keep him with me. . . . He is a very advanced man and very well conversant with the subject and possesses the critical faculty. . . . I shall speak to my Kathiawar friend about you. He, like your Guru, is a Sannyasi and it will be the right thing if he advises you. His knowledge of English is somewhat restricted but I shall try to help him there. I hope he will be able to show you a short-cut.

Kaviraj Narendranath Bidyanidhi was enthusiastic as well, telling Glen by the following August (1930) that "a Swamaji from Gujrat (in the Bombay Presidency) has come to meet our Mr. Ghosh, who we believe has profound knowledge in Tantrik Texts as well as our own Rasa Shastra (Books dealing with Metallic medicine)."

Maintaining their correspondence, Bidyanidhi continued to try to answer Glen's questions about ayurvedic medicine, reiterating the difficulties of doing so in letters. He went on to apprise Glen of the situation in

Calcutta and—in a not too subtle manner—expressed his concerns for the medical tradition: "My sons are studying Sanskrit well. Even now they are not sufficiently grown for Ayurvedic Teaching: My only hope if I get a good student from the west, to whom true shastric teaching in practical form can be taught, he will be the man to convey our ideas to your country."

Bidyanidhi continued to encourage Glen to come out for all these reasons as well as to work with Atal Behari Ghosh:

> I cannot speak too highly of Mr. Ghosh our esteemed friend for the research he has been doing. It is indeed a treasure that he leaves behind for the succeeding generation. It is indeed much to be regretted that we find not a second man to follow his steps. May the Almighty Mother (Maha Shakti) give us why one but a number of worthy sons, to complete his task!!!

He tied this to praise of Glen himself, saying, "I must say that your love for knowledge is admirable indeed and your solicitude for bringing relief to the suffering humanity is simply astonishing." But Glen was simply unable to travel, as the economic depression in the United States grew worse and worse. Finally, in the fall of 1932, Ghosh made one last appeal:

> I note that you are roaming all over the continent and can only surmise that it is for something to help you settle down and perhaps to restore you to me. I can give you a suggestion. You know I am the director of a company that owns the most agreeable site in the busiest center of the city. An offer of a million pounds Sterling was not entertained by us the year before you were out here. If there were any American Syndicate willing to make an offer . . . and if you can tackle it yourself, ask the party to send you out to settle terms.

While he had endeavored to pursue these avenues, Glen had not been idle in his own activities. For several years, he had been accepting and teaching students in both Saṃkhya philosophy and yoga under conditions of absolute secrecy.[14] A few years earlier, in the spring of 1930, through Ghosh, he had been able to meet Walter Evans-Wentz. Glen and Evans-Wentz began corresponding, and Glen was keenly interested in the Tibetan presentations of tantric yoga. Evans-Wentz kept him informed of his progress and research, often discussing the value of Tibetan sources. He told Glen of his aspiration to establish an ashram in California at his Barrett estate, plans that were temporarily derailed by the depression.

By 1934, as Theos and Viola were about to be married, Theos and Glen began discussing plans for a trip to India together. The problem foremost in their minds was how to avoid giving the impression that they were exploiting Viola. Given her suspicions about P.A., Theos was anxious to introduce Viola to "another teacher" but worried how she would react if she discovered that it was his father.

They decided that Glen's true identity was a secret that Theos should keep from Viola—at first, as part of his efforts to remove her from his uncle's influence. Fortunately, P.A. had spoken highly of Theos and his family when Viola's mother had first asked about them:

> He was telling us about his talks with her mother who asked if he knew my father & mother and what kind of people they were. He told us what he told her: My father was a man of excellent character—very studious— well read—and had an excellent mind. My mother was well educated and also of strong character. I was glad to have him say this in front of Vi—now if he changes his mind it will cause more suspicion on her part after she meets both of you—she will be still more dubious about him. She need not know who you are—but if she likes you and he does attack you, and then it is all revealed to her, with her attitude he will cut his throat.

Nonetheless, in order to keep their secret, Theos and Glen discussed possible pseudonyms before Glen and Viola ever met, including the name he had been given in India, Swami Bodhananda, and others.

> As for your names—they are grand—can't pronounce them—but that is alright—however Vi has heard & seen so much humbug connected with this stuff that she might become skeptical again—she has a keen head which she uses too damn much. She has heard of you—as my teacher—(not an Indian) so consider an impressive name more adoptable to this Caucasian race—just yourself—I only offer this suggestion for consideration. I want us to consider suggestive values—but this one is *so* suggestive.

In the end, they settled on the rather unimaginative name, Ted Wheeler.

Another complication was the financial situation. Despite more than ten years of effort to fund a return trip, Glen still had no money with which to travel to India, and Theos had only Viola's. Still, he was confident that he could pay Glen's way.

> We have been working on the will lately—she is changing it since there was half that she originally left to P.A. and the other half to DeVries—Her first step away from P.A.—Years will take us away from this hellish environment. It makes me sick to see this girl made such a sucker—she has had so damn much money that she does not know what it means to figure it in dollars—it has always been with thousands. She actually wants to be broke—& earn her own—she thinks it would be easy. She once offered to give all she had to P.A. & he refused it—she said she knows why now—she was under 21—she says he was just clever not kind—so she does see things. I hope I can send you to India. If she is going to give it away—so am I—so 2,000 for a trip should be easy—if it keeps coming as it has this last week.

Feeling confident that his son would succeed on his behalf, Glen began making preparations for a second trip to India. He contacted Hans Nordewin von Koerber, professor of Oriental Studies at the University of Southern California. Having spent four years in Tibet, von Koerber was just then completing a short book on the Tibetan language.[15] He gave Glen a list of contacts in India who might be able to help him with his research and offered him the use of an address at USC should he need to ship any items back to the States prior to his return.

During this time, Theos and Glen decided that Glen should begin corresponding with Viola—undisguised as her father-in-law—but that they should never meet under those terms. By fall 1934, Glen and Viola were deep in correspondence, discussing yoga and the broader spiritual dimension of the Indian approach to life. Praising Viola, Glen repeatedly impressed upon her the value of her relationship with Theos—a far cry from his earlier objections to their marriage.

> The innate joy I get out of this union, you cannot appreciate and will not until you yourself have spent many hours in the more practical efforts of yoga. . . . I don't believe there is a more lonely individual living than

the well-trained yogi. Yet just as he is capable of the greatest loneliness, he is also capable of the greatest happiness. So to put it in a few words a companion in yoga is a blessing rare to be found.

Instead of having to be deceived, however, Viola—with some encouragement from Theos—suggested to Glen that she fund his travel to India to prepare the way for their own trip the following year. Theos had impressed upon her the urgency of this, for he doubted his father had long to live.[16] In January 1935 Viola wrote to Glen,

I have been mentally revolving ways and means since appreciating the urgency [of] your immediate personal plans, and feel that we must, and can, find it possible to supply what is needed. I am sure Theos could not be at peace within, using for relative trivialities that which you require for your fundamental purpose, feeling about you as he does.

Thoroughly appreciative, Glen responded to Viola with "a word about your most gracious offer":

Such an opportunity for me will be another great event in life, it will enable me to clear up some matters I had to neglect when I was in the Orient, it will enable me to gather—I hope—considerable more material along the line of our cherished ambitions, will enable me to develop more tangible a life long hope, that of sowing the seed of yoga in this soil and nourishing it until it will survive of its own strength. . . . I am getting well along in this active stream of life and cannot hope to do very much toward the expansion of the art of yoga, I will need most of the time left to put my own house in order, but, in that, I have given the greater part of my life to this one end. I have had some experiences, have learned some things, that should be of material worth to others who seek the same path. It is with this thought that I want to busy myself with this work before my usefulness is gone. From this you may understand how I appreciate your sincere interest in yoga, and I add that I am hopeful that both you and Theos will someday be the active means of making yoga an Art of the highest regard and respect in this New World. . . . My going to India will be based entirely upon this one thought and every act, every move will be to collect and make material for this work.

Convinced, Viola wrote a check to cover the expense of sending Glen to India and his support while there. Upon receiving Viola's letter, Glen applied for a new passport and informed his students of his imminent departure.[17] By the beginning of April, with passport and money in hand, he obtained the necessary visas from the Chinese and British consulates in Los Angeles. Having shipped several trunks on ahead, on April 22, 1935, Glen set sail on the *President Johnson* bound for India.

FIVE

On Holy Ground

Yoga has a complete message for humanity.

It has a message for the human body.

It has a message for the human mind, and it has also a message for the human soul.

Will intelligent and capable youth come forth to carry this message to every individual, not only in India but also in every other part of the world?

—SWAMI KUVALAYĀNANDA[1]

ON THURSDAY, JUNE 13, 1935, Glen Bernard stepped off the gangway of the S.S. *President Johnson* and passed under the yellow basalt arch of the "Gateway of India," walking out into the streets of Bombay. It had been close to ten years since he'd last set foot on the holy ground of India, and Bombay was the last known home of his friend Sukumar Chatterji. But unbeknownst to Glen, Chatterji had since returned to Calcutta. Locating associates of his old friend, Glen sought out publishers of Indian classical literature. While in Bombay, he made contact with Raj Bahadur Singh, a local publisher of Sanskrit texts at the Shri Venkatesh Steam Press, from whom he acquired a number of books and began to gather information about other publishers and ashrams in the area.

Glen managed to locate Swami Kuvalayānanda, founder of the Kaivalyadhāma Yogic Institute in Lonavla—self-described as "an Institute for Scientific Research in Psycho-physiology, Spiritual and Physical Culture"—which had a branch in Bombay.[2] Beginning in early July, Glen began making requests to meet the swami but was repeatedly rebuffed, being told that "the Swamiji" was "extremely busy at present." Finally, after two weeks,

Glen received word that Kuvalayānanda had consented to see him, but their meetings proved brief and uninformative.

Not discouraged, Glen attempted to contact others in the Bombay area, including Dr. Ashutosh Roy, whom he had been told was working on a comprehensive treatise entitled "Hindu Yoga Systems." A few weeks later, Glen received a response to this inquiry, informing him that Ashutosh Roy had died the previous year with his work unfinished.

Spending the next several months in Bombay, Glen alerted Atal Ghosh of his arrival and followed up on their previous correspondence, inquiring about swamis and yogis he had met in America and might meet and seek instruction from while in Bombay. Ghosh, showing a more extreme attitude in his responses, told Glen to beware of what he might have heard from Indians in America, for "I do not know much about the swamis and yogis who visit your country but from what I can gather in a casual way I do not think very highly of them. It is against the fundamental principles of the Brahmanic faiths to proselytise by any overt act."

Glen's other correspondent in India, Evans-Wentz, likewise advised him not to be overly hopeful: "To find in India a master of *yoga* is a task of extreme difficulty. Even if one were met with, he would refuse to exhibit phenomena to any save a disciple who had been well tested and then probably only at a time of secret initiation."

Other than suggesting that Glen ask Atal Ghosh, the only other recommendation he made was to visit Ramana Maharshi's ashram in Tiruvannamalai, where "many of the sadhus speak English" and where Evans-Wentz had stayed the year before. But a trip to South India would take Glen far out of the way and interfere with what he was hoping to accomplish in the coming months. Having exhausted his contacts in Bombay with very little to show for his efforts, by the end of July he began making his way to Calcutta for a reunion with Atal Ghosh. Ghosh himself had been very busy. Aided by "an old Swami," he had just completed editing more Sanskrit texts for publication while the swami continued working on new ones.

By the beginning of September, Glen was in Calcutta and busily looking for "Tantrik Yogis" with whom he—and later Theos—could study. The responses he received, however, were the same ones he had heard many times before: "yogins in India generally do not proclaim themselves and it is very difficult to approach them." Still, he was able to get some recommendations for potential contacts with yogis in the tantric tradition. Glen reached two professors, Pramath Nath Mukhopadhyaya and Gopinathji

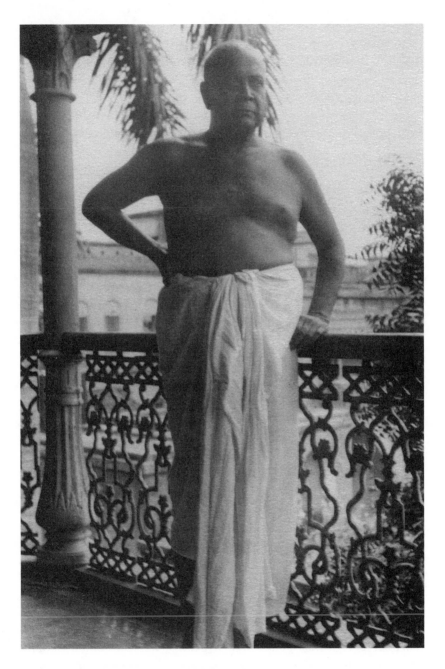

Figure 5.1 Atal Behari Ghosh, Chaibassa (BANC)

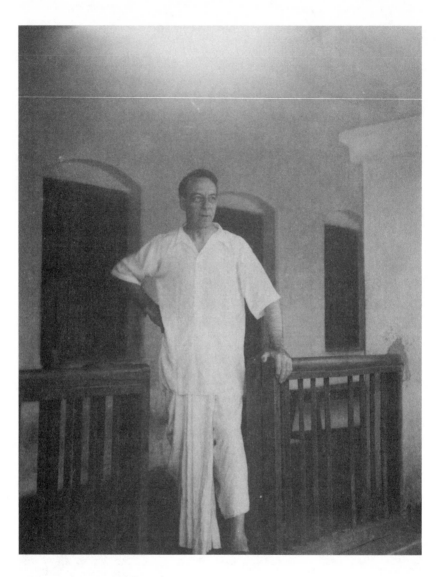

Figure 5.2 Glen Bernard (BANC)

Kaviraj of the Sanskrit College. He also reestablished contact with the ash-ram of his old guru, the Kalikâshram at Belur Math in Howrah. The swami then in residence, Swami Bhairabananda, replied immediately with an in-vitation to meet, but Glen had just taken ill and was unable to visit or at-tend the festivities to which he was invited.

Nonetheless, Glen contacted other old acquaintances in the Indian medical community, including Brahmanand Dixit in Agra, inquiring about the specifics of mercury-based medical compounds and asking for help locating tantric yogis. Dixit spoke of the wonders of mercury, and while he too claimed to know "not a single man who can be rightly said to be a perfect yogi," he also gave recommendations for men to contact, in this case a "Gurukul" practitioner in Chittargarh City.

Running to and fro around West Bengal, Glen took advantage of his occasional presence in Calcutta to contact Sukumar Chatterji, who was then attempting to form his own film company with a friend. Chatterji recommended a new book, a translation of the *Parad Saṃhita*, which explained many of the virtues of ingesting mercury compounds. "There is no question," he wrote, "about certain mercurial medicines with gold, arsenic, etc. and how mercury becomes not merely a disease destroyer but builder of youth and vigor." Above and beyond curing ailments, he explained, these compounds had extensive "aphrodisiac" qualities. He sent some sample medicines along with similar treatments for balding, all of which Glen began ingesting and which, not surprisingly, made him quite sick. After recovering, Glen eventually was able to visit Swami Bhairabananda at Belur Math—to whom he identified himself as Bodhananda—as well as others in the Calcutta area, such as the Swami Paramahansa Yogananda, whom he had known in California.[3]

Of greatest significance during this time, Glen was finally able to meet up with Walter Evans-Wentz, who had returned to Ghoom Monastery in Darjeeling the previous August and was due to pass through Calcutta in October. Over the months that followed, Glen and Evans-Wentz met and when apart, corresponded on various issues. Evans-Wentz felt that America was at a turning point in its history and that the economic depression was actually a great opportunity—a wake-up call for Americans to consider a new way of life.

Poor America seems unable to consider the great ideal of simple living and high thinking. The bubble of the theory of "God's Country" and the highest standard of life on earth has burst and America is as bewildered as a child when its own pretty soap-bubble has vanished. From latest advice, there is little or no improvement in the unemployment, and now everybody waits for the outcome of the Presidential Election, and the Bonus Group are jubilant over their Congressional banditry. They are now planning—while the getting is good—big pensions. How little brotherhood and real desire to subordinate selfishness to the greater needs of the nation there are!

Here the old fashioned life of the Hindu goes on untroubled by a world mad with armaments, machinery and exploitation. I hope it will ever be so.

While Glen and Evans-Wentz were so engaged, however, on February 2, Glen received word that Atal Behari Ghosh, his friend in Chaibassa, had died—ironically, just four days before his collaborator, Sir John Woodroffe, would die many thousands of miles west in Beausoleil, a suburb of Monte Carlo. Following the funerary (*śradh*) rites a few weeks later, at the request of Ghosh's son, Glen assumed the presidency of Ghosh's Āgamānusandhānasamiti (Agamas Research Society) and began a concerted effort to fund the last round of publications and distribute the remaining unsold texts to libraries around the world, even making a personal appeal to the Maharaja of Darbhaṅga, Kemeshwara Singh, for assistance with distribution and republishing out-of-print volumes. Glen was able to place copies of volumes of the "Tantrik Texts" series in the U.S. Library of Congress, as well as at the University of Pennsylvania, the University of Chicago, and Johns Hopkins University, and continued his efforts to reach other American libraries and universities as well.

Despite the loss of his friend and informant, Glen continued to acquire books[4] and cultivate contacts in the Indian yoga world, trying to locate tantric yogis and swamis near Calcutta—indeed, all across India—who could be considered authentic and knowledgeable and would be willing to instruct himself and Theos in the quickly approaching fall. It was a challenging enterprise that met with only limited success. In Mysore, he was told, "there are institutes where the yogic exercises or postures are also demonstrated or taught," but it was unclear "how far they conform to the standards of haṭha yoga." Still, he received recommendations for further inquiry:

You must have come across the "Yoga Mimamsa"—a journal devoted to Yoga. Sannyasis are also yogis, in a way, and are concerned with their own concentration and penance. Such an one is Ramana Maharshi near Tiruvunnamak (S.I.Ry); the Sage of Sakkoi may be another. . . .

The gentleman in Mysore is about 48–50 years of age and is a professor in the Maharaja's Sanskrit College, called the U.P. Krishnamachar. He seems to teach about 200 students. It is said that His Highness is favorably impressed with his teaching and demonstrations.

Glen continued recording all of these notes in planning the itinerary for the trip that he, Theos, and Viola would take in the months ahead.

Finally Glen's hard work paid off, and with help from Evans-Wentz, he made contact with two yogis in Bhurkunda, a seventy-two-year-old named Trivikram Swami and his younger disciple, Swami Syamānanda Brahmachāry, who had helped both Evans-Wentz[5] and Ekai Kawaguchi[6] years earlier. Relocating to Bhurkunda, Glen entered into a three-month yoga retreat, studying and practicing the various *āsanas*—attempting to master the most important practice of all, the *vajroli* mudra—and promised to teach Theos everything that he learned. Although deeply involved in his retreat, Glen continued to write to Viola and Theos regularly. At the same time, he continued to follow up on his contacts from Ghosh and Evans-Wentz, and contacted S. K. Jinorasa, the founder and director of the Young Men's Buddhist Association (YMBA) in Darjeeling.

Receiving his letter, Jinorasa praised Glen for his spiritual ambitions, though cautioned him about his motivation.

I am very glad to learn that you are greatly interested in the Yogi life in the jungle, and that you have made pretty good progress at it. Religious life is nothing but it entirely depends upon faith, and if you have great faith in it you are sure to succeed. In my own experience religious life is good for purification of self's mind if we can really have faith in it and practise it well. But at last it is a selfish thing in broad sense because he wants to purify himself and get salvation. It is just the same worldly people are doing, they are toiling day and night to earn something and to live happy life, so the ascetics go in jungles and try to purify their minds and get happiness of the mind. This is good for an individual no doubt but still the self exists there and he could not forget the self. When the self is there he must practise this and that darsanas to keep good morality of body, words and thought and when we forget our own existence where is then that self who observes all these rules and to purify whom. When we can forget our own existence then I see nothing in this world but only remains the "duty" and the "universal love." Desire of any fruition is evil and continuation of self or existences. Absence of desire is Nibbana. He who seeks for Nibbana shall never get, because there is the self or desire. Nibbana is for him who does not seek it.

Having helped Evans-Wentz in his research, Jinorasa made a similar offer of assistance to Glen, with one caveat:

I am glad to learn that your son and his wife will be coming to India in September and that they would also visit the Himalayas and would spend some time here. Yes, I shall certainly help you by introducing you to the learned lamas here. By the way I am very sorry to inform you that we have missed a great lama who could have helped you very much. He died a week ago in Sikkim. Regarding your tour in the Himalayas we can talk over the matter when you come up.

Glen, who through his contact with both Hans von Koerber and Evans-Wentz was already beginning to see the potential value in exploring the Tibetan side of yoga, took up Jinorasa on his offer, discussing the logistics of research in Sikkim and Tibet. That the Tibetan man Jinorasa referred to had just died in May 1936[7] was a problem, since highly educated Tibetans (in religious matters, at least) were not common in Kalimpong—or any other English-speaking areas. Nonetheless, Jinorasa promised to help locate individuals who could help Glen and Theos in the months to come.

While such plans were afoot, Glen continued in his efforts to amass literature and resources. From the editor of the *Kalyana-Kalpataru* he obtained copies of their published journal as well as copies of educational posters and pamphlets being produced by Swami Sivananda's main Western student in Latvia, Harry Dikman. Similarly, he was able to acquire a complete run of the *Yoga-Mimaṁsa* journal being published in Lonavla by Śrīmat Kuvalayānanda.

By July, Glen had returned to Bhurkunda in the Hazaribagh district of Behar, west of Calcutta, to continue his studies with Trivikram Swami. As he continued to consult with Kaviraj Narendranath Bidhyanidhi on mercury-derived medicinal compounds, Glen began to close in on what he saw as universal health prescriptions, hearing reports of life-extending procedures.[8] More significantly, however, while he had begun to develop proficiency in the practice of the *vajroli* mudra, he began to notice repeated references to it as a key yogic technique for the attainment of immortality, but could find no explanation of its application in any text.[9] Contacting Sukumar Chatterji, Glen asked for assistance in locating texts or individuals who could explain it to him.

In addition to recommending a new treatment for gonorrhea and suggesting that Glen "have some strychina [strychnine] beans and arsenic and tin and mica made there—for your future use," Chatterji responded, explaining all in detail as well as he could.

There is no book which gives any detail but there are instructions imparted by word of mouth which I have carefully collected. . . . Regarding Bajroli—This is what I have—one school claims that it is not for women and only men, specifically celibates should practice it. Another school known as Weerachari Tantriks, claim that it is specifically meant for married persons who practice it with their wives thereby interchanging each other's powers. The blowing [of air into the bladder] is meant for the beginner and occasionally when proper function does not take place of suction owing to some watery or slimy liquids in the canal. Just as water is sucked with or without Naoli through the rectum and a tube is used, but when sufficient practice is done no tube [is] required but if the water does not go in then finger is inserted to clean the passage. Same purpose is served by blowing in the bladder. Also there is an involuntary muscle which causes seminal discharge after Wajroli, that muscle becomes voluntary and brain can control it. . . .

The blowing of air in urethra as well as in the rectum is mentioned in one place to enable a person to control the air (Wayu) there with the breath. As shown Wayu is situated below, it must be controlled by breath or Mudras or naoli & such. It is to be practiced like all processes early in the morning and it takes from 3 to 6 months to complete it. The completion means the sucking of mercury. After which one can suck water milk honey etc. without a tube and even when erection takes place. Another mention is made of introducing filtered oily medicines in the rectum and bladder for various purposes. Main function tho seems to be to be able to suck one's own and the wife's semen back into the urethra, both the semens being reabsorbed into the body from the pores. Also a mention is made to practice it just before discharge and how on doing it, so that no semen is discharged at all.

The followers of Gorakshanath practice it early in the morning and at midnight, as they sleep early in the evening and at noon and keep awake all night to forenoon.

Chatterji recommended other practices for Glen to try out, including the suspension of cardiac activity.

The Sanyasi who was due has come.... Here is a thing that I wanted from some time. Stopping of the heart action. That man was here for a couple of days and he very freely showed me everything. It is taking the stomach back to the backbone and up towards the chest contracting rectum meantime and holding the breath out and suspending. 4 to 7 seconds of complete heart stoppage takes place and stethoscope even cannot record it. This should be easy for you to do. Only warning is, at the time of restarting the heart everything should relax very very gradually and no abrupt breath or relaxing is to be done. While holding thus an upper suction in the gullet is also practiced. Gorakshanath's Jalandhar & Uddyan Bandh is quite similar.

Glen and Chatterji continued their correspondence on many topics, including astrology, which Glen took quite seriously. In addition to horoscopic aspects of the field, Chatterji shared his notes on the crucial nature of astrological knowledge for medicine.

I have met a Kaviraj who has met a real yogi, as he claims, in north of Hardwar and saw him practice levitation. But he says the date fixed to see him is 2 years hence, when the Kumbha, which comes every twelve years, takes place.... [The Kaviraj's] medicines are remarkably efficacious from the first dose.... He has another method of making mercury [compounds].... He explains that encapsulating the metals and fermented juices, all herbal preparations lose their quality after one year and are useless after two years.... I am now trying out a process, very old one, which is difficult to understand because it is written in code words. Such as 305 is written as Ram-Kha-Wam. There were 3 well known Ram, so figure 3. Kha means akash which means cypher, hence 0. Wam means the five arrows of Kama god, our cupid. I know these so solved it, but I do not know all the codes, hence the trouble. Our astrologer also knows nothing about it but he has [a] book that I am copying out in portions.

Our astrologer says there are none who understand it. But I am sure we can find somebody who knows.

Chatterji likewise shared with Glen many of his theories on the physiological basis of the efficacy of these medicines, based on his readings.

In another place it is mentioned that in Wajroli when mercury is taken in and one has the power to open or close one of the dual passages—the one going to bladder and the other going to the prostate gland, then the mercury is kept near the mouth of the canal which carries semen and the passage of the bladder is closed. Most probably owing to body heat the vapour of the mercury goes to the semen canal!! Another passage mentions that milk, honey and mercury gradually should pass to the testicles and even to prostate but it is a bad translation because many other writings of the same book are quite humbug. In the Phallic Tantras it is written that there is an internal sexual cohabitation of the highest order which is the Divine Bliss and those only who have tasted it are empowered to add Ananda to their title. It takes place in the thousand petalled lotus between a small egg-shaped penus and the raised Kundalini. And this is the image of Shiva as it is worshipped today. . . .

The Kundalini wraps itself around the Shiva in the center and its tail tickles the Nadi called Puritat. Now Puritat is a Nadi where when mind goes we dream and make the inner world real.

The second copulation is of a lower-order and is Khechari which drops the liquid from the head of Shiva from the moon.

The third copulation is the worldly sexual one which gives temporary enjoyment but weakens life.

It is also mentioned somewhere, I do not recollect now, that when Kundalini is awakened all the 10 doors of the body must be closed. And something snaps inside and one faints and Guru helps. And thus the passage of spine is cleared and medula opens the third eye. There are three nadis in the spine—wajra, chitra and medhra, etc.

Although Chatterji had a certain degree of knowledge about the practices in which he and Glen were interested, they both still lacked a bona fide guru. The problem, as always, was how to finance such an exploration of the living tradition. Chatterji lamented, "If only you and I had money and time enough to go to Hardwar side, we might locate some fellow there who is on the way. On that side the path is known, found available, and a few lesser yogis known. While at Bhutan side, nothing is known. Only chance or luck can help." In the meantime, he was working on two projects that were very promising and could offer an answer to their financial situation. He wrote, giving Glen a glimpse, "Here is something to note. If mercury can be made to stand fire by the help of herbs only, i.e. no metal in it, then mixed with copper it can become gold. I am after these herbs information and if I find anything I shall write to you."

A second possibility that seemed to offer more immediate chances for success related to one of Chatterji's astrologers, who was convinced that by calculating the horoscope of animals, he could predict the outcome of horse races. A few weeks later, however, a rather disgruntled Chatterji was forced to report, "Our astrologer has miserably failed in Racing as I expected he might. The horses do not run on time as he expected, but there is always a difference of some 5 to 20 minutes in starting. So he has failed. But like all fanatics he is still hopeful, but I am not. So that is ditched."

Returning to their earlier discussions and responding to Glen's inquiry about the differing sects of "tantrikas" to be found, Chatterji described the basic difference between the two main groups, the Virācaryas and the Paśyācaryas.

Weera-achari Tantriks and Pashya-achari are two sects wildly differing in interpretation. Weera means the same root as Latin Vir, meaning life, heroism, pep, virility, etc. Achari means one who practices it and make it his second nature. So one who enjoys fullness of life and wrests every secret of life and enjoys it in every way is called Weera-achari.

Pashya-achari on the other hand, Pasya means grass eating animals and is a contemptuous word used by the Weera-acharis towards the other sect.

Weerachari goes through the 5 Ms that is the five words beginning with M. They are fish, meat, wine, mudra and sexual cohabitation. They take the meaning literally and figuratively both. Mudra has another literal meaning, i.e. money. It is for the worldly people. No temptation is to be avoided but should be sensibly indulged in without loss or injury but with decided gain.

Pashyachari on the other hand do not indulge in literal sense but have a figurative meaning—Fish means breath. Flesh means Khechari. Wine means the nectar. Mudra means the yogic mudras and sexual union means the union of soul with the universal soul. They are really yogis and are strictly celibate and vegetarians. It is the Weerachari Tantriks, who have invented Vajroli etc. They take both the meanings and while enjoying the outer, enjoy the inner also.

Much of this was already known to Glen (and Theos), having been covered in Woodroffe's book of essays on the *Śākta Tantra-śāstra*. Theos himself had described in his master's thesis the significance of the "ritual of the five 'M' aspects" as conveying the notion of complete engagement in transgressive behavior, taking care to make the further point that only the highest class of practitioner, a Vīra, would be qualified to engage in the rituals on a literal level.

Determined to pursue every possible avenue, Glen had business cards printed up, proclaiming himself just such a "Viracharya," a master of the Vira class of practitioners (*sādhaka*). Incorporating all that Chatterji had told him, with the three-and-a-half times coiled Kuṇḍalinī serpent—symbolic of the Mūlādhāra *cakra*—for a logo, his self-identification spoke volumes to those aware of its significance. Glen thus presented himself both as an adept of tantric yoga and as someone qualified to receive further instruction.

As their correspondence continued, Chatterji wrote at length about the interplay among the various yogic practices and the interpretation of the *pañcamākara* ritual by the "Weerachari" and others, himself citing the works of John Woodroffe and Arthur Avalon.

Fish increases ojah but also sexual inclination which destroys ojah. They eat fish but do not allow the effect to go to the sex center in its outward expression. If it does by chance, they practice vajroli and couter-act the effect. Meat produces restlessness but also nervous energy. They eliminate the undigestible portion of meat by Naoli and cool the bladder by Vajroli and by Khechari & breath make the blood of the pancreas, spleen etc. give nervous energy. Wine produces what is known as yogwahi i.e. which goes thru the whole system quickly. They drink it and by breath and special Naoli make it work upwards with no after effect on heart, stomach or nerves. Naoli according to them is to be practiced for special

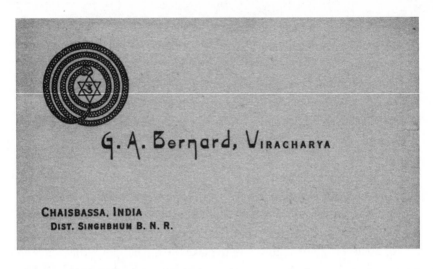

Figure 5.3 Glen Bernard's business card (BANC)

benefit to each function such as liver, kidney, pancreas, spleen, intestines. That is why the moving of the cord this way or that for special stimulation of specific place in the belly.

They also use alcoholic drinks made of various herbs, metals, shilajit, etc. and also take it thru the rectum or in the bladder as required . . . Mudra has two meanings, the money meaning the comforts of worldly life, ease, etc. and the yogic mudras . . . So is wine called Karan, meaning the great cause, the water of the cosmos. And here is a particular secret. The alcohol fermentation in the stomach of a particular nature produces suspension of that, samadhi, while of another kind, laziness or sleep. That is why by special breathing and help of these alcoholic fermentations, yogi sends forth the effect to whatever part of the body he pleases. Weeracharis make such special alcohol and use it thru rectum or bladder or mouth and help the stomach fermentation of that nature.

Arthur Avalon gives some information in English about them scattered thru his works. There is some in Asiatic Research Society but mostly denouncing them, written by so-called refined and virtuous people who are afraid to even talk of anything below the navel. Many idiotic degenerate fellows are secretly conducting the superficial rituals, and they call it "the Chakras." Kamroopa in Assam, Benares, and Orissa and Malabar section of Madras is their headquarters. Meherpur in East

Bengal near Chittagong way is a place of pilgrimage for them. After a little digging I can give you all the sects of the Tantriks.

You know these so-called "Twilight men & women" in the west creating new problems. Well, the tantriks recognized them and came to their rescue. They are known as "Karta-Bhaja" sect. They practice sodomy with vajroli, they also dress as women and interpret the world and nature as male and female sex. They eat semen of men and women and use menstrual blood for various purposes. Bunch of degenerates mostly, but at one time some very great men came out of them. Then there are Wam-margees—meaning the left-wingers. They even eat human excretion and sacrifice human beings, eat corpse, etc. That is their outer side. Their inner side is wonderful. They do not have any books of any kind. No record is even kept of anything. But handed down from mouth to mouth. Their explanation is wonderful and very feasible, which I will let you know some other time as it is too lengthy.

Despite his contempt for what he saw as ignorant interpretations of the tantric practices, Chatterji valued certain forms and had, perhaps, even more contempt for those who disparaged tantra outright.

As to why more persons do not practice etc. It is a difficult question. Why don't the humanity do the ABC of life? Then there would be less misery etc. All degenerate persons are prudish. Even speaking of penis is shameful. Everyone talks of higher things where they can talk at random and show off their study and never be found out. Such being the case, why practice Hatha Yoga which is very low, etc. God, religion, metaphysics, mysticism, forced celibacy, prudery, laziness, renunciation, all these bunk go as greatness. Nobody wants accuracy, facts, practical things, etc. but all want salvation. Until another Buddha or Shankar comes, no hope.

Even in the face of all these concerns and misgivings, he encouraged Glen to continue his study and practice, praising him as a true adept.

I am quite sure of all the Westerners, you certainly have a grasp of things more clearly and certainly far better than many Indian so-called Gurus. I am fortunate in having contact with some real ones while young. So I understand all the technical languages used and can trace others I do not know. So it is not so easy to fool me in yogic or Tantrik matters. By appearance alone, I can catch them. There is always an *a-sexual*, impersonal look on their faces who have raised the Kuṇḍalini.

Glen appears to have taken much of this to heart, and continued his yoga retreat with Trivikram Swami. In the meantime, he asked Chatterji to get in contact with Evans-Wentz for him, to let him know he was in retreat and that he still hoped to meet him on his return from Darjeeling. But Glen delayed his return until the last minute and missed meeting with Evans-Wentz one final time as he passed through the city en route to America. Instead, Glen made his way to Calcutta in order to meet Theos and Viola when they arrived in September. From there, the three of them could begin their adventures together.

SIX

Pretense and Pretext
Studies in India

My greatest difficulty has been in trying to find out what existed in the field so far as their literature is concerned . . . if I am able to organize the material to such an extent that others will be able to formulate their problems quickly and easily and start to work . . . I will feel that I have made a worthwhile contribution to one of the greatest storehouses of literature to be found in the world today.

—THEOS BERNARD[1]

AS THEY SET THEIR PLANS in motion for their trip across America and the Pacific to India in the fall of 1936, Theos and Viola began packing up their apartment in New York. Although it was only June, Viola was due to start her internship at the Jersey City Medical Center the following January and so had to prepare for it in advance. Placing their possessions in storage and their apartment up for sale, they organized one last "send-off" picnic party at the club in Nyack with friends and family. P.A. himself even gave Theos and Viola recommendations and suggestions for people to contact in India, including P. C. Bannerji, who had taught at his New York Sanskrit College in the 1910s, and S. L. Joshi, who had served as Secretary of the CCC. Similarly, Ruth Everett,[2] by then thoroughly enamored of all things Buddhist and Japanese,[3] gave Viola letters of introduction when she heard that they were traveling on a Japanese cruise ship and would be passing through Yokohama.

Saying good-bye to Columbia and New York, Theos headed west to Arizona to visit his mother and brothers, while Viola remained behind to complete her exams and spend time with her mother, who had been recently diagnosed with cancer. After driving across the country with a friend, Theos visited some of his old law school professors and friends from college, even getting his old boss at the *Arizona Daily Star* to write an article about his anticipated adventures:

> Theos Bernard, graduate of the University of Arizona in the 1934 class, is spending a short time in Tucson before leaving for India where he is being sent by the anthropology department of Columbia University for a year's study.
>
> While an undergraduate in Arizona Bernard majored in philosophy, but during the past two years at Columbia, where he has just been given a master's degree, he has specialized in anthropology. He has worked chiefly on ethnology with his interest centering about the philosophical in connection with primitive peoples. His study in India will be the relations or connections between the ethnology and philosophy of the people there. Columbia is sending him for a year. Mrs. Bernard will accompany her husband to India for the summer, but will return to New York this fall to begin her internship in one of the metropolitan hospitals. She has received her doctor's degree in medicine from Cornell medical school in New York City.[4]

Suitably embellished—"sent by Columbia" as opposed to "subsidized by his wife"—Theos was already beginning to lay the groundwork for his return in two years' time by portraying himself as an Ivy League scholar.

Heading on to Tombstone and traveling in style,[5] Theos took the opportunity to revisit the lands of his childhood, spending time with his mother and brothers out at the old family mine. Although he was some three thousand miles away while Viola went through the final formalities of her education, Theos reminded her that he was with her in spirit:

> This afternoon you are to receive your degree—which represents the completion of a chosen task and the first preparation for a future. There are endless ways in which this training can express itself and the job of the next four years is to find out which direction will lead to the greatest amount of happiness for you and at the same time keep whatever treasures you may possess today. Your friends will be about you today all telling you how proud they are and extending their sincerest congratulation, but no one will express their feelings with a heart any more sincere then [sic] my own. I come to this end with as much joy and feeling

of accomplishment as yourself—it was almost as though it was me who receives the degree. From my actions the past years, it may not have appeared as though I was much in accord with your efforts—but this is not true, and as we finally adjust the outward manifestations of our effort down the same narrow channel, you will realize all.

Despite his declarations of their same, singular goal in life, Theos remained nervous about Viola and her commitment to their plans. Preparing to leave Tombstone with his mother and brothers, he became worried when he hadn't heard from Viola in over a week.

Say, what happened to you—I have not heard from you since you left [Lake] Placid—or rather since you wrote last Sunday. Has something gone wrong . . . I want to know anything and everything when it concerns you—directly or indirectly—how about it—is it a go—that we always let the other party know? . . .

I do hope everything is all right and that my fear is groundless; for dear there is a great deal of love here, and I do not want anything to happen at anytime—especially when I am away—remember a wire will always bring me home—there is nothing on earth that will hold my attention if there is something of some consequence which affects you—I wish to be with you thru all things of this life.

Seeking Viola's reassurance that all was well with her, Theos let her know that all was well with his family and that he was the same as ever.

Everyone is well; so we should have a very enjoyable trip. . . . I dropped in to bid goodbye to several of my old prof. today and we had a few pleasant moments rehearsing old times and preparing thoughts for the future. Some of them I find beginning to fossilize already, others are as stimulating as ever before and are also making their growth within which this whole game is all about. I contacted the chap here in charge of the Archeology department—he has a law degree from Chicago and also has a Ph.D. in Anthropology; so you see there is one other nut in the world—but he doesn't have an M.A in philosophy—I still have them bested.

With his usual air of confidence, he advised Viola about his various stops along the way to their reunion in San Francisco. Departing from

Tombstone, Theos and his family then toured the Southwest before driving through California up to San Francisco, sightseeing along the way and visiting friends and relatives. After meeting up with Viola, they enjoyed the sights of the city for nearly three weeks. Seen off at the docks by his family, Theos and Viola finally set sail from San Francisco on July 14, 1936, on the luxury liner the *Asama Maru*, passing under the girders of the still unfinished Golden Gate Bridge out into the Pacific toward "the Far East."

An impressive ship for its day, the *Asama Maru* spanned close to 600 feet in length and was capable of comfortably housing over 800 passengers (more than 200 in first class). One of the two flagships of the Nippon Yusen Kaisha (NYK) fleet, it had set a new record for the fastest crossing of the Pacific Ocean on the Yokohama–San Francisco route shortly after its launch in 1929. As a luxury liner in the true sense of the phrase, it offered a full range of amenities on board, from exotic menus and a hair salon to a library and traditional Kabuki theater performances, and a main dining room outfitted in mahogany and adorned with marble columns. At the time, it was quite possibly the finest way to travel from America to Japan and beyond.

After more than two weeks of sailing at a leisurely pace, early on the morning of August 4, the *Asama Maru* docked at its first port of call, Honolulu, Hawai'i. Theos and Viola took the opportunity to visit with friends, tour the usual sites around Oahu, and have a quick swim at Waikiki before dashing back to the ship in time to make the departure that evening. The next day, Viola had tea with Captain Kaneko in his cabin, having presented him with her letter of introduction from Ruth Everett. As a result, she and Theos were invited to a sukiyaki party on deck that evening.

Spending another week crossing the wide Pacific may have lulled a few passengers into Melville's "unconscious reverie [that] takes the mystic ocean at his feet for the visible image of that deep, blue, bottomless soul, pervading mankind and nature,"[6] but Theos and Viola appear to have been focused instead on dining and socializing with the various other guests on board. Meeting a number of missionaries returning to China, they heard stories of fighting and even piracy near Nanking and began to reconsider their overland journey by railroad through China to Canton.[7]

Arriving in Yokohama slightly more than a week later, Theos and Viola immediately boarded a train on the Tokyo–Yokohama railroad, then settled into the Imperial Hotel in Tokyo. With three days allocated for sightseeing while the ship restocked its supplies, they took the opportunity to tour the country, visiting the Meiji Shrine and Imperial Palace in Tokyo

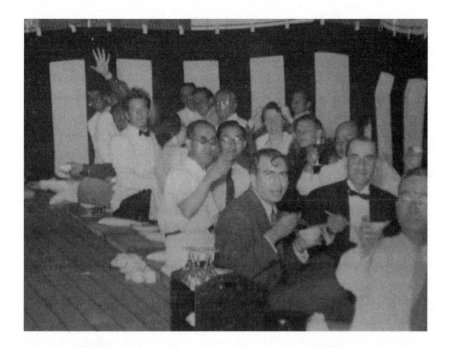

Figure 6.1 Theos and Viola Bernard aboard the *Asama Maru* (CUHS)

and the Daibutsu Buddha in Kamakura. From there they went to the Atami hot springs on the Izu peninsula to feast and relax before catching the overnight train to Kyoto, taking pictures all along the way.

Once in Kyoto, Viola and Theos followed Ruth Everett's recommendations and got themselves settled into the "Japanese House" at the Miyako Hotel—like "bulls in a China shop," Viola thought—to await the arrival of the abbot of the Shunkoin Temple, Sohaku Ogata. Guided by Ogata, Theos and Viola visited the various Shinto and Buddhist temples of Kyoto while discussing the history of Buddhism. They returned with Ogata to his home monastery in Shokokuji, where Theos was intrigued to learn that a "Hindu monk" from Calcutta was staying there, learning Zen. While Viola and Ogata continued their conversation on the metaphysical questions of the day, such as the effect of the mind on the body and the message of "the East" for "the West," Theos actively engaged the "Hindu monk" in his own discussion.

Taking the train to Kobe the next morning, Theos and Viola returned to the *Asama Maru* in time for its departure at noon. After a comparatively short two days at sea, the cruise ship sailed across the Yellow Sea—"which was yellow," Viola remarked—before sailing down the Whangpoo River and into the port at Shanghai. After disembarking, Viola and Theos headed to the local shipping office to send and receive cablegrams, as well as to arrange for inland travel for the next ten days before stepping out to explore the shops and restaurants along the streets.

The next day Viola contacted her friends in the city and attended to the various details of their jaunt through China—from making all the obligatory social greetings to purchasing plane tickets and ordering a silk pongee suit for Theos—while Theos himself remained bedridden, a victim of the previous evening's street food. Despite feeling under the weather, both figuratively and literally, Theos composed himself well enough to join Viola for dinner that evening at Marble Hall, the mansion in Shanghai belonging to Sir Elly Kadoorie, one of the most successful businessmen in Shanghai and a pillar of the Sephardic Jewish population in the city. Feasting on a twenty-five course dinner with enough wine to calm even the most tender of stomachs, Kadoorie entertained his guests with tales of his life and of other guests whom he had hosted, from Rabindranath Tagore and Halie Sellassie to the Thirteenth Dalai Lama, or so he claimed.[8]

After a long night and only an hour's sleep, Theos and Viola trundled off to the airport to catch a private plane they had chartered with three other Americans to fly to Peking with a leisurely airborne tour of the Great Wall and Forbidden City. By 9 a.m. they had arrived at the Grand Hôtel des Wagon-Lits—final destination of the famed Orient Express—where Kadoorie had already arranged a reception for them with guides and itineraries. Within a half an hour, they were off again, negotiating their way through the streets by rickshaw to the Forbidden City, followed in rapid succession by the Temple of Heaven, Winter Palace, and Lama Temple, with Theos's camera capturing shot after shot; their tour culminated in a multicourse dinner of bird's nest soup, roast duck, and other delicacies before they returned to the hotel.

Over the days that followed, Theos and Viola toured around the city before flying to Tsingtao and Nanking to board a hydroplane to Kiukiang, though not before having to exchange pleasantries with the ubiquitous Christian missionaries. "Do you know Lord Jesus?" one of them asked, to which Theos responded with a polite but succinct, "No." After more sightseeing, hiking, and socializing, they began making their way back toward the coast to resume their journey. On a leisurely boat trip down the Yangtze

River before boarding a train for Shanghai, Theos swapped camera tricks with passengers, pilots, and ships' captains—any Leica enthusiast he could find—while Viola caught up on the local gossip on Americans in China, including most notably Harrison Forman, who had been making loud claims about his recent expedition to Tibet.[9]

Upon their arrival in Hong Kong, Theos and Viola made arrangements to board a new ship, the smaller *Hakozaki Maru*. Spending one last day in Shanghai with their former pilot and new friend Chilly Vaughn while waiting for their most recent photos to be developed, they swam in the ocean and dined on the best local cuisine, from shark's fin in creamed crab soup to rum lobster and beer. After they set sail the next morning for Singapore, Viola sorted through their photographs, updated her diary, and wrote letters home recounting their adventures in Japan, while Theos remained sick and bedridden once again.

Recovering slightly the next day, Theos began reading William McGovern's *To Lhasa in Disguise*, an account of the experiences of the first American to reach Lhasa fourteen years earlier, achieved in contravention of both the Tibetan and British authorities. McGovern—who had succeed where his countryman William Rockhill had failed—offered his readers a role model for their own journey to Tibet in the form of an account replete with cultural cues and descriptions of potential obstacles. Lying in his bed, Theos studied McGovern's account avidly, reading through it in two days and gleaning as much information from it as he could before giving it to Viola to read.

Theos spent the next few days reading heavily, turning to Alexander Goldenweiser's philosophically reflective collection of essays on anthropological methods, *History, Psychology, and Culture*. Goldenweiser, although criticized by the more mainstream anthropology community for it, lamented the subjugation of creativity in research to normative methodological safeguards while encouraging the "incipient liberation of American ethnology from its methodological bondage." "The seeker of truths," he wrote, "is like the builder of roads; both must combine imagination with method, vision with technique . . . but unless there is vision first, there will be no road at all."[10] It was an appeal not far from Theos's own heart.

When the ship docked in Singapore, Theos and Viola placed their studies on hold and disembarked to tour the city and arrange transport by ship to their final destination, Calcutta. Registering with the local authorities, Viola sent and received her usual cablegrams to and from her sister as well as her close confidante, Blanche DeVries, who was beginning to experience marital difficulties with Theos's uncle, Pierre. Touring the botanical gardens, monkey groves, and amusement parks, Theos and Viola took more "vacation" photos of each other before stopping for dinner and a movie.

Despite the previous evening's "local cuisine" still playing havoc with them when they returned to their cabin, the next day they cruised through the backcountry roads of the city touring rubber plantations, taking more photos, and shooting film footage. Stopping in town to check for cablegrams and pick up supplies, Theos purchased a large supply of oversized cardstock on which to mount contact prints of his photos and label and categorize them, in order to more easily select prints for enlargement[11] before they both rushed to their new ship, the HMS *Karapara* bound for Malaysia.

Theos and Viola spent the next day on board the ship reading, and sorting and labeling their more than twenty rolls' worth of contact prints. Exhausted, they retired for the evening only to be awakened by dock workers unloading crates of copra and betel nut over their heads when the ship pulled into Penang late in the night. Braving the early morning monsoon rains—the fringes of a cyclone in the Bay of Bengal—Theos and Viola went into Penang to wire Calcutta for hotel reservations in anticipation of their arrival and to send DeVries a birthday telegram, before setting out to explore the city. With only a few hours before the ship departed again, they ran from the Chinese Snake Temple through the local botanical gardens to a Thai Buddhist temple, posing for each other and taking pictures, in 100+degree South Seas weather.

After three days of rough seas, the *Karapara* finally arrived in Rangoon, and Theos and Viola hurriedly disembarked and checked into a suite at the luxurious Strand Hotel.[12] After refreshing themselves, they ordered a chauffeured car and went to explore the temples, from the Shwedagon Stupa to the Reclining "Parinirvana" Buddha at Tharlyaung, spending the better part of two days being blessed by monks and seeing the sights. Reboarding the ship, they bided their time reading and sorting photographs for three more days until on Sunday, September 13, 1936, they finally arrived in Calcutta.

In an act of genuine kindness, P.A. had arranged for his old friend, P. C. Bannerji, to meet Theos and Viola at the dock. Arriving at the Great Eastern Hotel, they retrieved the mail that awaited them at the American Express office, but were somewhat dismayed to find that the letters they had sent ahead to Theos's father lay at the hotel unclaimed. Relying instead on Bannerji and his wife, they arranged the various mundane aspects of their impending trip, from ordering reprints of their photos to hiring reliable servants and finding Theos a dentist.

After two days in Calcutta, Theos and Viola finally received a phone call from Glen. While Bannerji entertained Viola by giving her a tour of the city, Theos and Glen sat down in their hotel room for a reunion and discussion of their plans for the weeks and months to come. Returning to the hotel after a few hours, Viola and Bannerji rejoined them, and all four went to Belur Math to visit the Ramakrishna Temple, where they were given a VIP tour courtesy of Bannerji's influence. Bannerji, moreover, gave them open letters of introduction to all the Ramakrishna centers across India, encouraging them to visit as many as possible. Parting company with Glen and Bannerji, Theos and Viola returned to their hotel later in the day. Only then did Theos take the time to fill Viola in on his discussions with his father and their plans for the coming weeks. Viola was not amused; she was, in fact, furious at what Theos was suggesting.

Far from a tour of scenic India, Glen and Theos planned a trip inland to Bhurkunda, to Trivikram Swami's ashram, where they would engage in a yoga retreat lasting several weeks, if not months. For the first time in a while, Viola blew up at Theos. She had not traveled halfway around the world and endured weeks at sea just to sit in a hut in the jungle for months on end while her husband and his father practiced yoga and studied with swamis. If such a "scheme" was Theos's idea of a good way to spend his time abroad, he could do it *after* she returned home.

The next day, Theos and Viola put the dispute behind them and caught the early morning train on the Bengal Nagpur Rail line south to Puri for a tour of the nearby tantric sites of great repute: the "Black Pagoda" Sun Temple at Konarak and Ramakrishna Math and Shankara Math, the first of the four "Shankara ashrams" recommended by Theos's uncle. Their first intended stop, the Sun Temple at Konarak, had been visited and praised unabashedly by John Woodroffe as a truly holy place:

[By] the ancient and desolate Temple to the Sun-Lord at Konâraka in Northern Orissa, a continuous rolling sound like that of the Mahâmantra is borne to me from afar. I heard the same sound many years ago at the Pemiongchi monastery when some hundred Buddhist monks rolled out from the depth of their bodies the mantra *Om.* Their chant then suggested the sea, as the sea now suggests the Mantra . . . the surf of the Bengal Ocean in great waves, marbled with foam with creaming crests, whipped into filmy vapour by the wind, ceaselessly beats upon a lonely shore. The waves as all else are Mantra.[13]

More notoriously (in polite Indian and British society, that is) the temple was renowned for the erotic sculpture adorning its outer walls, and was considered to be the site of "an ancient tantric cult" devoted to the Vedic sun god, Surya.

Upon their arrival in Puri, however, Theos and Viola learned that monsoons had washed out the roads to Konarak and the temple was accessible only by elephant transport—a journey that, despite its romantic qualities, would take two days. Instead, they decided to confine their trip to Ramakrishna Math and Shankara Math, two ashrams of equally great repute. Presenting the letter from Bannerji at Ramakrishna Math, they were treated to a tour of the temple by the resident swami, Sivaturananda, who accompanied them to Shankara Math as well. There they were disappointed to learn that the current "acharya," Bharadi Krishna Tirth, was away, although the acting head happily showed them around the complex, giving them information about where to find the other three "Shankarâcharyas" in Mysore, Bombay, and Hardwar. Consoling themselves with some shopping and tea, they returned to the train station only to discover that Theos had thrown away their return tickets, thinking them to be worthless stubs. After considerable negotiations, they managed to secure another second-class compartment on the evening train back to Calcutta.

After the previous day's somewhat botched adventure, Theos and Viola spent their time apart, Viola visiting local hospitals and medical colleges while Theos—annoyingly to her—insisted on attempting to get a refund for the tickets he had lost the previous day before visiting the Royal Asiatic Society of Bengal and the Mahābodhi Society with Glen. Arriving at the R.A.S., Theos and Glen were dismayed to find that the director, Johan van Manen, was out. Promising to return later, they went on to the Mahābodhi Society to visit the director, a personal friend of Glen's, for tea.

With Viola, Glen and Theos paid a visit to their travel agent in Calcutta, Gumbrill, to revise their proposed tour of India, the latter having informed them that their initial itinerary was unfeasible in the time allotted. When they expressed their interest in the Tibetan tradition, Gumbrill suggested that they contact Rai Bahadur Laden La, a man universally regarded as the most powerful individual in Darjeeling. While these plans were being made, however, the stress of Glen's agendas and opinions was beginning to wear on Viola, and the two of them got into a protracted fight over dinner.

Airing his opinion of the worthlessness of psychiatry since the field of study was nothing more than "a means to avoid work & to do very little with medicine," Glen provoked a heated argument over what constituted "medicine" and "real" research. The true crux of the argument, however, was what sort of research Theos would do while in India. Glen's opinion—which would soon become Theos's as well—was that anthropological field work (and anthropology in general) was a waste of time. Theos, he thought, should concentrate on creating a photographic record of his journey during the ensuing months and write a Ph.D. thesis drawing on sources "largely supplied by others." It was a debate that would not be settled quickly.

On their final day in Calcutta, they went out early to the Kalighat to watch the sacrifices at the temples. Only upon arrival, however, did they discover that the sacrifices would happen much later in the morning. As they made their way to the University of Calcutta, Viola took charge of the day's activities: meeting with the vice-chancellor, who arranged for a tour of the university's medical facilities, and with members of the archeology and anthropology departments to counsel Theos on possible research subjects in India—including the Todas of South India and various groups on the Tibetan border—none of which was of much interest to Theos himself. So, after a variety of pleasantries, they made a quick tour of some temples in the area before returning to their hotel to pack and catch the overnight train up through the jungles of Bengal to Siliguri and Darjeeling in the north.

Drenched by the monsoon rains upon their arrival in Siliguri, Theos, Viola, and Glen commissioned a private car to take them to Darjeeling, where they settled into the Mount Everest Hotel.[14] Beset with chills and a case of altitude sickness, Viola consigned herself to bed rest, while Theos and Glen immediately headed into the streets to find the first of their contacts in the area, S. K. Jinorasa and S. W. Laden La, in the hope of locating Lama Yongden, the man who had aided Alexandra David-Neel in her studies and travels. Unsuccessful on both counts, they were instructed to return the next day, when both men would be available.

Despite her persisting poor health, Viola awoke at 3 a.m. to join Theos and Glen on a trip up Tiger Hill to try to see Mount Everest. Though Everest was obscured by clouds, they chanced to meet a young fellow American from Illinois, Harry Espenschied, who had been traveling overland by bicycle from Germany through Greece and Afghanistan, down through Kashmir and Ladakh before ending up in Darjeeling. Sharing a cup of tea later in the day, Harry and Theos talked about his trip and shared the names of contacts along the route.[15]

Anxious to connect with Laden La, Theos and Glen called once more on his residence while Viola recuperated in the hotel. Although Laden La had still not returned, one of his sons, Willie,[16] met them and agreed—pending his father's permission—to take all three of them to meet Alexandra David-Neel's teacher, Lama Yongden, the next day. With time on their hands, Theos, Glen, and Viola arranged for doubly-manned rickshaws to negotiate the now muddy roads of Darjeeling in search of S. K. Jinorasa. Descending from the main bazaar and passing Bhutia Basti, they arrived at Jinorasa's YMBA (Young Men's Buddhist Association) school late in the afternoon, where they found Jinorasa with his brother, Gyaltsen Kazi, and a young Tibetan lama named Gedun Chöpel. Over tea, Theos showed the men "a yantra"—the Tibetan "Wheel of Life"—that he had purchased earlier that day. Jinorasa and Gedun Chöpel proceeded to explain the significance of the different symbols and general layout of the chart, from desire and hatred rooted in ignorance to the various realms of existence and the basic theory of dependent origination.

The next morning all three of them, accompanied by Willie Laden La, traveled to Ghoom Monastery on the outskirts of Darjeeling. After touring the temple and taking some photographs, Theos discussed the possibility of extended study should he return to Darjeeling. Cautioning him about the realities that that would entail, the monks advised Theos to try to contact another American who had been doing the same thing and had even reached Gyantse on one visit: a Yale alumnus named Henry Carpenter, who stayed at the Mount Everest Hotel every year.[17]

Heading back up to the Darjeeling markets, Theos and Viola did some last minute shopping[18] before packing and returning to Siliguri by car later that afternoon to catch the overnight train to Calcutta. Although she had planned to spend only a day and a half there, upon their arrival Viola discovered that her illness had progressed into full-blown pneumonia, and so, sensing the delay, Glen began making other plans for himself and Theos, including introducing him to his old teacher, Sukumar Chatterji, then living in Calcutta. Theos and Glen spent the next three days meeting off and on with Chatterji, who even played some rare recordings of Tibetan music and chants being pressed on the outskirts of Calcutta by the Gramophone record plant in Dum Dum. Determined to get a set of the records for himself, Theos made the journey across the city by trolley and rickshaw, which frustratingly took over four hours, only to discover that the records could not be had on the spot and would have to been delivered to his hotel.[19]

Viola was having her own troubles that day as well, having gone to the post office to send their film footage to be developed. When she returned to their room at the Great Eastern Hotel to start packing for the evening train, the stress of the day caught up with Viola and once again, she, Theos, and Glen got into a fight, this time over the simple logistics of their evening meal. The trip, for Viola, was not working out the way she had envisioned, from Glen's continual interference in their plans to the realities of life and hygiene in the Indian subcontinent. By the time they arrived in Varanasi the next morning, she had developed an abscessed tooth and an infection that began to make her mouth fester and bleed. With these many things weighing upon her, Viola's mood had soured dramatically, and little that transpired over the ensuing days would improve it. The burning ghats along the Ganges that Theos filmed with enthusiasm were for Viola nothing more than a place "where crap meets God," lined with royal edifices along the riverbank "for them to also have a place of sacred crap," and every expedition through the city seemed to proceed through "back alley ways of crap." Undeterred by such things, however, Glen and Theos pursued their research agenda, pressing on through the unrelenting monsoon rains to Sarnath and the Buddhist temples there before hurriedly returning to Varanasi for the night, then boarding their early morning train farther north and westward across the Gangetic Plain.

The weeks that followed were a nonstop whirlwind of sightseeing and shopping, with Theos alternately filming and photographing every exotic or artistic event and building he came across. Beginning the very next day, Theos, Viola, and Glen toured old Indian cities, from the Taj Mahal and Red Fort in Agra to the Man Mandir Palace in Gwalior. After dropping off a dozen rolls of film to be developed and more brief sightseeing, the travelers boarded a series of trains northwest from Delhi, only spending a night at various stops along the way, Peshwar, Rawalpindi, and Lahore, before embarking on their trip to Kashmir by private car, stopping along the way to visit with the Roerich family. Picnicking and camping, with their support staff of coolies cooking, washing, and setting up and breaking down

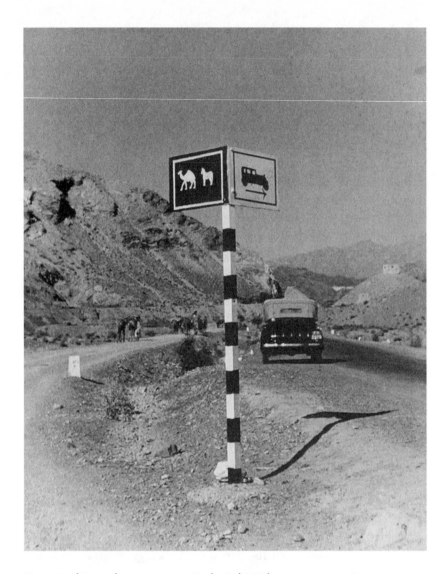

Figure 6.2 Chartered car en route to Kashmir (CUHS)

their tents and bedding wherever they went, shopping and shooting film
and still photos all the way, Theos, Viola, and Glen enjoyed themselves,
having escaped the heat and monsoon rains of the Gangetic Plain, traversing Kashmir and Ladakh and visiting sites from Hemis Monastery in Leh
to the Golden Temple in Amritsar. But while their adventures were finally

proceeding nicely, a drama of equal magnitude was playing itself out half a world away back in New York.

Having carved out an empire for himself in Nyack, Pierre Bernard was not above indulging himself in the opportunities his wealth and status accorded him. Since the time of their meeting in the early 1910s, Pierre and DeVries had been a couple in both their private and public lives. But even after their marriage, Pierre had his dalliances from time to time with the occasional young woman seeking knowledge of the "more advanced practices" of yoga, to which Blanche did her best to turn a blind eye, and by the 1930s, they had settled into a stable arrangement at the country club. A shrewd businessman and religious teacher, Pierre was well attuned to the needs and sensibilities of the club membership. He could see quite well that a rigorous course in religious theory and practice was something toward which few Americans were favorably disposed. What most of his clientele wanted was actual and vicarious excitement to relieve the tedium of their existence, so, like many a successful popular religious teacher, Pierre provided them with 10 percent religion and 90 percent entertainment, with the result being a rousing success. DeVries put her skills as a vaudeville entertainer, honed during the years of her youth in New York City, to good use, producing plays, musicals, and dance pieces performed on the grounds of the club. The days at the Clarkstown Country Club followed a strategic pattern of food, exercise, and entertainment, rounded out with an evening lecture by Pierre himself.

By the mid-1930s, however, the strains of the depression were beginning to be felt even within the confines of the CCC. Educational and social organizations began to fold around the country as membership dues were deemed unaffordable extravagances, and the same fate seem to be in store for Pierre's club as well. Feeling the need to curb expenses, Pierre was growing increasingly unsympathetic toward DeVries's expenditures to maintain the artistic environment, even telling Theos just before his departure, "the situation around here is terribly strained on account of DeVries reaction to cutting out some of these bums who are dancers." In a ploy to shift the focus of the club away from her artistic vision toward a new direction, Pierre decided the time had come to oust DeVries and began to elevate his latest paramour in her place. It was a move that sent shock waves throughout the community and literally around the world.

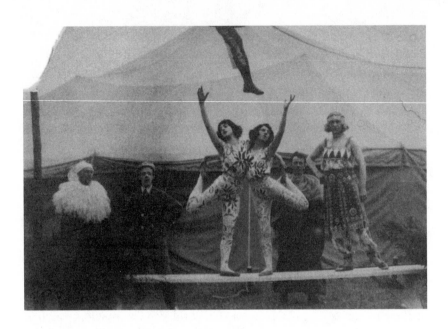

Figure 6.3 Blanche DeVries's "Theater of Much Discipline" (CUHS)

Distraught, DeVries had written to Viola, taking her into her confidence and seeking her advice. For the better part of three weeks, they corresponded about what to do, with Viola devoting much of her diary to her own thoughts and feelings about the events transpiring at home.[20] As one of Pierre's benefactors and longtime students, and DeVries's close friend, Viola was torn, unsure what course of action she should take, if any. In the end, she offered her advice to DeVries as best she could and decided to defer any radical actions until her return in two months' time.

Returning to Delhi in early October, Viola, Theos, and Glen began the next major leg of their all-India tour: a religious, scientific, political, and archeological adventure across the Deccan Plateau. From Delhi through Ajmer and Udaipur, Theos made the best use of his time, continuing to prepare for what seemed to be his inevitable trip to Tibet by reading Charles Bell's *Religions of Tibet*. Although more research would be necessary, Theos and Viola took the opportunity of a two-day layover in Udaipur to do some sightseeing. Throughout the weeks of their travels, their primary guide and manservant, Housseinie, had accompanied them on their various side trips, but when their car arrived the next morning, they found that the service came with its own guide, and Housseinie had to be left behind, un-

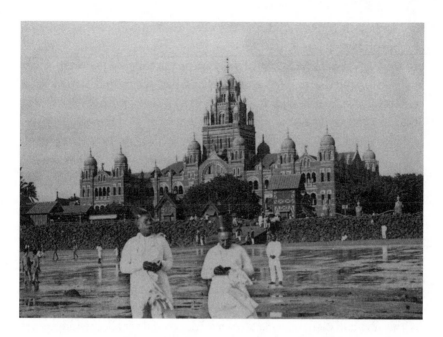

Figure 6.4 Church Gate Railway Station, Bombay (photo stereogram; private collection of the author)

derstandably upset, since the first stop on their tour was Akbar's infamous garden of slave girls. Traversing the arid climate of Rajasthan, even in the morning, was still tiring in October, and by the time they had reached the Juggernath Temple, Theos was feeling the effects of dehydration. Despite drinking water and eating a light lunch, by the end of the afternoon's visit to the Maharaja's residence, the Jag Mandir Temple, and a boat tour of the neighboring jungle, he was running a fever and showing the signs of sepsis.

Despite Glen's insistence on discussing the merits of the *Bhagavad Gita* for the study of yoga late into the night, they went early to the railway station the next morning to catch the only express train to Bombay. Arriving the next day at Bombay's majestic Church Gate Railway Station, in anticipation of an extended rest stop, the Bernards enveloped themselves in colonial splendor once more, checking into the five-star Taj Mahal Hotel, one of the last great hotels of the British Raj era, built in 1903 just opposite the Gateway to India and looking out over the Arabian Sea.

Wasting little time, they began to utilize another of their club contacts in India, Pierre and Viola's friend Dr. S. L. Joshi, the onetime secretary for the Clarkstown Country Club and then Professor of Comparative Religion and Indian Philosophy at Dartmouth College. Joshi had sent letters ahead of their arrival the previous July, and his friends and relatives were ready and waiting for the couple's arrival in Bombay, for having alerted their contacts in advance to their impending arrival, they found several letters awaiting them at the hotel, to which they immediately responded.

After weeks on the move and taking hundreds of pictures and feet of film, Theos and Viola made their way to the Kodak office to retrieve their negatives and contact prints and to preview their film footage. Daunted by the task of having to sort through hundreds of contact prints, then label and mount them, the sobering effect of their visit was compounded by the disappointingly poor quality of their 16-mm films, most of which appeared to be out of focus. Dropping their camera off to have the lenses realigned, Theos and Viola saw to their weeks of neglected grooming, though as usual, Theos got into a fight with a local man, this time with his would-be barber for trying to shave his head.

The next day, Glen's agenda took precedence and yet another adventure ensued, beginning with a long drive from Bombay to Poona via Lonavla to introduce Theos to Swami Kuvalayānanda in the hope that he would be more forthcoming than he had been the previous year with Glen. However, their plans became immediately more complicated by ongoing riots in Bombay. Eventually escaping the city and arriving at Kuvalayānanda's Kaivalyadhāma Institute, they were disheartened to find the Swami gone for the day and scheduled to return only later in the evening. Noticing, with some amusement, a copy of Pierre Bernard's *Vira Sadhana* on a table, they pledged to return in the evening as well and continued on to Poona.

Following a lunch of dubious quality, they tried to find another one of Joshi's contacts, V. S. Sukthankar, at the Bhandarkar Oriental Research Institute. Although this provided Theos and Glen an opportunity to buy more books, Viola was more intrigued by the possibility of visiting with a local Kaviraj, Dr. Sardesai, and a tour of a pharmacological factory—but could only do so *after* indulging Theos's extensive photographic pursuits. Spending the afternoon in social pleasantries with Dr. Sardesai's family, Viola, Theos and Glen headed back to Bombay, not reaching Lonavla until nine at night. Fortunately, Kuvalayānanda was there and took the time to talk with them; while Viola and Theos were entertained by the old man's thoughts on mankind, Glen was far less forgiving, pressuring the man on points of practice, from *kuṇḍalinī* to *vajroli*. Being intentionally evasive,

Kuvalayānanda responded with either vague generalities or tangential observations about whether or not such practices were engaged in at the Institute. Tired and feeling a certain degree of frustration, Glen accused Kuvalayānanda of remaining "silent" about the truth of the practices and their connection with sex and celibacy, a remark that ended the conversation as Kuvalayānanda got up and left the room in a flurry of half-spoken words, leaving Theos and Viola to pay their respects to the other temple residents and resume the last four hours of their drive back to Bombay.

With little to show for the previous day's boondoggle, Glen resumed his role as third wheel in the party as Viola set the agenda for the day ahead. After a return visit to Kodak, Theos and Viola were encouraged to see that the film they had shot of Udaipur was much better than the others they had taken thus far. Still, their film stock appeared to be suffering from the effects of heat and humidity as they traveled around the subcontinent, as well as some more technical fumbling on Theos's part. Resolving to fix the problem, Theos spent a great deal of time and money picking out new equipment for the camera before sidetracking Viola to another bookstore, with Glen sulking in tow. Having deferred meeting with Joshi's family the day before, after a few calls earlier that morning, they had settled on a plan to meet for tea in the afternoon with Joshi's friend, M. R. Jayakar, and as the time approached, Joshi's daughter and her husband called to escort them up to the Malabar Hill Ashram, where Jayakar stayed.

A respectable scholar, lawyer, and politician, Mukund Ramrao Jayakar held pride of place as a close supporter of Mahatma Gandhi in the ongoing struggle for Indian independence, not only against the British Raj—having abandoned his lucrative law practice in answer to Gandhi's 1921 call for a boycott of British law courts—but also against the prejudices of Indian society. Working with the noted advocate for the rights of the "untouchables," Dr. B. R. Ambedkar, Jayakar had been one of the first candidates in the joint electorate following Gandhi's 1932 "fast unto death" to protest the British government's declaration of separate electorates for "Depressed Classes." A contender for a position of national power against his more hard-line opposition colleague, Muhammad Ali Jinnah, by 1936, Jayakar was still enmeshed in the political scene, though occasionally he found time for religious pursuits in the study of Vedanta.

While Theos and Viola soaked up the insights Jayakar could offer on modern India, the British Raj, and a host of other concerns, Glen was far more concerned with resuming his own personal quest. Having been given

Śrī Yogendra's contact information in Poona the day before, he vowed to meet the man the next day, so after the obligatory social calls in the morning, the three of them went in search of Yogendra.

Offering India's answer to "Muscular Christianity,"[21] Śrī Yogendra claimed to have learned yoga as a teenager when became the disciple of Paramahansa Madhavadasaji, a Bengali yogi then reputed to be 119 years old. Glen was familiar with Yogendra from his earlier contact with Paramahansa Yogananda and Swami Dhirananda in the 1920s. Lucky in his research this time, Glen found Yogendra to be an engaging and open man, thoroughly conversant in yoga and quite willing to discuss it. For the better part of two hours, he and Glen talked about the different aspects of yogic practice as well as the politics of research. Yogendra had struggled, he said, to maintain his independence in the face of would-be supporters and collaborators seeking to exploit and "prostitute" yoga for their own ends; he even made a point of informing the Bernards how he "told the theosophists to go to hell." Finding camaraderie between them, Yogendra shared with Glen the insights of some of his unfinished works, including a comprehensive "History of Yoga."

Contrary to the populist presentations of yoga then being disseminated, Yogendra stressed the religious dimension as the only true motivation and goal, over the sensationalistic "street stunts" so often associated with yoga. The abilities resulting from proper yoga practice, he told them—from walking on water to controlling one's breath and heart rate and generating "yogic heat"—were merely the side effects of an accomplished yogi's true attainments. Such physiological changes could be recorded by scientific measurements, but they could never be understood by such means since the true heart of the matter was a spiritual transformation, not a physical one. Yogendra was in many ways the mirror image of Swami Kuvalayānanda's scientific yogi. Nonetheless, he displayed his own innovations in yogic theory. Denying the necessity of celibacy, he had caused much controversy a decade earlier when, having married, he began instructing his wife in yoga—something that traditionally was not done. Proclaiming the health benefits of yoga for all, Yogendra pioneered "simplified" *āsanas* and a systematized presentation of the different branches of yoga.

Hoping to explore these in detail, Glen asked for advice and contacts who could instruct him in specific breath control (*prāṇāyāma*) practices. Yogendra gave him the name and address in Bombay of his good friend

H. V. Kurthkoti, as well as the contact information for a seventy-one-year-old yogi in Bangalore, Swami Paramahansa Yogeeśwarar. Eager to follow Yogendra's advice, Glen began making phone calls and arrangements immediately upon their return to the hotel. Concerned that they not lose the momentum of the day, he called for a car to take them to Kurthkoti's residence, though Viola was becoming increasingly worried about too much travel in Bombay given the ongoing riots and curfews. With his typical "great air of final knowledge," Glen declared that Kurthkoti's residence was nowhere near the disturbances. When the car arrived, however, the driver refused to leave, explaining that their destination lay right in the center of the riots!

Taking charge, Viola placed a phone call to another of Joshi's friends, Dr. Vasant Rele, head of the Nair Hospital and Medical College. She made arrangements to meet him forthwith, and with Theos in hand and Glen in protest, they left the hotel again. They found Rele at home lounging in a dhouti, and this time Viola took the lead in their discussions. As a medically minded man, Rele believed in interpreting all the ancient Vedic scriptures and mythology in terms of physiological metaphors. Having written several books on the subject, he autographed and presented copies of several of them to Viola. According to Rele, *kuṇḍalinī*, the fierce fire described in yogic texts, was nothing more than the vagus nerve that ran from the brain stem to the pelvic region. Animated and overjoyed at the opportunity to discuss such matters, he spoke at length for several hours before Viola had to beg his pardon to leave, citing a prior engagement for tea. Insisting on being dropped off at the hotel, Glen returned to his room to sulk while Theos and Viola went out to socialize with more of their Bombay contacts, ending the evening with their first private dinner without Glen in weeks, which Viola insisted on celebrating with champagne and good food.

On their last day in Bombay, Theos and Viola spent their morning running errands, picking up clothes and photographic prints before being entertained by Joshi's daughter and her family over an extensive lunch. Returning to the hotel to pack, they were immediately joined by Glen, who began discoursing on the arrogance of so-called Indian "authorities" on yoga, asking why every single individual they'd met insisted on dismissing everyone but themselves as ignorant of the true meaning of yoga. To make matters worse, Glen observed, none of them knew anything, let alone as much as he already did, not even his own guru. Viola, despite being preoccupied with the curious silence from DeVries, found the irony of Glen's own statements, lost on him, to be yet another item on her list of annoyances with Theos's father. It was a list that would continue to grow.

The following week, they were back on their itinerary of chauffeured cars and trains, to the first-millennium cave temples of Ajanta—which Theos dismissed as pointless until he saw them, after which he couldn't stop praising them, sounding "as tho he'd built them"—to Ellora—where Theos succeeded in insulting the curator and, after the latter stormed off, rapidly shot a dozen illegal photos—to the Dasara Festival in Mysore as guests of the Maharaja. Once again, thanks to more letters of introduction from S. L. Joshi, Theos and Viola returned to their purely leisurely pursuits: more medical surveys and social banter. With Theos and Viola so occupying their days, Glen was left to bide his time—something he did not do well—and with the slightest passing comment from Viola, the two of them would once more be in a heated argument, usually over whatever ayurvedic theory Glen felt trumped Viola's observations. Thus, as the trip proceeded southward, the tempers of all three seemed to rise along with the temperature, leaving Viola angered, Glen sullen, and Theos nervous.

Patient by nature, Viola was always the first to regain her composure and perspective. With several more weeks of travel together ahead, Viola made repeated efforts to soothe her companions, enticing Theos with photographic opportunities and locating yogis to demonstrate various feats for Glen, including the legendary Kṛṣṇāmācarya, while she tried again to reach DeVries back in New York for an update on the situation unfolding there. Arriving in Madras, the three of them spent a day visiting the Theosophical Society in Adyar before going their separate ways, Viola returning to her discussions with various members of the medical community while Theos and Glen went in search of Swami Paramahansa Yogeeśwarar.

In Chennai, Glen and Theos found the elderly man at ease in his study and after a brief meeting, concluded that here finally was a man with substantial yogic attainments who might be able to help them and, more importantly, would be willing to talk with them at length. Glen and Theos promised to return in a week, when they could devote the necessary time and effort to study with the man. Rendezvousing with Viola back in Mysore after a quick side trip to the Nilgiri Hills to film and photograph the Todas—a subject of anthropological study that might earn Theos another trip to India—the three of them went shopping for books and souvenirs before returning to the hotel to pack for the evening train, the Indo-Ceylon Express bound for the southern tip of India.

On her last day in India, Viola remained determined to see as much as she could at every chance, be it on a brisk walk through the Minaksi-Sundaresvara temple complex during a train stop in Madurai or in opportunities for photos or film of locals while on their way to Mandapam for health inspections prior to leaving the country. Passing through customs without incident, they boarded the ferry at Danushkodi Pier, and arriving at the docks of Ceylon some six hours later, settled into a first-class compartment on a train bound for Colombo.

As Viola prepared to reenter the world of medical training and personal drama that awaited her in New York, she was more and more preoccupied with the latest news from DeVries, who had begun to send her cablegrams again, though infrequently. Dealing with the mass of mail awaiting them, starting the monumental task of sorting, mounting, and labeling the hundreds of additional contact prints they had amassed, verifying the shipment of trunks, furniture, and books purchased along the way, and settling their accounts, they faced the realities of the end of their trip. Ignoring Glen while attending to these various issues, Theos was far more concerned with making sure he and Viola parted on good terms without a last-minute fight, as they were on the verge of spending a long year apart. Glen, of course, took this personally and although they were surrounded by opulence in the Galle Face Hotel, he once again began to sulk.

Nonetheless, Theos paid all attention to Viola's needs—swimming in the hotel pool, sightseeing at Buddhist temples, a visit to the Mahābodhi Society to follow up on some of Roerich's recommended contacts, more visas for Egypt, Italy, and so on—as well as some quiet time alone. Finally, with all the details sorted out, on November 5, 1936, Viola boarded the *Katori Maru* steamship in Kandy back to the States, with obligatory stops for her own sightseeing along the way. Glen and Theos, alone and undistracted at last, returned to India to commence their research together.

SEVEN

A Well-Trodden Path

Studies in Darjeeling and Sikkim

Men who leave behind their weeping sweethearts to practise asceticism—
and those who have done so in the past, and those who will do so in the
future—they are doing something very difficult indeed, and so it was in the
past and will be in the future.

—AŚVAGHOṢA[1]

PARAMAHANSA YOGEEŚWARAR entered into the religious life at the
age of twelve when, after he prayed (*manasika puja*) to the local deity of
Kanchipuram in Tamilnadu, Ekambareeshwar Pritivilingam, the god appeared to him in the guise of "an aged saint by the name of Nithyanandar
of Vettaveli Paramparai," who initiated him and taught him yoga, bestow-
ing upon him the name of Śrī Paramahansa Sachidananda Yogeeśwarar. By
the turn of the century, Yogeeśwarar had disciples throughout India, Ceylon (Sri Lanka), Southeast Asia, and South Africa, and had gained fame for
his perfection of the practice of the "suppression of water" (*jalaṣṭambha*)[2]
through breath control (*prāṇāyāma*), often lecturing while in a full lotus
posture and floating effortlessly in water.

Back in Chennai in early November, Theos and Glen lost little time returning to Yogeeśwarar's ashram. For the better part of the next week,
they met with the swami and persuaded him to demonstrate some of the
basic *āsanas* used in yogic practice. Unfortunately, while Yogeeśwarar
could explain many of the practices and their purposes—being far more
forthcoming and pleasant than Kuvalayānanda—his girth prevented any
useful photographic documentation of the practices, and Theos believed
that he himself could give a better demonstration of haṭha yoga *āsanas*,
even if Yogeeśwarar's mastery of *kumbhaka* was impressive.[3] Discussing the

situation, Theos and Glen decided to return to Calcutta and from there journey to Bhurkunda, where Glen had done his retreat six months earlier, to see Trivikram Swami. Arriving in Calcutta a few days later, they quickly got settled and began making preparations to travel inland again. Contacting his friends to make the necessary arrangements, Glen received a letter that had been waiting for him with news from Bhurkunda: "Trivikram Swamaji breathed his last on the 17th Sept."

Decamping in their hotel while they decided what to do, Theos sent off a telegram to Viola, who by then had reached Italy. Her response was that the situation between DeVries and P.A. had degenerated further, culminating with DeVries moving out and leaving the club. Convinced that she should take some time away from New York, DeVries had followed Viola's advice and boarded a steamship from New York to rendezvous with her in Paris. Feeling too far from the situation to make an informed judgment despite Viola's description of the events, Theos suggested that Viola make decisions on both their behalves regarding their relationship with P.A. and the club, and he would wait and see what she decided. In the meantime, Glen had come to his own conclusions, and suggested that they still make the trip to Bhurkunda the following weekend since it offered their strongest chance for success.

Consequently, Glen and Theos packed their bags and camera equipment, caught the train from Calcutta to Ranchi, and traveled to the ashram by train, rickshaw, and bullock cart and finally on foot—a journey Theos thought was a nightmare. "It is hell," he wrote to Viola, "unless you just don't give a dam [sic] and then it is on the threshold of hell." With Trivikram Swami gone, Swami Syamānanda had assumed the lead role at Bhurkunda and with the company of Glen's tantric brothers and sisters, he and Theos arranged for a meeting with Swami Syamānanda. Without hesitation, Swami Syamānanda agreed to allow Theos to photograph and film his and his students' demonstrations of the various *āsanas* connected with *kuṇḍalinī* yoga, and provided them with diagrams of the *cakras* as well.

Returning to Calcutta a few days later, Glen and Theos spent some time reorganizing their materials and planning the next steps of their trip. When he went to have his latest round of photographs developed, Theos got into an argument over the quality of service he was receiving at the Kodak office in Calcutta. The Bombay office always seemed to work just fine, but there was always, it seemed, a problem in Calcutta, from poor-quality prints to out-of-stock supplies. With the most crucial phase of his research looming ahead, Theos could not afford such uncertainties, so despite promises and offers of special consideration, he negotiated a new deal with the Agfa company, garnering a discount on film and services while preordering a large supply of 16-mm and 35-mm rolls of film for his cameras and buying a large assortment of accessories, including filters, lenses, and magazines. But Theos was anxious to head north, for even in the course of accomplishing what he wanted to do, after having "walked ten miles in this city under the blazing sun of the fall, and having knocked around with the rest of the hordes on the street cars" he was in one of his typically foul moods. Less deterred by the atmosphere of Calcutta, Glen in the meantime attempted to contact the various individuals they had missed on their previous stay in the city, especially at the Royal Asiatic Society.

The president of the Royal Asiatic Society of Bengal at the time was the noted Dutch Tibetologist Johan van Manen.[4] He had arrived in Calcutta in 1919, following an interest in Indian and Tibetan religion instilled in him by his early contact with the Theosophical Society in the 1890s as a young man in the Netherlands.[5] In was through the study of Theosophy that van Manen came not only to his interest in Indo-Tibetan religion but also to his own deep-seated religious convictions. Working closely with two English-speaking Tibetans in India, he had studied literary and spoken Tibetan as well as Tibetan sectarian doctrines, rituals, and histories. He became a member of the Asiatic Society in early 1918, and by the end of the year he had taken the position of librarian at the Imperial Library in Calcutta, bringing his Tibetan friends with him. Three years later, he was the General Secretary of the society.

Over the next fifteen years, van Manen pushed the acquisition of Tibetan materials and the study of Tibetan Buddhism within the society, surveying the literature of Tibet and writing numerous articles. By the end of 1936, he was suffering from recurring health problems, and the last of his Tibetan manservants, Nyima, had left, replaced by a Chinese boy—the son of a Chinese soldier who had settled in Calcutta when the brief Chinese occupation of Lhasa ended twenty-five years earlier and the defeated soldiers were sent back to China, humiliatingly, via India, where many chose to remain. Twan Yang, who, like many Chinese, held Tibetan culture in high esteem, served van Manen well in those later years and even remembered the visit from Theos Bernard[6]—even if the opposite was not true. Having missed van Manen in September when they were last in Calcutta, Theos and Glen made a point of meeting with him this time, in December.

Visiting him at his home just opposite the Calcutta High Court House overlooking the Hooghly River, they sought van Manen's advice on the direction that Theos should pursue for his dissertation. As early as 1918, van Manen had articulated what he saw as the best approach to Tibetan studies, which required laying a sound basis for future Tibetan scholarship. This must be done, he thought, "by way of painstaking, laborious and to a certain extent inglorious and humdrum drudging away at small texts with scrupulous attention to the smallest minutiae for a secure fixing of illustrative examples by coordinating corrections of text, full discussion of meanings, sharp formulation of definitions and subtle analysis of all questions and problems involved."[7]

What Theos should do, van Manen thought, was follow in Evans-Wentz's footsteps: as Evans-Wentz had done with the notable figures of Padmasambhava and Milarepa, he should explore the subtleties of Buddhist philosophy through the lens of one person's life. Van Manen stressed, however, that he should not envision his dissertation as "something complete in and of itself" but rather as "only the foundation for future work and also so as to encourage others who want to work in this field." Already feeling that a trip to Tibet would be necessary, Theos began to allude to it in his letters to Viola, though he wrote only of "new plans in the air" that were "still a little premature to go into . . . for things may happen in Sikkim which will again alter them." Theos could take van Manen's advice, recognizing its value, but he was determined to remain ultimately concerned with only "the one particular philosophy that is to be found here," gently suggesting to Viola that he would "inevitably be lead [sic] to such people who have attained this development of understanding." Nonetheless, he assured Viola, his world-traveling days would soon be over and he could settle into "a sedentary life of reading, writing, and translating"; to that end, he was starting to "hunt manuscripts for future work" and "learning a language completely" to make life easier for Viola and their life together. Theos thought he could make considerable headway by retracing the footsteps of those he had read about, beginning with Alexandra David-Neel. To that end, he and Glen set out for Darjeeling with the ultimate goal of reaching Lachen on the Sikkim–Tibet border, home to David-Neel's informant, Lama Yongden, about whom he and so many others had read.

If Calcutta and the heat of the jungles were oppressive to Theos ("this stinking swill hole"), the foothills of the Himalayas had precisely the opposite effect. As they arrived in Darjeeling, Theos's spirits were immediately on the rise. "Each day is filled with beauty and inspiration," he told Viola. "It is impossible to look thru the azure blue of the Himalayan valleys and catch a fleeting glimpse of those majestic ranges of the distant north shoving their noses up into the heavens and not be effected [sic]; I tell you, it does things to you—you want to run, fly, jump and love all at the same time." Even while riding through the mountains in a rickshaw, the views were inspiring. "Why a mountain should inspire one is hard to say," he wrote to her, "but one glimpse of what can be seen in any direction from this point is almost more than the insides can take. No wonder Milarepa could do things. If I was practicing in a land like this, just the view from my cave would throw me straight into samadhi." For Theos the Himalayan mountains were truly, as Jung had remarked, "that metaphysical fringe of ice and rock away up north, that inexorable barrier beyond human conception."[8]

Best of all, Jinorasa was by Theos's side the moment he arrived back in Darjeeling and expedited everything that Theos needed in order to leave as quickly as possible for Lachen. Indeed, Jinorasa was amazingly capable at affecting the outcome of any political process in the area. Where so many had met with bureaucratic obstacles at every turn, the people Jinorasa helped had doors opened to them without hesitation, for in addition to being a key player in the revival of Buddhism in the area, Jinorasa was also a relative of the Sikkimese royal family with cousins filling the administrative ranks of the government and a very powerful brother who would one day become the first Chief Minister, Kazi Lhendup Dorji. Consequently, in all that he asked for, Jinorasa's name carried the authority of his entire family's reputation.

Making his way to Gangtok, Theos was reluctant to travel to Lachen during the depths of winter. The private secretary to the Maharajah of Sikkim gave him a solid history of his many predecessors and fellow adventurers in the area, and impressed upon him that no amount of friendship or influence would allow him to circumvent the man who actually held the keys to the door into Tibet: the British Political Officer for Sikkim, Sir Basil Gould. Armed with this information, Theos left Gangtok and returned to Darjeeling briefly before going on to Kalimpong, the economic gateway to Tibet and home to a community of expatriate Tibetans and peddlers of British influence. Once there, he and Glen settled into the Himalayan Hotel, the former residence of David Macdonald and his family, a stately hill station establishment overlooking the center of town. The translator for Younghusband on his 1904 expedition to Tibet and subsequently the British Trade Agent in Gyantse for twenty years, David Macdonald was famous in the area, particularly for having turned down a knighthood for saving the life of the Thirteenth Dalai Lama in 1910, asking in exchange only a small parcel of land in the heart of Kalimpong for himself and his family. His children grown, the old family home had been turned into a luxury hotel, then being run by his son-in-law, Frank Perry.

Theos and Frank immediately became friends, and Frank began talking with Theos at length about the mishaps and misadventures of all those who had gone before him—including Edwin Schary, whose unpublished book manuscript he gave Theos to read[9]—speaking quite highly, in particular, of Alexandra David-Neel. Within days of checking in, Theos met another guest, Gordon T. Bowles, a Harvard-Yenching Fellow conducting an anthropological survey of the Tibetan borderlands.[10] Quizzing Bowles on his experiences in and around Tibet, Theos discovered that he had traveled at one point with Harrison Forman, of whom Theos's erstwhile pilot in Shanghai, Chilly Vaughn, had spoke quite highly. Bowles was of a decidedly different opinion. Theos noted Bowles's views without revealing anything, leaving the mystery of differing opinions for Viola to puzzle over in his letters to her.

No sooner had Theos and Glen settled into their hotel room, however, than Theos received word from Jinorasa: Lama Yongden was coming from his retreat cave in the mountains down to Lachen and would be available for an interview there if Theos could come quickly. Already envisioning the broader context of his activities, Theos realized that the greatest amount of time would be spent "in bringing the problems down to something concrete," and yet, "from the looks of things so far, the specifics have been found or rather decided upon and if they ever come to pass, I will feel that I have left a real addition to the culture of this old world for someone to dig it up in the next millennium." As always, though, for Theos "the job that presents itself at the moment is being able to get ahold of the mss."

Pinning their hopes for success on a meeting with Lama Yongden, Theos and Glen made the trip to Lachen, convinced it was the only way "to get a line up on the literature and secure the right manuscripts." If the previous weeks had proven boring, on a cinematic level at least, the trip to Lachen from Gangtok was anything but. "We have taken many trips together in the mountains," he wrote to Viola, "but this so far surpasses everything that we have ever seen together that it is impossible for me to describe it to you by making a comparison." He continued,

On the trip coming up one finds everything from the grandeur of the tropics to the splendor of the frozen north. One passes over endless swinging bridges which span the gorges out by the foaming rapids far below, thru jungles of ferns and orchids constantly being lighted up by the reflecting misty veils thrown over this luxuriant growth by the rushing waters above in their efforts to find a way to their kind which are constantly passing by perpendicularly below. This entire country is built on end with all the trails carved into the side of walls. There are places where trails have been hung along sheer cliffs hundreds of feet above the rapids. What one does when they near one of these pack trains, god only knows. Luckily I rounded the more dangerous corners alone, but there have been a few tight squeezes.

Although Theos never missed a chance to practice his narrative skills, he had a slightly stronger motivation on this occasion for practicing his eloquence: he had "completely run out of film . . . and as for the Leica," on his trip to Lachen he was "left with only two rolls," so had make "every effort to make each frame count." While Theos did his best to document the trip, he was still overcome by the scenery—from tea gardens to mountain ranges to the sight of his first yak—and shot the better part of both rolls on the trail.

Upon reaching Lachen, Theos continued up the mountain behind the small village to Lama Yongden's monastery, where he spent the winters away from his cave retreat, to obtain the audience he sought. "He spent hours relating the mental aspects to the problems of the investigation," he told Viola. Lama Yongden, having devoted "the years of his youth . . . to make [an] inner develop[ment], having attained some perfection in this direction . . . he is now in his eighties and his mind sparkles as a fountain ever flowing under the sun of understanding." More importantly, however, "the great meditator of Lachen"[11] gave Theos very pointed advice on how to pass himself off as a Buddhist pilgrim—just as he had advised David-Neel.

Half a world away, unfortunately, Viola was having no such comparable experiences. Besides coping with her mother's ongoing battle with cancer and her sister's impending divorce, she was still dealing with the after-effects of the blow-up at the CCC between P.A. and DeVries. Discussing the matter with her, Theos resolved to support Viola's decision that they should renounce their membership and sever all ties with the club out of loyalty to DeVries and convince others to do so as well, since "like a child playing over an area charged with dynamite—it is our duty to remove it even tho it has no way to realize why." Anticipating the worst for the future with P.A., Theos suggested that they take their decision one step further and dispense with their apartment in Nyack, suggesting that they could easily use the excuses of financial constraints and logistical inconveniences with Viola in New Jersey and Theos in India, Tibet and—he felt sure—soon studying at Oxford. Feeling more and more confident that he was embarking on research in unexplored territories, Theos had decided to abandon Columbia; neither the anthropology nor the philosophy department suited his needs and goals since the former was filled with people he didn't like, none of whom could "see what I wish to do," and the latter could only be considered a fall-back solution at best. Indeed, Theos felt assured of his ability to get accepted into the Ph.D. program at Oxford with Evans-Wentz, not just because of their now shared interest in Tibetan studies and his personal connection with the man through his father, but in particular, because he could bring to the field precisely the aspect that Evans-Wentz lacked: firsthand knowledge of the yogic tradition. It would be a challenging application to make, but if he had learned anything from traveling in social circles with Viola, it was the value and strength of a skillfully offered handshake and smile in the right quarters.

First, however, Theos needed sources—texts—and lots of them. Arriving back in Gangtok, he chanced upon a meeting with one of Jinorasa's cousins, who informed him that he could halve the Rs. 4,000 expense of copies of the Kangyur and the Tengyur in Calcutta by buying his own paper and shipping it up to Tibet to be printed there. He and Viola decided that it would be a worthwhile expenditure and placed the order with Jinorasa's cousin, who thought the manuscripts could arrive as early as mid-February.

Returning to Kalimpong, Theos began following up on recommendations in the area. He had asked for help in learning Tibetan when he was in Darjeeling, and Jinorasa recommended that Theos meet the one man in Kalimpong who could best assist him—a young man known as Tharchin Babu, who had taught Tibetan to many in the area already—and provided Theos with a letter of introduction. At the same time, through Frank Perry Theos met the Pumsur brothers, distant relatives of a Lhasan aristocratic family who ran a wool trade operation in Kalimpong. Always eager to negotiate a business deal, they also offered to assist Theos in obtaining a copy of the Kangyur, the same new redaction recently printed in Lhasa, through one of their brothers there. For Theos, all of this was nearly overwhelming, but it was just the tip of the iceberg in Kalimpong.

Like Tashkent a thousand years earlier, Kalimpong was a cultural juncture—the meeting place of age-old civilizations and a crossing-over point between radically different worlds. Below and to the south lay the jungles and lowlands of British India and most prominently of all, Calcutta, the commercial port for hill stations such as Kalimpong where the whole population of India—Lepchas, Nepalis, Bengalis, British, Chinese, Malaysians—and a host of traders, missionaries, soldiers, and bureaucrats daily swarmed over each other in pursuit of their lofty and not-so-lofty goals. Above and to the north lay Tibet, perched atop the high Himalayas, stretching from the narrow valleys of Ladakh and Guge near Kashmir in the west to the wide-open plains of Amdo and the Chang-tang on the border of China to the east. It was a kingdom like no other and a monastic haven far above the mundane world, a place that six million people called home, whose natural borders were visible from space. Kalimpong was where these two worlds met.

Called "Da-ling Kote"[12] by the local Bhutias after the old fort on the 4,000-foot ridge line, for most of its prehistory, Kalimpong was little more than the stockade (*pong*) of a Bhutanese minister (*Kalön*).[13] Only after the annexation of the area by the British in the late nineteenth century did the small village formed around the ruins of the old fort begin to grow. In the wake of the 1904 Younghusband invasion of Tibet, Kalimpong took on greater significance as a trading post as the wool trade shifted from the administrative capital of the region, Darjeeling, to its new economic capital, slightly closer the Tibetan passes of Jelep-la and Nathu-la, with easy transport south to Calcutta for shipping to the textile mills of England, and eventually America.

Though still in many aspects a trading post and missionary enclave, by the 1930s Kalimpong had much to offer a Tibetophile. Most notably, it was home to the only Tibetan language newspaper in the world, *The Mirror* or *Me-long*, as it was known in Tibetan. It was also home to the newspaper's editor and the de facto center of the Tibetan expatriate community in Kalimpong, Dorje Tharchin, known affectionately as Tharchin Babu.

Born in 1890 in the village of Pu in the Khunu region of Spiti,[14] Tharchin was the son of one of a handful of Moravian Christian converts in the western Tibetan borderlands of Spiti, and had spent the early years of his life in Khunu, being educated in missionary schools (taught in a mixture of Tibetan and Urdu[15]). When his parents died in the early years of the century, Tharchin finally left his village at the age of twenty and decided to try to go to Tibet in order to properly study the Tibetan language. Relocating several hundred miles south to the soon-to-be British capital of Delhi,[16] Tharchin sought work to earn money for the trip. After a brief bout of malaria, however, he returned north to the British "summer capital" of Simla at the mouth of the Kulu valley, close to his old home in Khunu. Upon recovering, he went to work as a common laborer on the construction of the Hindustan–Tibet road. Spending his time between Simla and Delhi, by the late 1910s Tharchin was fully ensconced in his identity as a Christian and could often be found preaching in one of the local bazaars.

On one occasion, Tharchin reported, he was preparing to preach in a bazaar in Delhi when, looking at the last page in his Bible, he saw the phrase "Printed at the Scandinavian Alliance Tibetan Mission Press, Ghoom, Darjeeling." Discerning its import with the help of a friend, Tharchin saw an opportunity to get closer to Tibet and immediately wrote a letter (in Tibetan) to the press in Ghoom asking for an apprenticeship. To Tharchin's disappointment, the response informed him that the press had been sold, although he could be considered for missionary training as a Tibetan and Hindi teacher in the Ghoom Mission School if he knew Hindi—which he did not. Nonetheless, Tharchin did not want to miss his opportunity, so, accepting this offer, he hurriedly bought a primer on Hindi grammar and after the Delhi Durbar of 1911,[17] left for Ghoom in early January 1912.

For the next five years, Tharchin remained at Ghoom teaching Tibetan and Hindi (while learning Nepali) at the Christian school belonging to the Scandinavian Alliance Mission. There he met the onetime Christian convert Karma Sumdhon Paul, then acting as headmaster.[18] Although Tharchin tried his best to proselytize to visiting Tibetans and the local residents of Sikkim and Bengal, he met with only mixed success. Nonetheless, he continued as a lay preacher, interacting from time to time with his cohorts in the region, including the increasingly influential Dr. Graham, who ran an orphanage for Anglo-Indian children in Kalimpong. While some of Tharchin's missionary companions often earned the ire of both the British and Tibetan authorities for routinely flouting administrative restrictions on their activities—making reference to a "higher calling"—Tharchin actively cultivated the friendship of both the Tibetans and the British, and benefited greatly from it.

By 1917, Tharchin had managed to secure a government scholarship and so relocated to Kalimpong to enter the teacher training program operated by the Scottish Union Mission. Having recently published two small Tibetan language primers, a *Tibetan Primer with Simple Rules of Correct Spelling* and *The Tibetan Second Book*,[19] he had sufficient knowledge of the language to capture the notice of W. S. Sutherland, a missionary who had spent the better part of forty years in the Kalimpong area running a combination orphanage and missionary school. He quickly put Tharchin to work teaching Tibetan to a mixture of Bhutia and Tibetan boys in the orphanage. Although claiming to offer a complete education, Sutherland's schools integrated Bible study as much as possible, offering a curriculum of "Grammar, Geography, History, Arithmetic, Euclid, Physics, . . . Old and New Testament History, Church History, Pastoral Theology, and Apologetics with special reference to Hinduism."[20] After graduating two years later, Tharchin was asked to remain in Kalimpong as permanent teacher of Tibetan at the Scottish mission.

Despite all these activities and events, Tharchin continued his proselytizing trips throughout Sikkim during these years, as well as serving as a Tibetan translator for embassies to Bhutan and Sikkim. During this time, he had the opportunity to visit Tibet for the first time, in 1921, accompanying the wife of the British Trade Agent at Yatung, Mrs. David Macdonald, to her husband's post just over the Tibetan border. Tharchin stayed in Yatung for the next four months, assisting Mrs. Macdonald with her English and Hindi school for the children of British officers stationed there, before pressing on deeper into Tibet toward Gyantse, the first major city between the Tibetan border and Lhasa. No sooner had he arrived than word of his activities in Yatung reached the ears of British officials stationed in Gyantse, and they requested that he open a similar school there. Despite the lack of funds, Tharchin obliged and began instructing the children of British officers and Tibetan aristocrats—as well as a few Tibetan officials[21]—in English and Hindustani (Hindi). The school was initially a success, but Tharchin's construction of an unabashedly Christian curriculum—including morning prayers, Christian hymns, and Bible readings—would eventually doom it to closure when its thinly veiled proselytizing enterprise became apparent to the Tibetan government,[22] which then opened a new school in Gyantse with British help (though similar charges would shortly doom it as well). Though not invested in the schools financially, the British authorities viewed these closures as a bad sign, with one officer remarking that the Tibetans "will regret this decision one day when they are Chinese slaves once more, as they assuredly will be."[23] Nonetheless, Tharchin remained in Gyantse for two more years, teaching and assisting in the translation of Hindi and English military manuals into Tibetan for the newly formed Tibetan army.[24]

It was during this time as well that Tharchin began to forge friendships with many of the high-ranking Tibetan and British dignitaries who passed through Gyantse on a regular basis, including Sir Charles Bell; the renounced King of Sikkim, Taring Raja; and various current and future members of the Tibetan government, including members of the cabinet and national assembly,[25] as well as relatives of the various aristocratic houses. Although this period would prove crucial to Tharchin's future, granting him access to all levels of government and rendering him famously influential, his proselytizing behavior was not always appreciated, least of all by the British, whose reactions ran the gamut from nervous tolerance to outright contempt.[26]

Satisfied with the level of language instruction they were receiving, the Tibetan officials under Tharchin's tutelage invited him to return to Lhasa with them, and in September 1923, Tharchin made his first trip to the capital city as their guest. It was there, while living across the street with Dorje Theiji, that Tharchin met his wife, Karma Dechen. Within a few months, Tharchin had secured her parents' permission to marry; shortly thereafter, they returned to India via Gangtok, where Tharchin served as translator for Dorje Theji while the latter attended military school.[27] Tharchin would later speak glowingly of this time; far more significant, however, was that in the midst of these activities he began work on what would be his greatest achievement and eventually earn him worldwide fame.

In August 1925, while working for Sutherland's successor at the Scottish Union Mission, John Graham, Tharchin noticed "a Roneo Duplicator lying idle" and asked if he could take it, thinking to produce his own newspaper in Tibetan. Graham offered it to Tharchin, though with little encouragement, saying that his office staff had failed to get it working the entire time they had had it. Nonetheless, Tharchin began tinkering with the duplicator and after two months of effort in his spare time, finally got it to work. On October 10, 1925, Tharchin produced the first issue of his very own Tibetan language newspaper, *The Mirror—News From Various Regions.*[28] After a brief hiatus, he commenced regular publication the following February with monthly issues. Although he received encouragement and advice from all around, his first real commendation came a year later, when he received a letter from His Holiness the Thirteenth Dalai Lama, accompanied by a gift of twenty rupees, stating that he was receiving Tharchin's newspaper, "was very glad and added to continue it and send more news which would be very useful to him."[29]

Encouraged by this, Tharchin began to think of himself more and more as a newspaperman, expanding beyond the simple relaying of news from other sources to the production of news content himself. He petitioned the Tibetan government for permission to visit Lhasa as a reporter, and on August 20, 1927, accompanied by his wife and two British civil servants, headed for Gyantse, and from there for Lhasa to conduct the first important interview of his career—with the Thirteenth Dalai Lama. Arriving in Lhasa a month later, Tharchin remained self-conscious about his broken Tibetan—the result of having grown up in the borderlands of Tibet—and spent the better part of the next three months attempting to improve his speaking abilities before finally applying for an audience with His Holiness in mid-December.[30] Tharchin and his wife returned to India the following February (1928), receiving 100 rupees along the way from the British Political Officer at Gyantse, Arthur Hopkinson, to support the continued publication of the newspaper. By June, the Scottish mission had received a new litho press, which Dr. Graham made available, sending Tharchin to Calcutta to receive training in its use and allowing him to use the press to produce his newspaper as part of his official duties at the mission.[31] This clear link between the newspaper and missionary activities was not lost on some, and Tharchin's good fortune proved to be a mixed blessing, as many came to disregard and even dislike the newspaper.

Tharchin had begun his newspaper with only fourteen subscriptions, and by the third year his subscriptions were close to fifty. But he was still sending more than a hundred free copies to officials in the Tibetan government, although more than half were usually "lost" along the way by the Tibetan post office. These, however, were the least of Tharchin's troubles. Greater difficulties during these years came from more hard-line missionaries who would soon appear in Kalimpong, in particular, Dr. Graham's replacement at the mission, the Australian Reverend Knox. Despite the often prominent "articles" on Christianity that regularly appeared in the pages of *The Mirror*, Knox was not favorably disposed to Tharchin's activities as a newspaper editor, and shortly after arriving in Kalimpong brought an end to the subsidization of the paper in terms of both material resources and Tharchin's time.[32] By the early 1930s, Tharchin had managed to stabilize the publication of his newspaper, although he was constantly in search of new subscribers and advertising to underwrite his costs.[33] It was thus with a certain degree of trepidation that he rejoined the Scottish Union Mission under Rev. Knox as "Tibetan Catechist,"[34] agreeing to accept strict limits on his official activities in exchange for a salary. While there was little love lost between Tharchin and Knox, the position allowed Tharchin to continue publishing his newspaper. In the process—though unintentionally—he was building a community around him that would significantly alter the face of Tibetan politics, for better and worse. Just as Kalimpong was growing, his reputation seemed to grow along with it, and Tharchin finally began to benefit from this.

In 1931, the French Tibetologist Jacques Bacot arrived in Kalimpong, and making inquiries at David Macdonald's Himalayan Hotel, was directed to Tharchin as a potential assistant in his research. Bacot's interests, however, were very specialized: the recently recovered cache of eighth- to tenth-century manuscripts from the Silk Road town of Tun-huang. Having just recently edited and published Tse-ring-wang-gyel's *Tibetan-Sanskrit Dictionary*[35] as a follow-up to his translation and study of a Tibetan grammar treatise,[36] Bacot was eager to apply what he had learned to translating the early Tibetan documents now in his possession. To his disappointment, deciphering their contents was a far greater challenge than he'd thought, and without the help of a native Tibetan scholar he could proceed no further. Bacot enlisted Tharchin to help with his translations, paying him handsomely. Although together they made some additional progress, many of the passages were well beyond Tharchin's abilities too. Bacot had limited time in India and knew that it would be hopeless to attempt to finish the translations in isolation back in Paris. So although he would most likely never return to Kalimpong, he left his photographic reproductions of the texts with Tharchin, who promised to enlist the aid of others to complete their translation. Ironically, as Tharchin and Bacot struggled over the manuscripts that fall, several hundred miles north in Tibet, another would-be scholar of ancient Tibetan manuscripts was likewise in search of material and human resources to aid him in his research—and his own work would affect Tharchin's dramatically.

Born in the late nineteenth century, Rāhula Sānkṛtyāyana had grown up in India, but was very much a product of the British educational system rather than anything indigenously Indian. Fixating on Tibet as a repository of untapped knowledge, in the summer of 1929, Sānkṛtyāyana embarked on his first trip in search of Sanskrit manuscripts brought there close to a thousand years earlier and presumed to still be extant in the great monastic libraries. Sānkṛtyāyana knew that prior to the rise of the "Three Great Seats"[37] of learning in the early fifteenth century, the center of Buddhist knowledge and translation activities was Sakya, a small, secluded valley retreat located several hundred miles south and west of Lhasa. It was there that in the early thirteenth century the faculty of the great Buddhist university of India, Vikramalaśīla, had fled, seeking refuge from the Muslim invaders who had razed their university and put all its inhabitants to the sword, ending the Buddhist intellectual dominance of the Indian subcontinent. It was also at Sakya that the last abbot of Vikramalaśīla, Śākya Śrībhadra, and his entourage began teaching and collaborating with Tibetan scholars on the next great wave of translations and oral transmissions on the Tibetan plateau. For Sānkṛtyāyana, this was the logical place to look for Sanskrit manuscripts. But after many months, he came home disappointed, having found only Tibetan manuscripts.[38] Sānkṛtyāyana had begun attempting to "restore" the Sanskrit version of one text of interest from the Tibetan, Dharmakīrti's *Pramāṇavarttika*, when he learned that the Sanskrit original had recently been discovered in Nepal. Reinspired, he began planning a second trip.

By 1934, Sānkṛtyāyana was better informed, and having identified Ngor and Shalu monasteries as likely places with Sanskrit manuscripts, he was ready to visit Tibet again.[39] This time, however, he was searching not only for rare manuscripts but also, just as important, for a scholar or two who could assist him in his studies, so he went first to Lhasa. While staying there, he developed friendships with various members of the aristocratic families and ruling officials of Tibet. With the assistance of the sons of the house of Surkhang, Reting Rinpoche, and the Kalön Lama,[40] Sānkṛtyāyana's second trip achieved success before even setting foot in a monastic library, as he was also able to acquire photographs of manuscripts from Kundeling Monastery right in Lhasa itself.

Not without justification, Sānkṛtyāyana thought of himself as a scholar of the heyday of Buddhist India, the "Buddhist millennium" spanning from the time of Nāgārjuna in the second century C.E. to the destruction of the great centers of learning in the early thirteenth century. Although many of the oral traditions from this time still survived in Tibet—a difficult source to access—the literary legacy of Buddhist India was encapsulated in the second half of the Tibetan Buddhist canon, the Tengyur.[41] In the early twentieth century in Tibet, one man stood out as the foremost authority on the canon, having earlier been deputized by the Thirteenth Dalai Lama to redact the first half, the Kangyur,[42] for publication in Lhasa: Dobi Geshe Sherap Gyatso.[43] Before even meeting him, Sānkṛtyāyana thought that Geshe Sherap Gyatso would be the ideal collaborator in his research. A scholar at Drepung Monastic University west of Lhasa, Geshe Sherap Gyatso was not only one of the greatest scholars of the twentieth century produced by that institution but also a key political figure of the day. Although Geshe Sherap Gyatso was unable to help Sānkṛtyāyana personally in the way he wished, he recommended instead that Sānkṛtyāyana consider working with his most promising—and at times, most troublesome[44]—student, a young man from northeastern Tibet (Amdo) named Gedun Chöpel.[45] Just how confident Sānkṛtyāyana was in Geshe Sherap Gyatso's recommendation is unclear, since he also sought out the help of another recommended scholar, the tutor to the house of Tsarong, the Mongolian Geshe Chödrak[46] from the great monastic university of Sera, just north of Lhasa. Geshe Chödrak also declined Sānkṛtyāyana's offer to come to India, but Gedun Chöpel accepted, and together the two men traveled south and west toward Nepal with formal letters of authorization, stopping at various monasteries and temples along the way, such as Ngor and Shalu, in search of Sanskrit manuscripts.

By the time they reached Nepal in November 1934, Sānkṛtyāyana and Gedun Chöpel had amassed a considerable collection of Sanskrit palm-leaf manuscripts[47] that they could study. Settling in Kathmandu, for the next five months they worked on cataloging and examining their finds, then left for India the following March. Abandoned by Sānkṛtyāyana, who embarked on a trip across Southeast Asia to Japan, Gedun Chöpel was left to fend for himself for more than a year in Darjeeling and greater Sikkim. Only when Gedun Chöpel met Tharchin, who was still looking for someone with scholastic training to help him decipher Bacot's Tun-huang manuscripts, did his fortunes take a turn for the better. Seeing an opportunity to secure a more stable environment, Gedun Chöpel agreed to help Tharchin and moved in, living and working with him on and off for the next eighteen months, translating the early Tibetan histories from Tun-huang for Jacques Bacot.[48]

Despite his reliance on Tharchin, however, Gedun Chöpel did not suffer for company in Kalimpong. As the economic fortunes of the Sikkimese-Tibetan border towns fluctuated, Kalimpong was slowly taking over Darjeeling as the wool-trading capital of northeast India. More than 50 percent of the wool traffic of central Tibet passed through the small town, and the economy of Lhasa became linked to the price of wool in Kalimpong. As a result, Kalimpong was quickly becoming home to a growing merchant and expatriate Tibetan population. This fact hadn't escaped the notice of Jacques Bacot; nor did it escape the notice of another would-be Tibetan scholar, the British researcher Marco Pallis. Arriving in Kalimpong, Pallis had sought out his own Tibetan scholar to aid him in his research and found the Mongolian lama Ngawang Wangyal, whose own goals and interests had led him south as well, via Peking and Lhasa in the company of the British representative Charles Bell, for whom he had served as translator for several months.

When Theos Bernard stepped out into the streets of Kalimpong in early January 1937 with his father, this was the world he walked into. A town that in many respects marked the northernmost limit of success in the Christian missionary assault on Tibet, Kalimpong was also the staging ground from which Tibetan scholars and their Western disciples were beginning to launch their own assaults on the countries of Europe and the Americas, bringing the insights of a Buddhist worldview to the Western world, and Theos Bernard was determined to be one of them.

That January, Theos settled into a routine of studying Tibetan with Tharchin. While this was a fine arrangement for Theos (and a financial boon to Tharchin[49]), Glen saw it as a waste of time, and his annoyance began to wear on Theos's nerves even more than before. Within a week, Glen decided that it was time for him to leave. "It would be absolutely wrong for him to remain," Theos explained to Viola, for

he is about at the point where he is going to kill every Hindu in India, not saying anything about the rest of the lives he is going to terminate. If he met one in his dreams he would throw himself completely out of bed trying to get at him. When you saw him he was an angry child; so multiply that by ten and double the total each day for every day since you have been away and you will have some idea of his present state.

As glad as Glen was to leave, Theos was even more happy to get away from his father. In addition to the trip having taken a toll on his health, Glen had a problem, however—beyond the usual financial one. Although he had a return ticket for a ship in the Dollar Line, there was a strike on and ships were only leaving India every four months. As usual, Theos had to ask Viola to bail his father out, in addition to maintaining their "continued arrangement" for his support. Even though Glen was preparing to leave Kalimpong, Theos assured Viola that their research together would not end. Indeed, with Viola's support, Glen would be hard at work upon his return spending "all of his time wiping [sic] together some literary data that I want in order by the time I return." Just as important, Theos told Viola, with her support Glen "will also be able to continue on with the laboratory experiments which are necessary to finish up this work on Mercury which is needed for our future practice."[50]

"Practice" was indeed on his mind, and all other concerns were quickly falling behind, barely worth a casual remark to Viola. Theos believed they were moving into a phase of their lives together that was centered around their work and that "life is always going to be a pace like this and there will never be enough time to find that home and have children." Having renounced that possibility, he reiterated to Viola his feeling that they should dedicate their lives to finding "some way so that others may better help themselves, and so forget that as an entity we exist," and along those lines had some recommendations for her career. Although this was only a passing comment for Theos, it was an unexpected shock to Viola.[51]

Oblivious to the deep impact those statements would have on Viola as a reversal of his earlier promises, Theos was caught up in his world of studies, having settled into a stable routine at the hotel:

5 am: Awake; practice yoga/prāṇayāma
7am: Tibetan lesson with Tharchin; followed by mile walk, a light breakfast of oatmeal and milk, and studies
Noon: Lunch and errands, followed by studies
4pm: Tea time and review
5pm: Tibetan lesson with Tharchin again

6:30pm: Washing, more yoga exercises, and study
9pm: Reading, or writing to Viola
11pm: Sleep

With Glen finally gone, there was little to distract Theos, and he remained confident that he could master Tibetan with ease, and since it was "only a matter of time and routine," he soon "would have a working knowledge of it." This was important, because beyond gaining the ability to access the content of Tibetan texts himself, the ability to claim knowledge of Tibetan would be crucial in gaining admittance to Oxford University. William Mc-Govern's observation that learning Tibetan meant learning three different "languages" because "there is not only an ordinary and an honorific language, but also a high honorific language used in addressing high dignitaries"[52] was, in fact, quite true, and Theos feared that he would have little time for letter writing to anyone besides Viola.

Although he thought that he could easily lose himself "here for the next fifty years in work and never know there was an outside world," nonetheless, she shouldn't worry too much about him losing his perspective:

> Do not take it that I feel that the purpose of life is to learn a language or become versed in the Tibetan literature—those two things are just as worthless as a million other things that man is playing with so far as his real purpose is concerned. I only dabble with this form because I believe that behind it there is some information that I can use to better enable me to continue on with my other work.

This was the real reason, he told her, that he never had done "a great deal of talking about the real inner development to be derived from Yoga" because he "did not want to talk without having had first hand personal experience with it." But in the absence of direct guidance and authentic commentaries, getting that experience would prove difficult. Nonetheless, Theos took encouragement when and where he could, even being allowed to photograph a Tibetan text belonging to Tharchin, with figures illustrating different yogic exercises.[53]

But many of these issues, Theos recognized, were long-term concerns. In the short term, he had received most of the knowledge that he needed from his father, and the rest was clearly explained in the pamphlets they had gotten from Kuvalayānanda. Solidly engaged in those exercises, he was pleased to tell Viola that in addition to his language studies, his practice of the yogic exercises was progressing; working on his breathing exercises (*prāṇayāma*), he had gotten to the point where his *uḍḍiyāna bandha*[54] was "up to its highest form of perfect"—something Viola had yet to see—and he promised he would demonstrate it for her on his return. While all these developments provided positive reinforcement to Theos,

> one of the thrills of the entire adventure has been the following of the footsteps of those that I have read about for so long—David-Neel, Mc-Govern, Sir Charles Bell, David Macdonald who I have come to know as a real friend, and all the members of the Everest Expeditions. . . . The field is so vast and those who have been combing it are of such a variety and interest that there is yet an unlimited quantity of material for me whose background is so entirely different. They have all told what there is to find, but no one has revealed what lies behind that which exists, and here is my task.

His challenge, as he saw it, was to "prove to others the real concrete aspects of this philosophy which is nothing but an explanation of the functioning of nature." But Theos thought all of this was exciting because he found it a stark contrast to his life in America and the obligations imposed on him by American society. It was an inner conflict that was causing him to waffle between excitement and frustration:

> I am out for a Ph.D. and for some God for known reason I have chosen the most remote thing that we know of for its subject; so now that I have started, I must see it thru to the bitter end regardless of how much it hurts . . . that is why I am here—to work and find out how much of what I believe really exist[s] . . . [but] if I did not have to have a degree, I have my doubts as to how long I would stay here. I do not care as much about the degree, but the public does, and I care about the public to a certain extent, therefore it is essential that I come up to what they call a standard, before I tell all to go to hell and do as I please about anything and everything. All I want to do is meet their requirements. Mine are much higher, but they do not understand them; so again, I must do the adjusting. And then to top off the distrust of the public, I have its nest in my home, for Viola doesn't give a dam [*sic*] about it, just as I don't give a dam about medicine.[55]

For Theos, this was a wonderful thing—the fact that they were "separate individuals" and yet had a love that couldn't be found elsewhere, with only "minor differences" between them. But when Theos's letter arrived, Viola was not amused by his comments. Minor differences? "Like hell they are!" she thought, and as fast as the mail could travel, Theos had Viola's response and once again had to work to repair the damage to their relationship. "There is nothing that hurts me worse to feel that I have in some unknown way brought you a hurt," he wrote back. Trying to convince her that she had taken his statements "all wrong," he reassured her that "if you only knew all the love there is for you in me, you would never misinterpret things." Just the same, Theos couldn't hid his anger:

> I suppose you think that I get a kick out of living away from you—what in the hell did I change the course of my life and marry you for if I wanted to get away from you. You also indicate that you feel that my whole choice of action is a bit queer—well, I have to do something in this world, we all cannot be doctors.

But venting at Viola would solve little, he knew—even if that realization didn't stop him—so he suggested, "I feel that it is best for us to dispense with the writing and know that we have a complete understand[ing] over all of these things," while attempting to assuage her anger by saying that if they persisted in their long-distance argument it would be "likely to cause us a little trouble which is quite unnecessary, for our adjustment is perfect and will more than carry us on thru a life of continual happiness." Turning philosophical, as he usually did at such times, he reminded her that "our whole society is pretty rotten and that civilization on the whole is man's most highly perfected machine for his own destruction."

Theos sent his letter immediately, but by the next day had decided that a further apology was probably necessary, telling her, "I have been having my mood." More important, Theos tried to convince Viola that not only was it bad for their relationship in the long term for her to misunderstand him, but also it had an adverse effect on him in the present: "you always read or listen to my words and never hear what my heart is crying out," and "it is a hell of a feeling to have everything shot to hell and then realize that the only place that can be called home is the ground that you stand on for the moment." For without her, he told Viola, he was lost, but even with her, the future remained uncertain. "I wonder if there is any way of telling what on earth I will be doing five years from now," he wrote. "Hell, I bet that I do not even die regularly—probably alone someplace, mad as hell at myself for being there." But, having run the gamut of his all too typical range of emotions, in the end, as always, he reaffirmed his undying love for her—as Theos always chose to expressed it, "I lub OO OOoo."

How, precisely, all of these concerns would play out, Viola could not tell, so she chose to respond to all of Theos's conflicting signals, the expressions of his "dammed good for-nothing emotional nature," by putting such discussions on hold—at Theos's request—for the benefit of his state of mind until such time as they were reunited. After and despite it all, Viola reminded herself that she *did* love him, and he did seem lonely and very miserable.

As the weeks passed, Theos's spirits slowly recovered and his mood began to improve as the Tibetan New Year approached. When he met Tharchin for his daily morning Tibetan lesson, the comings and goings of various people for the holiday meant that Theos was introduced to many new faces. One man who stopped by to convey his greetings to Tharchin was a young Kalmyk Mongolian lama, Ngawang Wangyal. Wearing a traditional Mongolian monk's robes and a somewhat incongruous homburg hat,[56] Wangyal made an immediate impression. He was, as Theos would find out, a brilliant scholar who had already played many roles over the course of his life.

Born to Mongolian parents in the Kalmyk region of Russia[57] at the turn of the century, Wangyal had entered his local monastery at the age of six, joining his older brother, Kunsang, who began tutoring him. By the time he was sixteen, his interests had turned to medicine and he relocated to a medical college in Outer Mongolia, where he began studying the Tibetan medical tradition. After a year, however, his teacher suddenly passed away, and he was left stranded and directionless, for in the absence of his teacher, his interest in medicine quickly faded. To his good fortune, the Bolshevik revolution had just taken place in Russia, sending a group of Buryat Mongolian Buddhists south to attempt to secure sovereignty for the Mongolian peoples. Among them were the abbot of the Petrograd temple, Sodnom Zhigzhitov; the notable Buryat intellectual Badzar Baradinevich Baradin; and the foremost Buddhist in all of Russia, onetime tutor to the Thirteenth Dalai Lama, and advisor to Tzar Nicholas II, Agwan Dorjiev— whose presence in Lhasa at the turn of the century had made the British Raj so nervous. Although he hailed from Mongolian Buryatia in Siberia,

Dorjiev had maintained a commitment to the Kalmyk Mongolians and was famous among them, often visiting Kalmykia and even establishing two colleges there for the study of Buddhism. Hearing of Wangyal's abilities as a student, Dorjiev took him on as a disciple and eventually decided to bring him along to Lhasa to ensure that his studies continued.

Thus accompanied by Buryat Russian political spies and secret emissaries,[58] Wangyal arrived in Tibet and settled into Drepung Monastic University, home to many Mongolian monks in Lhasa, and, like Dorjiev and so many other Mongolians before him, entered its Gomang College. Trained well by his teachers, the young Ngawang Wangyal completed his studies in half the time of his fellow Tibetan students by doubling his lessons. When his studies were finished, feeling homesick for Mongolia, by the late 1920s Wangyal was ready to return home for a while. Making his way to Peiping (Beijing), he had the good fortune to meet some Buryat monks who advised him to proceed no further. The Bolsheviks had begun to exert their complete authority over Russia and his Mongolian homeland and in every area under their control Buddhists—and monks in particular—were being persecuted. He was advised not even to contact his family, since doing so could put them at risk. Although he had no way of knowing, such difficulties had already touched his family. Kunsang, his older brother who had been such a formative influence on him as a young boy, had risen to the post of abbot of his monastery, only to be arrested by the Bolsheviks. Already in prison before Wangyal had even completed his studies. Kunsang would die there without the brothers ever seeing each other again.

Heeding the advice of his fellow monks, Wangyal decided to stay in China. Finding work as a translator for Russian scholars and as a teacher among his fellow Mongolians, he learned English in the process, and was sufficiently fluent in so short a time that he was able to serve as translator for the British Political Officer, Charles Bell, when he visited Mongolia, China, and Manchuria. Although Wangyal's studies in Tibet were completed, one of the requirements for the geshe degree was the obligation to feed one's home monastery for a day. As Drepung had a population of over 7,000 monks, this was no small feat, especially for a Mongolian far from home. With the money he earned in China during those years, Wangyal was eventually able to return to Lhasa, but initially did not want to fulfill the final obligations to his monastery in order to obtain his degree, even if he'd had the money, which he didn't. Feeling that the system had become corrupt, he, like his teacher Agwan Dorjiev, thought than too many monks and geshes weren't really studying. Worse yet, men he considered to be the really great teachers—like Geshe Sherap Gyatso, who had been driven out of Lhasa for daring to edit the canon, or his own teacher, Geshe Jinpa, who, poverty stricken, was living in the basement of Gomang College—were not receiving the respect and support that they deserved. Consequently, Wangyal felt that a geshe degree was no longer a hallmark of knowledge and attainment, but rather proof of having bought a lot of tea and made good aristocratic connections. The Pha-la family, however, who had been his friends, insisted that he go through with the process, going so far as to cover the cost of feeding his monastery. Even so, Geshe Wangyal eventually left Lhasa and made his way to India. At thirty-five, he was only a few years older than Theos when they met in Kalimpong. Having mastered Tibetan and Russian over his native Mongolian, Wangyal had English fluency that, though limited, was more than good enough for most conversations.

Theos and Geshe Wangyal immediately struck up a friendship, which Theos's interest in Tibetan literature only strengthened. Relaxing in Tharchin's home, they had a long conversation about the Tibetan canon and the educational system in the great monastic universities. Geshe Wangyal explained that he had agreed to work with Marco Pallis and would return to England with him at the end of his visit in a few months. Eager to learn about potential research partners for when he returned home, Theos quizzed Geshe Wangyal at length about where and in what texts he could find the answers to many of his research questions, and was duly impressed by the answers. "He is a fine chap," Theos wrote to Viola, "but now he is pretty naive so far as the world is concerned but he has covered a vast amount of literature in his own field and I have found him extremely helpful in telling me where certain kinds of information can be found."

Although Geshe Wangyal had only agreed to go to England with the tentative possibility of guiding Marco Pallis back to Tibet, he would rather return to China, he told Theos. "His favorite stop is Peking and he wishes to eventually get back there to do more studying." Since such a journey from England would be more easily accomplished by traveling via America, without hesitation Theos invited him to visit him (or Viola, at least) should he actually reach the United States. "I have given him your address," he told Viola, "and told him by all means that he is to call you once he arrives and that you will do whatever is possible for him. . . . He may never turn up, or I may be there before he is. This is just all in the way of a warning that someday a Lama might come into your life."

At the end of Tharchin's impromptu tea party, thoroughly warmed up to Theos, Geshe Wangyal insisted that he accompany him to his home to attend *his* New Year's party, where a number of Tibetans were gathering. Far from the sort of restrained event that British decorum imposed in Tharchin's household. Geshe Wangyal's party was host to a contingent of guests freshly arrived from Tibet—a group of dignitaries traveling en route to China via Calcutta, along with many local well-wishers.

No less prominent than the Three Great Seats of Learning that were homes to the scholars of the Lhasa valley, the great monastic university of Tashilhunpo in Shigatse, some hundred miles southwest of Lhasa, boasted many brilliant minds and political figures as well. Not the least of these was the Panchen Lama, whose political machinations had proven too much for the central government and who as a result had spent many years in self-imposed exile in China. Political instability seemed to be the theme in Europe and the rest of Asia in the 1930s, and Tibet was no exception. While the Bolsheviks to the north, the Chinese communists to the east, and the British to the south fought their opponents in both the physical and political arenas, all eyed Tibet as the key to controlling central Asia. Seeing the potential for the downfall of his beloved country, the Thirteenth Dalai Lama—the "Great Thirteenth," as he came to be called—had tried to modernize Tibet while maintaining its independence from the three surrounding empires.

With different factions in the monastic and aristocratic ranks all clamoring for influence, there was a constant power struggle among pro-British, pro-Chinese, and isolationist groups in Tibet throughout the first few decades of the twentieth century. The Panchen Lama and Tashilhunpo Monastery, always having had strong ties to China—from which they benefited financially—had supported the brief Chinese occupation of Tibet and seizure of the Lhasa government from 1909 to 1912. As the situation continued to heat up, ten years later the Ninth Panchen Lama would have to flee for his life. But the sudden death of the Great Thirteenth in December 1934 left a power vacuum at the highest levels in Tibet, and with a contingent of three hundred Chinese soldiers and the backing of the Chinese Republican government, the Panchen Lama was trying to return to Tibet and in particular, it was feared, to Lhasa to take control of the government. Having thrown out a failed Chinese invasion of Tibet twenty-five years earlier, Tibetans talked of renewed Chinese aspirations to take Eastern Tibet (Kham) and convert it into a Chinese province.[59] There were rumors that the Panchen Lama had his own candidate for the Fourteenth Dalai

Lama, whom he had identified himself and had traveling with him in his entourage. Even if all these things were untrue, fearing the leverage that any of them would give the Chinese government over Tibet, the Tibetan government chose active opposition, and by 1937 the Panchen Lama and his party had been stalled on the other side of an active skirmish line on the Tibetan–Chinese border. For several years he had been biding his time, awaiting resolution of the dispute.

Eager to see the situation resolved, the British Mission in Lhasa had been advising negotiations between the Lhasa government and the Panchen Lama, the latter choosing as his intermediary his associate in self-imposed exile, the Tā Lama, Ngak-chen Rinpoche. Quite a few notables had joined him on his circuitous trip to rendezvous with the Panchen Lama in Kye-gu-do, including the semiofficial Republican envoy to Tibet in Lhasa, Madame Liu Manqing.[60] Sitting in that small room with Theos in Kalimpong were Ngak-chen Rinpoche, Geshe Sherap Gyatso, and various members of Ngak-chen Rinpoche's entourage—a formidable party.

Tā Lama Ngak-chen Rinpoche, Losang Tenzin Jigme Wangchuk,[61] was a descendant of the family of the Tenth Dalai Lama, educated at Tashil-hunpo Monastery. When the Ninth Panchen Lama had fled Tibet in 1923, Ngak-chen Rinpoche had accompanied him, and they traveled throughout China giving teachings and empowerments. He had returned to Lhasa in 1931 and again in 1933, but by 1937 little progress had been made in resolving the stand-off between the factions, and so Ngak-chen Rinpoche had left Lhasa—some say he was dismissed and recalled—in the company of the Chinese representative, to rejoin the Panchen Lama on the Tibetan–Chinese border.

Traveling with him was a close friend of the late Thirteenth Dalai Lama, Geshe Sherap Gyatso, the scholar from Drepung who had been the editor of the most recent redaction of the Buddhist canon. Following the death of the Great Thirteenth, his political enemies had moved against him and he had decided to abandon his life in Tibet and go to China, ostensibly to translate his redaction of the Tibetan Buddhist canon into Chinese.[62]

Finally, Theos thought, he was making real progress; finally, he was beginning to interact in real Tibetan circles. For although the Tibetan expatriates and traders who populated Kalimpong were a pleasant enough group, the relentless proselytizing by the local missionaries had reduced many of them to a less than respectable state. Writing to a friend who had recently professed his belief in Christianity, Theos informed him that the

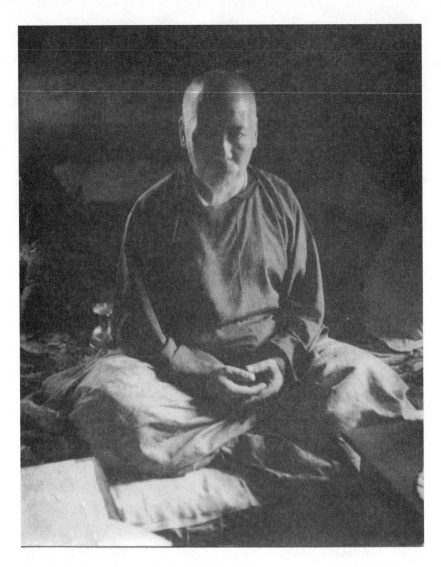

Figure 7.1 Ngak-chen Rinpoche (PAHM)

faith "had reduced itself here to a handful of Devil Chasers preaching in elegant stone houses of superstition to a congregation of Money Christians," for that was about what it amounted to in Kalimpong in Theos's eyes. "The Tibetans are good Christians as long as there is a chance to make a little money or have something nice given to them," he continued, "but they all have their Buddha at home." Here now, however, were Tibetans with no such pretenses.

From the positive impression he made on the assembled notables, a few days later Theos received an invitation to dinner from one of the aristocratic families that maintained a house in Kalimpong. Tsarong Lhacham—Lady Tsarong—the wife of the famous Tibetan general and former cabinet minister Tsarong Shapé, was in Kalimpong, and hearing about Theos, she invited him over for a meal. Although Theos thought little of it at the time—beyond the details of the food itself and how it "played havoc" with his diet regimen—this meeting would prove his most important connection within Tibet.

A couple of weeks later, the entourage of Ngak-chen Rinpoche was on the move again, south to Calcutta to board a ship for China. Though he did not plan on doing so, Theos would soon be reunited with them in Calcutta, for one morning a passing report in the morning newspaper sparked his imagination: a conference was scheduled to take place there soon. But this was no ordinary conference.

"To keep count of thousands of paces," the semifictional Hurree Babu explained to his pupil, there was "nothing more valuable than a rosary of eighty-one or a hundred and eight beads, for it was divisible and sub-divisible into many multiples and sub-multiples."[63] When it was first published at the opening of the twentieth century, Rudyard Kipling's *Kim* was both hailed as a wonderful piece of literature and derided as the ultimate testament to the colonial fantasy, an idealized representation of life in "the Great Game." To those in the know, however, *Kim* was little more than a lightly fictionalized account of the actual sort of intrigues afoot in British India, such as those of Sarat Chandra Das ("Hurree Chunder Mookherjee"), Tibetan scholar and British spy.[64] Das, a slightly rotund Bengali like Kipling's Mookerjee, had employed the very techniques described in Kipling's work in the early 1880s, traveling with a Tibetan lama[65] from an outlying monastery as part of his disguise while laying the groundwork for a military invasion being planned by the more ambitious elements within the British Raj. "We had given ourselves out to be pilgrims," wrote Sarat Chandra Das,[66] and though published within years of each of his trips, his works were not widely available, their circulation having been restricted by the Indian British authorities as a security risk.

Only slightly more than twenty years after Das's initial surveys of the southern passes and valleys, India's Viceroy, Lord Curzon, sent an army into Tibet, ostensibly to secure the release of two British Sikkimese spies captured there. As a result, in December 1903, the recently promoted Colonel Younghusband led his small army—2,000 infantry, 10,000 coolies, 7,000 mules, 4,000 yaks, and five newspaper correspondents[67]—up over the Jelap-la Pass from Sikkim into Tibet, and after fighting a series of embarrassing and regrettably bloody battles,[68] proceeded north toward Lhasa. Though aimed at stabilizing relations with the nation of Tibet, ironically, this confluence of events—Agvan Dorjiev's emissary to the court of the Dalai Lama, British fears of Russian penetration into that Himalayan kingdom, and the obvious irrelevance and ineffectualness of Chinese representation in Lhasa—produced levels of colonialist paranoia that served to mark independent Tibet as doomed, a prize destined to be swallowed by one of her aggressive imperialist neighbors.

Younghusband himself viewed his activities at the time entirely within the scope of his duties to the empire, remarking shortly after his return that he and his comrades "may have nasty jobs to do but it is the game and they will play it through."[69] In February 1937, the Younghusband who was about to arrive in Calcutta was a very different man from who he had been in those days, for the years had transformed him—like the occasional few who saw too closely the toll of death their campaigns had taken—from unrepentant man of war to unrepentant man of peace. Younghusband himself attributed this change to the influence of a Tibetan lama he had met while in Tibet, the eighty-sixth Regent of Ganden Monastery (the Ganden Tri-pa), Tsang-pa Lo-sang-gyal-tsen,[70] who had assumed the Regency of Tibet when the Thirteenth Dalai Lama fled the advancing British army and had served as the Tibetan government's chief negotiator. Comparing the Regent to the Tibetan lama in Kipling's *Kim*, Younghusband remarked that he was "an old and much respected Lama . . . a cultured, pleasant-mannered, amiable old gentleman, with a kindly, benevolent expression." On his last full day in Lhasa, Younghusband was visited one last time by the Ganden Tri-pa, who presented him with a small bronze statue of the Buddha, telling him, "when we Buddhists look on this figure we think only of peace, and I want you, when you look at it, to think kindly of Tibet." Recounting his time in Tibet, Younghusband later wrote that he took some time for himself just before leaving and "went alone up onto the mountain side and in the holy calm of eventide I chewed the cud of all I had just experienced."

I was naturally elated at the successful ending of a critical mission. But suddenly, as I sat there among the mountains, bathed in the glow of sunset, there came upon me what was far more than elation or exhilaration . . . I was beside myself with an intensity of joy, such as even the joy of first love can only give a faint foreshadowing of. And with this indescribable and almost unbearable joy came a revelation of the essential goodness of the world. I was convinced past all refutation that men at heart were good, that the evil in them was superficial, that the main impulse in them was to the good—in short, that men at heart were divine.[71]

Rising early the next morning, he carefully placed the statue of the Buddha in his saddlebag, and looking out over the early morning skies and distant peaks of the Himalayas, headed out calm and contented in the wake of his deep religious epiphany.

By the spring of 1937, while most of Europe braced for another war, it was *this* Younghusband, a religious man of peace, who was organizing a "World Congress of Faiths" in Calcutta. Following the 1893 World Parliament of Religions in Chicago, the theme of religious ecumenicalism spurred a number of gatherings and conferences over the subsequent decades, and now Younghusband himself had taken up the challenge of promoting world peace and interreligious dialogue. "The aim and purpose of this Congress," it was declared,

is to promote a spirit of fellowship among mankind through religion and develop a world-loyalty while allowing full play for the diversity of men, nations and faiths. The Congress does not emphasise that all religions are alike, nor does it wish to formulate a synthetic faith out of the various elements contributed by the different religions, but seeks to engender a spirit of fellowship between the religions as they are, in their common attempt to solve the problems of humanity.[72]

Having hosted a similar meeting in England the year before, Younghusband set his sights on India, hoping to return to those lands for the first time in decades.

Excited by the prospect of meeting Younghusband, Theos prevailed upon David Macdonald to accompany him to Calcutta to attend the conference, offering to cover any and all expenses if he would introduce him to the esteemed knight.[73] Not having seen Younghusband in many years and with little likelihood of any future opportunity to do so, Macdonald accepted and the two men headed south for Calcutta. After they checked into rooms at his favorite abode, the Great Eastern Hotel, Theos began strategizing for the days ahead. Just as they arrived in Calcutta, the newspapers were announcing even more exciting news concerning the conference: not only was Sir Francis Younghusband returning to India, but he was also being transported and accompanied by his friend and neighbor, Charles Lindbergh. Seizing the opportunity before him, Theos suggested to David Macdonald that they invite their old and new friends for lunch just prior to the start of the conference. Eager for a reunion, Younghusband accepted the invitation, and Ngak-chen Rinpoche, having shaken Younghusband's hand as a young man in Lhasa in 1904, looked forward to meeting the man again. So one evening in late February there assembled in a restaurant in Calcutta an impressive gathering of men and women of power, influence, and intelligence—Sir Francis Younghusband, Charles and Anne Lindbergh, Madame Liu Manqing and the Chinese representative accompanying the party to China, David Macdonald, Ngak-chen Rinpoche, Geshe Sherap Gyatso, and Gedun Chöpel—and in the middle of them all was Theos Bernard.[74] He was beside himself, overjoyed at having met Younghusband *and* having struck up a friendship with Lindbergh on top of it all:

> How and why did I ever have Lindbergh dining with me in Calcutta with a Lama from Tibet is just as much a mystery to me as it is to you and even he—for he expressed the same thoughts—why should I from Arizona, meet him in India. As it turns out he is much interested in some of these things. He expresses the desire to have a longer chat so that we should go into many of the details—this may come to pass—hard to say—for we are both anxious to leave Calcutta.

Although he enjoyed his time with the Tibetan company, Theos lamented his still inadequate language skills. Writing to Viola, he complained that while he could talk to David Macdonald in Tibetan and be understood, "when a group of Tibs all get talking at once—I hear one word here another there" though he regrettably had "no clue what they are talking about in particular."[75]

Although the conference was to last a week, Ngak-chen Rinpoche's party would only be in attendance for a few days, as their ship was departing before the conference's close.[76] The first day, all would be in attendance to give their opening remarks, wishes, and congratulations to Younghusband and one another. Seeing an opportunity, Theos had a brilliant idea, and he described it in all its glory to Viola:

> The right hand man of the Tashi Lama from Tashilhunpo was in town on his way to China . . . I got Mr. Macdonald to bring him down—we did good as it turns out—he took a liking to me so now we are one. Never before has Buddhism from Tibet been represented at a Congress of World Faiths, so an invitation was extended and except then, I up and got ahead of them to put Ngak-chhen Rinpoche on the program representing Tibet. With this we were all guests of honor—and in my estimation he was the finest of the entire lot. . . . Mr. Macdonald interpreted the speech which I had written for him to present—it all happened in five minutes, mind you—he didn't know that he was to speak until he was in the taxi on the way to the Congress. It was given to him, he read it over and delivered it without notes in a most humble fashion.

Standing at the dais, with Younghusband seated nearby and his bronze Buddha statue from Tibet displayed prominently, Ngak-chen Rinpoche gave his brief speech:

> It has afforded me a great pleasure to be present at this World Congress of Faiths. I bring good wishes to this Congress from all the Buddhists under Tashi Lama of Tibet. I heartily wish it all success in its universal call to bring peace and goodwill and happiness to mankind. I offer my blessings to the World Congress of Faiths on this auspicious occasion of the celebrations of the Centenary of Sri Ramakrishna, one of the greatest spiritual geniuses of India.

As author of the speech, given his familiarity with its content, Theos volunteered to serve as Ngak-chen Rinpoche's "translator" for the event. And so, the official conference proceedings read: "Mr. Ngak-Chhen Rimpoche, Prime Minister to the Tashi Lama . . . interpreted by his Secretary Mr. T.C. Bernard."[77]

When Theos talked about translating the Tibetan canon with Ngak-chen Rinpoche and David Macdonald later that day, the lama offered his insights into the various problems associated with such an endeavor. As a final gesture, Ngak-chen Rinpoche recommended that Theos visit Tashil-hunpo Monastery and extended a formal invitation to visit him in September,[78] when he hoped to return to Shigatse in the company of the Panchen Lama.[79] "So there will be another opportunity for further works," Theos told Viola.

> Isn't this all the making of my good fortune—he is enshrined as one of the Masters of Tibet—so I return to Calcutta to find in one of the filthiest, darkest and most remote holes of Chinatown the one individual that many people would go to any extreme to meet—it is all because of friendship and interest in their teachings—what would Paul Brunton do with a chap like this or Lachen Rinpoche—such it is and I am trying hard so as to be able to take advantage of every opportunity that comes up.

Such opportunities were increasing, Theos noticed, and in addition to a personal invitation, Ngak-chen Rinpoche offered to secure a copy of the Tibetan canon—Kangyur and Tengyur—for Theos "at a reasonable figure" for, as a representative of a monastery, Ngak-chen Rinpoche could get a set "for the asking" and told him that he was willing to help Theos, since "he feels that it is wonderful they are for the Western world."

The next day, Theos's good fortune continued, as he and Lindbergh were able to meet and converse yet again. "Had a long talk of several hours with Lindbergh," he told Viola.

> He is as keen as a child on all of my work here—it is arousing his interest. He has been working for many years with Rockefeller Research in N.Y. on atmospheric effects on blood, mind, etc.—for aviation purposes—so he is eating a lot of these things up—he is anxious that we get together and plan some experiments . . . we are having lunch together today and then are going to see if we can find . . . a place where I have had some good fortune with books.

Despite his profession of interest for the sake of his aviation research, there seemed to be more behind Lindbergh's fascination with yoga. At the time, his wife, Anne, was more than amused at the conference by "seeing her agnostic husband in front of banners declaring 'Religion is the highest expression of man'" and watching him blush when "an Indian poetess . . . compared him to 'Buddha, Galileo, and other spiritual figures in the world,'" with an "intense embarrassment . . . visible to all."[80] However, in 1937 the pain of the kidnapping and murder of their son was still fresh, and Lindbergh continued to struggle with depression. He had tried to occupy himself with a series of "enthusiasms," some more superficial than others. When it came to yoga, Lindbergh hoped that it might offer a permanent solution to his problems.

Indeed, when he had contacted Francis Younghusband a year earlier, Lindbergh had asked for his help in researching "supersensory phenomena" and his assistance to "find fakirs and fire-walkers and 'squat with a yogi' . . . while stressing the need for total secrecy."[81] When he met Theos Bernard, however, Lindbergh seemed to feel that his interests and research met these needs exactly, and they agreed to correspond and collaborate on a series of experiments upon Theos's return to America.

As the conference drew to a close, Theos was anxious to turn as many of the ideas he had discussed with different people—yoga experiments with Lindbergh, obtaining copies of Sarat Chandra Das's then out-of-print *Tibetan Dictionary* and *Grammar* from his son, and arranging the purchase of a Kangyur and Tengyur through Ngak-chen Rinpoche, among other things—into concrete plans. Meeting with Ngak-chen Rinpoche one more time with David Macdonald's help and interpretation, Theos settled on a price of Rs. 1200 for a copy of the Kangyur recently printed in Lhasa and offered to the Thirteenth Dalai Lama. Since it was "even a better buy than any other possible with Jinorasa's cousin in Sikkim" and Ngak-chen Rinpoche's entourage had the copy "here, packed, and ready to leave for America" in an instant, it was a deal he simply couldn't pass up. Cabling Viola for an extra five hundred dollars, Theos purchased the copy from Ngak-chen Rinpoche and the next day had it taken to the docks at Calcutta and loaded on a ship bound for New York, advising Viola to "have them stored anyplace but at the Club," for they could strategize upon his return about where to put the "325 vols. of Tibetan mss. . . . [so he] can have a monastery as a den to study in." Overjoyed at his luck in getting this set of books to America, Theos thought "nothing could be better except to have a lama over there to help me carry on my work." But he had plenty on hand to deal with before pursuing that idea any further. Seeing Ngak-chen Rinpoche and his entourage off as they boarded their ship, Theos and all assembled were treated to *bon voyage* speeches by both Younghusband and Macdonald at the docks.[82]

After a few more visits with Lindbergh, Theos was certain "we'll be doing things one of these days." Having met "Sir Francis"—who promised to help him make contacts at Oxford, including Sir Charles Bell and L. Austin Waddell—the Tibetan lamas, and the various other delegates in attendance, Theos felt that the "trip and stay in Calcutta has hit me pretty hard, but it is one of the best investments for friendship I ever had." As he prepared to return north to Kalimpong, his luck held true: the day before he was to leave, Sarat Chandra Das's son arrived at his hotel, bearing copies of his father's grammar that one otherwise "can't buy for love or money" and a promise to try to get him a copy of the dictionary as well, while van Manen provided him with a rare copy of Csoma de Körös's 1834 Tibetan grammar. All in all, the week was proving unbelievably profitable for Theos, not only in terms of his resources but also in his state of mind.

> I will notice the effect of all of this on my work next week—gee, I am going to have to buckle down still harder, because there is now going to be half enough time to complete this joy—Never in my life have I enjoyed work so much—If you were like me, you would forget that there was a world—really I spend every waking hour in a state of glowing enthusiasm—regretting that I have to leave it for sleep. I wish I could live on two hours a day— maybe someday. I have so much planned to do that it makes me tired carrying the thoughts around and the pressure is so great that I cannot act fast enough to keep from being almost smothered under it.

On his last evening in Calcutta, Theos had a final meeting with Lindbergh and his wife, Anne, "going into various aspects of Pranayama that hold an interest for him." The meeting reaffirmed that Lindbergh was "about the best chap that I have ever met," for Theos had "the strongest feeling for him—just because of the way he thinks—he actually sees the problems involved and their practical significances," as Lindbergh explained, for "high altitude flying."

Nonetheless, once back in Kalimpong, Theos had to settle back into his routine of study and practice. As he communicated all his adventures and thoughts to his wife, Viola took the opportunity in responding to raise some of the more practical issues about their life together. When she hinted that she didn't mind all of his expenses and running around, so long as it would help him get his fill of the experience and settle down afterward to "something more sane to the general run of the public," Theos responded in his typical half-flippant manner: while he thought visiting India and Tibet "once in a lifetime is enough," still he felt the need to justify himself by saying "you had better get to know what is really on the inside of me." Unfortunately for Theos, Viola was already beginning to, and his idea of a future was not her "life plan" at all. Nonetheless, Theos *could* take a hint, if not sensitively, and suggested that he indeed had plans for financial stability. Reiterating his eagerness to maintain a source of income for the years to come, Theos informed Viola that he was investigating opportunities connected with the wool trade passing through Kalimpong.

No sooner had Theos returned to Kalimpong, however, than he heard that the British Mission's cameraman, Freddy Chapman, had just returned from Tibet with color films of places and events and had gone down to Calcutta to develop and cut them. Given that he planned to do the same with his own films, Theos felt obliged to see what he had obtained. This would prove worthwhile, confirming the importance of color film in Tibet and leading to a solid friendship between Chapman and Theos, but more crucially, Chapman was the personal secretary to the British Political Officer for Tibet, B. J. Gould, who had returned to Gangtok but was very ill and likely to be shortly sent to England for medical treatment. If Theos was to obtain the all-important letter of permission to enter Tibet from Gould, he would have to act quickly, so he began packing up to visit Calcutta again, with the knowledge that he would most likely head to Sikkim immediately afterward. Hedging his bets, however, Theos decided to also ask Viola to contact her friends at The Explorers Club for a letter of introduction to Suydam Cutting, the researcher from New York's Museum of Natural History recently approved for travel to Tibet.

Although she remained supportive of Theos's studies in India, over the months since her return, it seemed to Viola that he continued to place extra demands on her time irrespective of her obligations in her pediatric internship—something Theos rather insensitively called "baby business . . . one of those necessary evils in order that man can remain on the globe." Because of statements like that, at times it seemed that Theos was actively trying to enrage her. To make matters worse for Viola, by then beginning preparatory work for her psychiatric internship, Theos kept hinting that he was having experiences beyond the normal range of most— semireligious experiences that were the result of delving deep into his own mind.

In this little adventure of mine into the hidden corners of my unconscious I have uncovered a few things that I would not trade for all the power and money on earth, and if I can but continue furthering deeper and deeper into those almost unfathomable depths my passing is sure to be a happy expression of this cycle of living.

Just as disturbing for Viola, Theos was also beginning to have what he saw as broad insights into the problems confronting human civilization, which he unhesitatingly shared with her as well.

There is no difficulty in being able to see why our constant buzz of this jittery night life, etc. is an essential part of the present civilization. It is not that the machine is wrong; it is because man is shot to hell—If we changed the character of man all of this other turmoil and unrest would disappear—so would even war vanish—but such is not the case—for now we have the machinery and the vicious circle is at play. I know that you think that I am going mad, but after [all] the actions believed by almost a billion people cannot be laughed at lightly. You always wanted to come forth and know the message of our ideal man—true enough say all works of man—there do exist those who live in that rich world of their inner conscious and there is where we must go to find true solace.

To Viola, these were more than just academic speculations in his graduate work, they were clearly ideas that he was taking on a personal level—far more than ever before—all of which she found more than a little disconcerting. Worried, Viola expressed her concerns to Theos, subtly suggesting that she thought it best for him to "have someone around" while he was away from home for so long. Initially interpreting her comments as nothing more than loneliness, Theos reassured her that he felt the same way, and reminded her how much he was relying on her for emotional support. "If I really felt that you were not with me in feeling on this adventure of mine," he told her, "I could not carry on as I am so far away, yet way down deep in the heart, the little man tells me that he and your little man know exactly what we are doing and how much we are as one in our conscious feeling . . . for you and I are really as one even when you say that you are skeptical about what is supposed to be the true workings of this part of the world on that unfathomable problem of being." Not to take such things too seriously, he reminded Viola, these ramblings were just his way of telling her "I love you and am mighty glad of it." Even when she made her concerns more explicit, Theos dismissed them, reassuring her that "what may be happening to my consciousness during my stay in these parts" was only producing "a richer feeling for living" that would make him love her more and more. When she pressed him for "details," however, Theos finally responded,

It is impossible for me to go into the details of these "unconscious adventures" which I have been referring to, for it takes a certain time and mode; so you will have to wait until I have returned from Tibet when I will be settled again and at the job of trying to climb onto one of the dips which are more or less analogous to a rubber ball striking the floor no sooner than it hits, it is up again, and your job is to learn to hit and not return; so the big job first is that of changing the regular function of the system—and it is towards this end that the various Yogic exercises come into play once the body has been thoroughly cleansed. I must say that it is one of life's richer experiences to hit bottom once even though it is impossible for you to remain—you at least return knowing that there is something rich deep within you which you have never tasted before and to which there seems to be no external substitute. . . .

After the first stage of development has been reached in the hot house of external activity, and little more internal cultivating can be carried out after which another rest period must follow for those seeds to develop and so on is the process. . . . Here is where the next life comes into play—the individual will never be able to carry on his work of this life, but the Chit will continue in its path of development. However we do not have to talk about any metaphysical speculation, for there is more than enough right here in the material to hold the imagination of anyone and prove to them that there is a way to gain control of these finer forces. I am so anxious for the day to come when we can be continually together, and have endless hours on our hands during which we can live to a fixed discipline of hard work and thereby both have these experiences together, for never until you have tasted of such will you ever have any faith in my doings.

Although Viola promised that she would try "one of these days to get under a bush and let the tides of consciousness rise and fall," still Theos's attempt to attain a permanent alteration in his consciousness gave her much to think and worry about. Having promised not to disturb him with her concerns, she wrote at length about them to their mutual friend, Ashbel Welch, instead.

Despite what Viola may have thought, to Theos, his ideas seemed perfectly sane and rational. He could see what true madness was—the materialism of the world—and it was most irritating to him. "There is nothing that becomes more maddening to me," he told Viola, "than these people who live wholly [sic] on this material plane, and from such a group I have just returned." While he had admired Chapman's films in Calcutta—"several thousand feet of colored Tibetan pictures which were wonderful"—and while he liked Chapman on a personal level, Tibet, in Theos's opinion, had slightly unhinged the man.[83] Chapman was, Theos felt, a "youngster of about 30 . . . he doesn't know where he is or where he is going or why."[84] Nonetheless, Theos was confident that he could "be friendly with all sorts and conditions of men and they are never the wiser about me, so we have got along wonderfully and thus still learning more about new conditions of the human beast." Chapman as well seemed to take a liking to Theos, and later even invited him to return to Tibet with him in a few months as part of his expedition to climb Chumolhari, whose peak approached 26,000 feet. Although Theos declined, citing his wife's concern for his health, his time spent with Chapman in Calcutta was very productive and led to his meeting not only a close friend of Suydam Cutting but also another resident of Kalimpong, Raja Dorje, and his brother, the King of Sikkim. Hurriedly returning to Kalimpong from Calcutta, Theos prepared to head straight to Darjeeling to meet with Gould, who was coming down from Gangtok. At the last minute, however, Gould's trip was postponed, leaving Theos in Kalimpong to resume his studies.

Informing Viola that he was trying to maintain modest goals for his studies and subsequent work, Theos reassured her that he had no delusions about what he thought he could accomplish.

I have secured some manuscripts which give the lives of Padma Sambhava, Tilopa, Naropa, Marpa, Mila, and his 100,000 songs. It is my aim to have the life of Padma Sambhava translated before I leave here, and also to have made a start on the others. . . . All I want to be able to do here with them is to paint a picture so that others can see the relationship and what each added to the line of thought, leaving it to future students to sound the depths of what lies here. One going into such a field for the first time can hardly be expected to do more than organize the material. I know that my greatest difficulty has been in finding out what existed and what was worthwhile; so with this as a start, others will be able to strike to the heart of things much more quickly.

With the biography of Padmasambhava already "in the process of being translated,"[85] Theos laid out his approach to the materials before him systematically. First he would work through the Abhidharma treatises—which had already received some treatment by the Pali Text Society—and from there, he would engage in a study and translation of materials related to the "Wheel of Life" (srid pa'i 'khor lo), followed by an exhaustive study of the collected tantric works associated with Padmasambhava.

One of the problems Theos faced was the sorry state of scholarship in the English language. "I have read eight books since coming up here ... all on Buddhism," he told Viola, but they were far from useful, as "these authors in most instances are not so well informed ... they seem to think that there is hardly anything here but a lot of ignorant inspiration." But from reading and studying the primary source materials himself, he exclaimed, "my mind is constantly filled with the things that I really get a real thrill out of [and] never in my life have I ever lived in such a perpetual orgy of inner happiness."

Nonetheless, Theos tried to remain focused on his main task—learning the Tibetan language. Even with a vocabulary of slightly more than a thousand memorized words, listening and speaking were difficult for him. In addition to his classes with Tharchin, he was lucky enough to be able to spend time with Geshe Wangyal. "He can speak a little English," Theos wrote to Viola, "but is anxious to improve it and since I want to become fluent in Tibetan there is no reason why we should not be talking." For Theos, talking with Geshe Wangyal was an enjoyable distraction—if not also a challenge, as the geshe forced him to drink cup after cup of tea—even if the subject of tantra was not open for discussion.

> He is a very quiet and modest sort of chap and we have some fine chats at odd intervals, for we see each other several times a week ... from him I am able to get an excellent line up on the literature which exists in the country. As far as knowledge on the subject of my interest he is of little value, for they do not allow them to begin the study of the Tantras until they have finished their geshe, and he having just secured this recently—a

few years ago—he has not had the time to go any further, for he has been too much on the move since that time. A couple of times to China, twice back to Lhasa and a long trip all over Mongolia and Inner Mongolia outlines his peregrinations; so you can see that he is familiar with Asia. He possesses a wonderful sense of humor so I am constantly at him for being such a sophisticated monk or rather Lama, for he has that title. . . . Really, I have a lot of fun out of him.

All in all, their talks were of benefit to Theos on many levels—from the information Geshe Wangyal could impart to his simple encouragement.

He is most tolerant with my broken speech, but always tries to encourage my attempts which I am a bit hesitant to use with him. With the bearers, traders, etc. I do not mind spitting out broken sentences, but with these fellows I seem to feel that I should say nothing unless I can say it perfectly which is never the case. . . . I am at least getting my vocabulary large enough that I can grasp what others are talking about which is something and if he keeps on giving me encouragement I may be able to answer them in the course of time.

Throughout that time, Theos's study of Tibetan seemed an unending series of complications, with grammar and spelling rules compounding one after another. He persisted in trying to read the biography of Padmasambhava with Tharchin and "every time that I am able to recognize a word," he told Viola, "I jump with more glee than a five-year old with an ice cream cone." Still, he realized that at some point he was going to have to "bring my teacher home with me so that I can continue my study of the language and translating . . . for it is obvious that one cannot learn to read a language of this nature fluently with only one year's study."

But far from just an extravagance for his own benefit, Theos was planning on a much grander scale. He had the idea, he told Viola, "of someday having an institution or what have you of my own where I can personally guide and try to inspire all the research that I would like to see done in the world on this subject that seems to hold an undying interest for me." Theos assured Viola that there would be a role for her to play in the institute as well. For, having studied ayurvedic medicine at length, Theos thought the next step would be running clinical trials in the United States to validate ayurvedic principles, with "large clinics and hundreds of patients and endless clerks to keep the necessary records." As soon as Viola finished her medical internships, Theos informed her, she would be in the perfect position to spearhead such a research project. "There is a great deal that awaits you," he told her, "and no one but you can do it and it must be done, for the ideas must be added to our present culture."

Theos let Viola know that he was pushing himself on the physical side of things as well, and by the beginning of April, having continued with his yoga practice, he had gotten to the point were he could perform his controlled breathing techniques (*kumbhaka*) for up to six minutes. While proud of his accomplishment, he knew he had a long way to go, remarking that a yogi in Kalimpong he had met could maintain *his* control for up to two hours. He lamented that "its technique he does not know how to convey to another, because of his lack of knowledge on the laws involved," despite long talks and practice sessions together.

By early April, preparations were well under way for his journey to Gyantse with Tharchin, including the purchase of a second camera. Still weighing on his mind was the fact that he still did not have the all-important permission letter from Gould despite having set May 15 as his target date for departure. Continually reassured by his friends, Theos felt confident that it would come since "several friends in these parts have extended themselves in writing to him and talking with him personally," including David Macdonald and the Raja of Bhutan.

While Theos bided his time waiting for an opportunity to meet Gould, as luck would have it, he again met Tsarong Lhacham, the wife of Lord Tsarong, this time at a long Tibetan afternoon meal hosted by the Macdonalds—along with Rai Bahadur Norbu Dhondup, his wife, Frank Perry, and the Macdonald daughters. Although they had met a couple of months earlier, this time Theos was able to make a somewhat better impression. At David Macdonald's suggestion, he had letters of petition written and addressed to the four cabinet ministers, the Regent, and the prime minister of Tibet, seeking permission to visit Lhasa. When Theos and David Macdonald arrived at Tsarong Lhacham's home to present the letters and gifts for delivery to the officials, she gave them a tour of the family home. While showing her guests the family shrine room, she unwrapped one of the Tibetan books on the altar, and to her amazement, Theos managed to read the title out loud. Having never met a Westerner who could read Tibetan, much less scriptural Tibetan, she was duly impressed by his admittedly "blundering attempts" and promised to do what she could for him. But unless he could meet Sir Basil Gould, the British representative in Gangtok, no amount of assistance from her would help, for Gould was the only man who could guarantee his entry into Tibet, and without him, Theos was lost.

Still, Theos couldn't let mundane concerns slow him down. Having fixed on a plan for his return, he began to envision different ways of promoting himself and his newfound knowledge. Being "anxious to set up my own monastery in N.Y.," he speculated on the possibility of overseeing the construction of one at the 1939 World's Fair, scheduled to take place in Flushing Meadows, overlooking Manhattan. Another possibility, he thought, was to use his recent acquisition of the Lhasa Kangyur for advertising, if he could get a photo article published in *Fortune* through their contacts. That way, he theorized, the books could "be advertised some way so that scholars and interested students will know where there is such a set and it will in turn help me get in contact with people who are interested in this field of research." This was the "first essential," Theos thought, in order "to give this material all the publicity that we possibly can, for the purpose of stimulating a strong creative interest in the field and thereby get students interested so that this work can be carried on for all time." To that end, Theos suggested that Viola show some of their earlier photos to their friends in the publishing industry and inform them that he would endeavor to take more. Even a Tibetan curio shop—possibly run by DeVries—was not out of the question, and he put all of this forth to Viola for her opinion.

Among some of his other concerns during this time, however, was the fact that since he had sent most of his extraneous belongings home with his father, the clothes Theos had were beginning to wear thin. Rather than simply being able to purchase clothes, Theos discovered, due to "some more of this dam oriental servitude, or rather Artificial English Importance," he would have to have them handmade. Consequently, in addition to having a pair of jodhpur pants and coat made by a regimental tailor, Theos decided to have complete sets of Tibetan-style clothes made for himself and Viola and set off to Darjeeling to commission them, taking the opportunity to drop in on some of his friends there.

Visiting Jinorasa, Theos met another one of his brothers, Rhenock Kazi, and together they discussed and explained to Theos several new viewpoints on Buddhism that he had not understood. "So you see," he told Viola, "I am far from being set" in this knowledge. Most useful, however, was his good fortune in being able to buy a copy of the rare out-of-print Tibetan dictionary by Sarat Chandra Das in Darjeeling for Rs. 10, compared with the Rs. 100 being asked for it in Calcutta. With Jinorasa's help, Theos was able to get a pass for Sikkim so that he could visit Gould in Gangtok, with "no trouble since they more or less knew me—I simply went to the office, had a nice chat about the inspiration of the century and walked away with the pass—no police enquiry or anything." Flushed with success, Theos returned to Kalimpong to wait for the right moment to make his petition to Gould, while accolades and offers of assistance continued to pour in. Even the Raja of Bhutan promised to speak to Gould on Theos's behalf after they played tennis together.

In the meantime, Theos continued to make his plans for the future, hoping to fulfill his "present ambition" of writing "an index to the Kangyur and Tengyur." Moreover, he explained to Viola that there was a man in Kalimpong who could play an important role in this undertaking. After several months of interactions at Tharchin's house, Gedun Chöpel began to truly live up to his reputation in Theos's eyes. "Do you recall the Lama that you met at Jinorasa's?" he asked Viola.

> Recall what a high reputation he held—well during these past months I have been finding that he can well live up to it, and it is my desire to eventually have him come to the States and perhaps my present teacher [Tharchin] and the three of us will settle down to a real constructive undertaking. I want him particularly for the Tantric aspects of these books, for he is so well versed in all of the esoteric meanings and it is more or less necessary to have one so trained, while anyone knowing the language could carry on the other job.

And so Theos spelled out his plan "as a definite proposal," asking Viola what she thought. It was, Theos felt, an absolute necessity to have someone like Gedun Chöpel by his side in America to work on this material, for although he had just completed working through two Tibetan grammars with Tharchin, his skills at reading literary Tibetan remained effectively nonexistent. He felt he could "read the stuff off in Tibetan as I can English," having memorized close to two thousand words, yet "the literary is too classical to be able to do anything with." So he resigned himself to spending the remainder of his time in the months to come focusing on colloquial Tibetan.

Viola, however, was deeply enmeshed in the obligations of her internship, her mother's ongoing health concerns, and managing the New York apartments. Unlike Theos, she was "in an impossible rhythm for planning, meditating, reflecting," while Theos was in an ideal one for engaging in endless "pipe dreams" that Viola could not consider "because of the pre-occupation with things of the moment." As a result, she was simply left wondering where her husband's inspiration was leading. While Theos awaited Viola's response to his questions and proposals, after months of antici-pation, he finally received word from Gould. Rather than having ignored Theos's letters and the appeals of several friends, it seemed that Gould had simply been delaying a meeting until he visited Kalimpong. Chapman, hav-ing arrived at the Himalayan Hotel to pay Theos a visit, conveyed word that Gould would be arriving the next morning. While fairly confident that the meeting would go well, Theos remained slightly apprehensive: "one never knows just how he stands because of all the petty intrigues and jealousies in this scatter brain corner of the disconnected British Empire."

Finally the next morning came, and meeting Gould for the first time, Theos succeeded in making a good impression; he and Gould "hit it off like a couple of old lovers after a twenty years absence." Gould had been hearing about Theos for some time now, and luckily for Theos, when they approached each other it was much less awkward than it could have been. The delay in meeting Gould had worked in Theos's favor, for as the weeks and months passed since he'd become a figure of public fascination, the stories of his abilities had grown as well. By the time they finally met, Gould believed Theos to be little short of a savant who had mastered Ti-betan and Indian philosophy in a superhuman fashion. Gould went so far as to defer to Theos's better knowledge, asking him to review his own work on the Tibetan language, the *Tibetan Word Book*,[86] that he was preparing for publication. Graciously, Theos agreed to come to Gangtok early and look over the manuscript. Downplaying his own abilities, and in a show of proper colonial etiquette, Gould offered Theos his assistance in helping him reach Tibet.

When Theos told of his desire to visit Gyantse, Gould suggested that he write a formal request, upon receipt of which he would send his official recommendation to the Indian authorities on Theos's behalf. But Theos had been told what to expect from Gould, and without a moment's hesi-tation, produced precisely such a letter from his pocket. With the sort of smile that a father gives an impetuous young son, Gould accepted the let-ter and composed a cablegram on the spot for Theos to wire down to Cal-cutta immediately. Theos had succeeded. That was the final piece of the puzzle, and with it in place, he was ready to leave. Gould cautioned him that his influence could only get him as far as the trading post in Gyantse— and then only for a six-week stay; to proceed any farther into Tibet, Theos would be on his own. Hurrying home after sending off Gould's wire, Theos tracked down Frank Perry, who began helping him acquire the clothing and gear he would need for the trip north. Overjoyed, he bragged to Viola about how he had succeeded where others had failed. Just last spring, he told her, "there was this chap from England studying Buddhism and who can speak the Tibetan language and he was refused permission to enter the interior, but I must confess that none of them use their heads."

But Theos had to struggle to keep his own arrogance in check. Even as Gould was helping him achieve his goals, while claiming to like the man personally, Theos resented every moment of dependence upon him. "Gould," he wrote, "is a man of about fifty five and stands a little over six feet of which every inch is ego and he feels very proud of the fact that he has the only existing colored pictures in the world of the country." Not be outdone, Theos bragged to Viola, "I have several thousand feet of such film and hope to produce a much better job than they did; I know when to let the other fellow have the show, mine will come when they have all died off."

But Theos's ambitions went far beyond simple adventure documenta-tion. "The so-called pillars of the 'United Kingdom,'" he felt, were blind to the enormous opportunities before them. "As the old saying is, the bigger they are the harder the fall, one might add that the bigger they are the deader they are, and a blind man could feel it," he told his wife.

The tragedy that seemed to be causing all the trouble was the fact that here, in one of the most beautiful spots in the world with the stimulation of centuries of thought, all that people seemed to be concerned with was the name and form of society which has eked its way into every notch of the social world. However, it is my feeling that I came out of the battle with a deeper understanding of the human personality and its apparent unintelligible purpose in this life.

Even for the other would-be students around him, Theos had nothing but disdain. "I am to be the first American Student of Tibetan Buddhism to visit Gyantse," he told Viola, but only because he had used his head. His British and American competitors—"glorified Himalayan heroes" he called them—were nothing but "a bunch of wash outs."

All delusions of grandeur aside, Theos was painfully aware of his actual abilities, at least on a linguistic level. For the past three months, he had been studying hard. He had managed to find dictionaries and texts, he had employed Tharchin Babu as his Tibetan teacher and routinely visited Geshe Wangyal and Gedun Chöpel, and consequently had made considerable progress. But it fell far short of what he would need in Tibet; he knew he would need a guide and translator—and if nothing else, someone to handle the finances and negotiate expenses with the locals en route.

It required little effort to convince Tharchin to take a leave of absence from his job at the Missionary Press in Kalimpong, for there was little love lost between Tharchin and the missionary Knox, who (when not trying to fire him) kept him working at a bare subsistence wage. It was better than no job at all, but Theos offered him a substantial salary for two months' work. So, obtaining assurances from his employers and a leave of absence (for only one month), Tharchin had already begun to pack his bags and prepare to lead Theos into Tibet.

Theos's only concern at this point was his age. Though perfectly acceptable as a scholar in America, Theos knew that as a young man in his late twenties, he was far too young to be given the sort of esoteric teachings he was seeking in Tibet. In the monasteries of Tibet, years of study and dozens of exams would have to be passed, putting a student well into their forties before they could request a teacher to bestow the tantric teachings. But Theos had neither the time nor the patience for such things. So in an attempt to *look* older, he decided to grow a beard. It would help hide his age, he told Viola, since "they all seem to think that only an old man should be doing this sort of thing." Hoping he could "pass off another ten years onto the beard," he sent her a picture of himself, promising he would shave it off before they saw each other again.

The logistical details, although foremost in importance, were least in Theos's regard. All of that had been left to the staff of the Himalayan Hotel, for David Macdonald himself actively promoted the hotel for just such activities in his guide, *Touring in Sikkim and Tibet*, published only a few years earlier:

> For most of the tours Kalimpong affords the most suitable starting point.
> In this town, transport, servants, stores, and all to do with touring, may
> be arranged much cheaper than in Darjeeling, and most important of

all, mules can be readily obtained for the carriage of kit. They are more satisfactory than coolies or ponies.

The Himalayan Hotel, in Kalimpong, caters especially for tourists in the hills and in Tibet, and the Proprietors, who have lived for years in Tibet and the Darjeeling District, can advise intending travelers, on receipt of enquiry, from their own experience.

They can give letters of introduction to Sikkimese and Tibetan notables and officials and prominent people, and thus afford visitors experiences which would otherwise be missed. They will make all arrangements for either short or long tours, with or without guides and interpreters. All the intending tourist need do is to take his ticket to Siliguri and the Himalayan Hotel will do the rest.[87]

Macdonald was still true to his word, and even as for weeks now, Theos, Tharchin, and their friends had been making their own plans and strategies for their absence, the staff of the Himalayan Hotel, under Frank Perry's observation, had been engaged in their own busy activities on their behalf. Theos was even able to purchase another 16-mm film camera, a Contax, one of the dozen or so brought back by the British Mission from Lhasa, which he decided to keep permanently stocked with color film.

But perfected logistics alone would not enable Theos to accomplish his goals. Cunning and precise timing would be equally crucial. In a few days, the wife of Lord Tsarong would be returning to Lhasa; having purchased a number of gifts of different quality and quantity for different Tibetan governmental officials, each "in accordance with his position above the others"—as McGovern had deftly noted was necessary—Theos was sending them on ahead to arrive shortly after Tsarong Lhacham, along with an enlarged and framed portrait of her taken by Theos a few weeks earlier. To be successful, however, Theos knew that he would have to work every possible opportunity for its maximum potential. Tharchin was well on board with his agenda, as Theos had convinced him to write a series of short articles about "a sahib who is out from America studying their religion." A month before their departure, the first article appeared in Tharchin's newspaper:

An American Sahib named Mr. Bernard, having come to Kalimpong, has been studying the Tibetan literary language. He, himself, [has] great faith in the Insider's Doctrine [Buddhism], and with his preliminary exceptional study of Tibetan, has expressed his wish for a means of spreading the teachings of the Insider's Doctrine [Buddhism] in America. From the depths [of such aspiration, he] ransomed a Kangyur, [and] with this established foundation, once [he] has also acquired a Tengyur, he has indicated that he definitely plans on founding a large temple in America. This is the news in brief.[88]

It was a good start for the campaign that Theos was waging to reach Lhasa, establishing his motivations and aspirations. But not to let the Tibetan government's attention lapse, Tharchin published another article in the very next issue, in the form of a sincere appeal for assistance.

We have received a request for advice for the next nine weeks. On this 3rd day of the 4th Tibetan month, having crossed the earth and the waters, the American Sahib named "Bernard" would like to ascertain if it is possible to depart northward to Tibet and if so, makes a formal request for any account of expenses and individual offerings per month for the duration of the fifth and sixth months, and makes a formal request to the newspaper readership, to anyone with a better knowledge of the costs, who has previously done so and is residing here.[89]

Having been granted permission to proceed into Tibet, Theos was quite self-conscious of the fact that he would be "the first American Student of Tibetan Buddhism that has ever been granted permission to visit Gyantse." To surpass this would require him to strategize at every turn and utilize every advantage.

A few days after his meeting with Gould, Theos had visited relatives in Kalimpong of yet another aristocratic family, the Pangdatsangs.[90] They would be valuable contacts in the wool trade, and getting to know them was part of Theos's larger plan to make as many friends within the aristocracy as best he could, to "get down to the true consciousness of the people . . . for it is a general rule that a traveler brings you back a study of the peasants and beggars of a country which is always a bad impression."

It was early one morning as he stepped outside the cottage barracks at the Himalayan Hotel, a room that had been his home for many months, that Theos looked to the north as he often did, and finally glimpsed in that morning light the first pass into Tibet. As the clouds cleared over Nathu-la

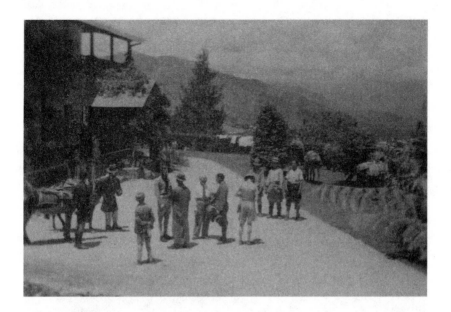

Figure 7.2 Preparing to leave for Tibet in front of the Himalayan Hotel (PAHM)

in the distance, he could see the blanket of snow left in the wake of a recent storm; at 16,000 feet, it would be a cold crossing. But the day had finally arrived and now as the full force of the journey that lay ahead sank in, he knew that his efforts of the preceding weeks and months had finally come to fruition. This would be the culmination of his "having spent the most of this short span of life in awakening the consciousness necessary to be able to encompass what is concealed deep within all name and form of this 'Penthouse of the Gods.'"[91]

But scarcely awake more than an hour, Theos could hear men rustling about outside, crating last-minute items and labeling the last of his boxes filled with 20,000 feet of 16-mm motion picture film and 180 rolls of 35-mm still film. Echoing over it all was the sound of Frank Perry's voice instructing the various coolies and tinwallas in their activities and overseeing the entire operation as he had done for many days. With a knock on his barracks door, Theos knew that Frank was summoning him for the final departure. Gathering himself together, Theos joined the crowd assembling on the lawn in front of the Himalayan Hotel, with Frank even taking possession of two of Theos's cameras to record the entire event both in still photographs and on film.

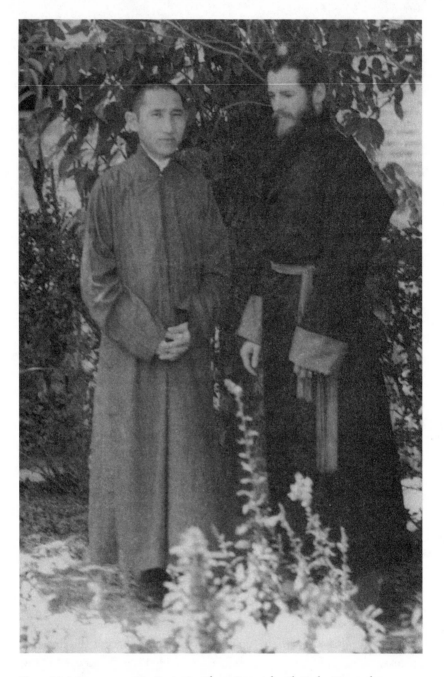

Figure 7.3 A Commemorative Portrait—Theos Bernard with Geshe Wangyal

A cheery crowd of well-wishers had gathered at the hotel that morning to see Theos and Tharchin safely on their way. At the head of everything was David Macdonald, Theos's host and advisor during those many months who, along with his son-in-law Frank Perry, had truly made the entire trip possible. The Macdonald daughters and the staff of the hotel had turned out as well to pay their respects to their long-term guest. Even Geshe Wangyal had come down to the hotel to bid Theos his fondest wishes, despite preparing to leave himself for London the very next day. After compliments were paid all around and he sent off two separate mule caravans—one to Gangtok, which would accompany them, and one to Phari, with provisions for his stay in Tibet—Theos stepped into his waiting car to make the first leg of his journey, leaving Tharchin behind to oversee the mules. As the car pulled out of the compound, Frank Perry ran alongside, giving him one last "running handshake" of support before the car sped off, taking Theos down the dusty road ahead.

EIGHT

Tibet, Tantrikas, and the
Hero of Chaksam Ferry

If one could but come here and stay for months on end, photographing
these treasures of divine conception, and noting down their esoteric aspect, the world of literature would be the richer. Perhaps by this contact
and acceptance into their faith as one of their own, I am laying the foundation for the work myself. I know that it is beyond the province of my
present undertakings, but having once gained this foothold such fruit may
follow, for only one of their flock would ever be allowed to enter these
reverend chambers; so I will continue to build the foundation.

—THEOS BERNARD[1]

"DON'T THINK PROUDLY, 'I am going to Tibet,'" a Mongolian monk once
told the young Ngawang Wangyal. Instead, he advised him, "remember,
even camels go to Tibet!"[2] Although Theos made no mention of any parting
words he received from his teacher that May morning on the grassy lawn
in front of the Himalayan Hotel, passing on such gems of wisdom would
not have been out of character for Geshe Wangyal. But irrespective of any
advice he may have received, compared to the flurry of activity that surrounded his departure from the hotel, the solitude and quiet of his lone car
ride to Gangtok was both calming and disconcerting. For weeks now he had
been filled with excitement and the "spirit of adventure," but the thought
of what unknown events still lay ahead filled Theos with a certain degree
of trepidation that he had no choice but to suppress.

As his days that followed in Gangtok were mostly spent waiting for Tharchin and the pack mules to arrive, rather than sitting around idly, Theos
took the opportunity to spend time with Sir Basil Gould, from horseback

riding in the mornings to fulfilling his promise to "look over" Gould's Tibetan grammar and *Word Book*,[3] while politely trying to obtain as much information as possible about his journey ahead. The epitome of British gentility, Gould allowed Theos to review the British Mission "Diaries" for the previous few years as well as all of their photographs and films, ostensibly to recommend material to Gould for publication. Although Chapman and other members of the British Mission had produced "hundreds upon hundreds of pictures portraying all of the physical realities of Hidden Tibet," nowhere did Theos see an image that conveyed any feeling or emotion; instead, he felt, "all they have done is to compile several albums of mental photography."

Although he had hoped to engage him in a philosophical discussion, to his disappointment, Theos discovered that Gould was of the typical British disposition concerning Tibet, Buddhism, and tantra, convinced that the latter was "more or less the undermining influence in all of Buddhism, being nothing more or less than some degenerate form of practice that came from 'nowhere.'" Talking late into the night, Theos did his best to convince him that "there may be something else behind those more or less debased forms that the outsider always observes," but what Gould thought or was "convinced" of after these conversations remains questionable.[4]

Determined to record every aspect of his adventure—with a certain self-awareness of his future readership, including his wife[5]—Theos forced himself to sit down at his typewriter every night to set down his daily account of events. For Theos, it was the ideal way to practice his writing and craft an informative, yet entertaining story that was philosophically reflective while incorporating knowledge from the books he had read to date. These diaries, he wrote to Viola, would form the basis for a lecture tour that he could give around the country after his return.

Still worried about permission to visit Lhasa, Theos remained convinced that a good fall-back plan would be to ingratiate himself with Suydam Cutting and casually suggest that he accompany him to Lhasa, and so began crafting a long, friendly letter to Cutting about their common interests and mutual friends. Before he could send it off, however, Theos received word from Viola that their mutual friend, Ashbel Welch, had already—and quite bluntly—informed Cutting of Theos's wish to accompany him to Lhasa, and the idea had been immediately rejected. Although she was upset at having "balled up the works" for her husband, Theos assured her that such secondary communications were easily reparable, reminding her that he could "handle most any situation and accomplish the majority of my designs if I can but have a personal interview."

After two days, Tharchin arrived in Gangtok, bringing word that there was already talk in Tibetan circles about Theos from the articles in *The Mirror*. Encouraged by this news, Theos rose early the next morning, but little sleep and a rough breakfast proved too much for his queasy stomach, and having vomited his breakfast almost as soon as it was eaten, he had no choice but to face the day of his departure in a less than satisfactory state. Heading down the hill as the morning light began edging its way through the valleys, burning off the night's mists, Theos and Tharchin with their syces, Norphel and Hla-re, set off toward the mountain passes.

Informed that the Sikkimese dak bungalow at Karponang that should have been their first stop was occupied, Theos, Tharchin, and their eighteen-mule caravan would have to do double duty the first day, traveling twenty-three miles—all uphill—to reach the second station, the dak bungalow at Changu. By midday they had reached Karponang, and after a brief rest pressed on with the mule caravan well ahead of them on the trail already. But the rains in Gangtok the day before had turned to hail and snow at the higher elevations and began to fall upon them as they climbed toward Changu. Still feeling the effects of his bad breakfast, Theos slipped into a painful half-sleep on the back of his pony as his syce led him up the mountain.

Despite the torrential downpour and the cold, there were moments for Theos as he drifted in and out of consciousness that lent the first leg of that journey a dreamlike quality. As they trudged directly into the clouds that had been raining down on them below, different images confronted him each time he opened his eyes. At one moment, Theos and his pony would be shrouded in mist, soaking the skin and forming droplets trickling off every surface, yet seemingly timeless moments later, when he opened his eyes, a gap in the clouds would reveal vast fields of blooming rhododendron trees towering overhead and tiny mountain flowers just barely jutting out of the otherwise seamless white snow. At other times, the trail wound around narrow cliff edges passing over streams and underneath roaring waterfalls, whose spray made the rain showers seem gentle and tepid by comparison. When the small party of wet travelers finally crossed the last ridge of the day, the sight before them struck Theos as the most beautiful he could have seen—a lake of pure crystal mountain water nestled high between mountain peaks, with the Changu dak bungalow at the far shore. All Theos could do was marvel at the sight—before stumbling off his pony to fall to his knees, dry heaving into the snow.

Awaking the next morning to the sound of Tharchin and the boys fixing breakfast, having lost twenty-five pounds since arriving in India, Theos could feel the cold mountain air bite deep into his skin even underneath his thick sheepskin cloak. A heavy snow had fallen during the night, and the clouds racing up the gorge toward the summits of the mountains ahead did not bode well for the coming day's weather. Although their next destination, Chumi-tang, lay only ten miles away, the snow and sleet had reduced the trail to the Nathu-la Pass[6] to a crustless mass of snow over a bed of mud. For close to four hours, the small caravan inched forward as the men spent more time picking up fallen mules and horses than actually walking. When they reached the pass, barren of all signs of life save the evidence of past travelers, all the men stopped to add small stones to the piles scattered among the prayer flags, paying their individual respects to the local mountain gods who had allowed them to live thus far and tread through their domain. As they descended the last two thousand feet from the pass, the landscape opened up once more to reveal vast forests of fir and rhododendrons cut through by tiny gorges of ice-filled streams.

Rising at four the next morning, the party left the bungalow early enough to have time to visit the Kagyu Monastery at Dro-mo,[7] sending one of their three coolies on ahead to the monastery to alert them to their approach. By the time Theos and Tharchin arrived at the Kagyu Gom-pa,[8] Theos's only meal in the previous thirty-six hours, a bowl of tomato soup cut with yak's milk,[9] had left him weak and dehydrated, and with a perceptible feeling of altitude sickness, he was not in the best shape. Nonetheless, hospitalities given required graciousness to be reciprocated, and after a cup of butter tea, a brief tour of the monastery, and the opportunity to offer a *khata*, a silk scarf,[10] before the central forty-foot-tall statue of Maitreya, Theos was led upstairs for an audience with the abbot, a Kagyu yogi reputed to be seventy-five years old, with an impressive topknot of matted hair. But mere moments after offering his *khata* to the abbot, illness, exertion, and possibly the tea caught up to Theos and he ran for the door, followed quickly by a young monk who held a small bowl under his chin. His stomach purged, Theos returned to the audience chamber; lying exhausted on cushions on the floor, he was allowed to put questions to the abbot—who, having read Tharchin's article in *The Mirror*, knew of his guest's professed Buddhist faith and offered answers via Tharchin as translator. From the abbot Theos learned more about the Nyingma tantras, the life and teachings of Padmasambhava, and the practice lineage of the Kagyu school stemming from Nāropa and Tilopa, through Marpa and Milarepa. Informing the lama that he had acquired a set of the Kangyur, the abbot informed him that these only represented the "later transmission" tantras, and suggested that if he was really interested in the Nyingma lineage he would need a set of the sixty-four-volume Nyingma "Gyu-bum,"[11] or collected tantras, and would want to consult Long-chen-pa's condensation of it into seven volumes.[12]

Proceeding to Yatung proper, the group decided to rest for two days and obtain fresh pack animals while Tharchin visited friends and Theos got caught up on his diary and letter writing. With a fresh pack of twelve mules, they headed for their next destination, Gautse, halfway between Yatung and Phari. Throughout the morning the going was slow, as their party encountered numerous oncoming pack trains loaded down with wool, attempting to negotiate the same narrow trails. On their ascent out of the cliff-hemmed Chumbi Valley, the view behind them was of early spring grass, dotted with the tents of nomads and yaks grazing; by the end of the summer, Tharchin told Theos somewhat nostalgically, "the grass is several feet high and reminds one of a quiet lake when the wind blows." As the day went on, one of the residences of the eighth-century Indian siddha Padmasambhava, Dung-kar Monastery,[13] slowly came into view in the distance. The abbot, the same famous "Geshe Rinpoche"[14] about whom Theos, Viola, and Glen had heard from Jinorasa, was still being mourned, and consequently the monastery was not open to casual visitors and tourists. Apprised that Theos was no British tourist but rather an American Buddhist on pilgrimage, the monks welcomed him but still forbade him to take any photographs.

For Theos, this small monastery—the southernmost in the Geluk lineage—was the most beautiful he had yet seen, and he could only speculate that if this increase in beauty continued the farther he proceeded into Tibet, it would be "beyond the powers of [his] imagination to visualize what [he would] see in Gyantse." As he toured the monastery, Theos was saddened by the death of the geshe, the architect of the monastery temple, because "one with enough feeling to have constructed [the temple] must know a little about the external forms of these things which are so arranged," but thought that "the grandeur of his work says that he held a greater religious feeling than religious understanding." For Theos, these two capacities—knowledge and artistic sense—seemed necessarily separate, despite the fact that from the monastery grounds the abbot's meditation retreat "many, many thousands of feet above . . . on the ridge of the opposite canyon wall" was clearly seen.

Dung-kar Monastery proved very inspirational for Theos, as the rich, vivid colors of the new murals and statues sparked ruminations on the nature of color, image, and religious affection. But Theos's speculations were interrupted when, having finished the general tour of the monastery's temples, he and Tharchin were informed that monastery's oracle was preparing for a trance and if they wished, they could stay for the event. Having spent several months reading various accounts of Tibetan customs and culture, as well as Buddhist philosophy, Theos decided to take advantage of the opportunity. As the ceremony commenced and the monk began to enter into communion with the spirit of the oracle, however, it was far more than Theos had expected.

We witnessed the entire performances of him entering the separate shrine where the spirit is said to dwell and listen to the chants and clashing of cymbals that are supposed to prepare him for his state and drive the spirit into him and then all of a sudden he started talking at a frantic rate of speed and writers were getting everything down just as quickly as possible and all of a sudden he ups and collapses, one of the attendants grabbing him in his arm and let him fall back into his throne gradually. They were all very attentive and appeared to hold the same consideration as we do for one who has just relaxed from the exhaustion of having purge of the stomach.

While everything else up until this point had proven to be grist for Theos's speculations and insights, this event was nothing he was even remotely prepared for, and so having recounted the experience, he could only remark, "That's that."

After some more tea and sightseeing, Theos and Tharchin resumed their journey northward toward the dak bungalow at Gautse for the night. As a result of the day's events, they ended up staying awake late, discussing various aspects of religion. There could not have been a stranger conversation for two men to have had at that time and at that place—an American Hindu-Buddhist convert discussing religion with a Khunu Christian convert seated in a British rest stop in the southern reaches of Tibet. Theos tactfully avoided the obvious issue of his own low opinion of Christianity when talking with Tharchin, instead discussing the broader themes of the purpose of religion and the universality of man leading on to the inevitable conclusion of the superficiality of cultural forms.

From his study of Saṃkya philosophy, Theos believed that life could be thought of as a "continual moving force and that part of that energy has been bound up in this body." "The mere fact that we can alter so many reactions of human animals by the process of conditioning," he argued, "shows that it moves, and that through the process of repetition it becomes hooked up with various external forms of stimuli which help to either move it in one direction or another," giving rise to "the fundamental emotions of love and hate," which are nothing more than vocalized expressions, "a formalized sound which is the perfected external form of that inner manifestation which can be infinite, and so can our words be infinite, for this energy can take on an endless variety of subtle shades." Begrudgingly acknowledging some truth to Franz Boas's idea that "all men on earth are the same," Theos felt that it would be simple for him to learn all he needed to in Tibet, for "one could know the Tibetan as well as a Tibetan knows himself as soon as one becomes acquainted with a few of his names and form of external expression, for in the end all man is reduced to a few fundamentals, and the only difference between them is in their culture patterns." For Tharchin, however, such emotions were not superficial forms and for him the issue was one of comparative "doctrines"—the "doctrine of love" (as he characterized Christianity) and what he perceived as being in opposition to it, the "doctrines of Buddhism and Hinduism." But such a conversation could only remain unresolved, and more importantly for both men, should end amicably, for by two o'clock in the morning each was looking forward to sleep, especially with a scheduled wake-up a mere three hours later.

After rising early, if slowly, as they intended the next morning, they found the next day's journey relatively slow going at first. For the first eight miles out from Gautse the path ahead was little more than a trail of strewn boulders that offered little foothold for man or animal. But having broken through the gorge, they could see ahead the plain of Du-na,[15] little more than a barren series of hills with a thin brown carpet of scrub, with the occasional herd of grazing yaks. Far more impressive was the sight of Chomolhari, whose icy peak towered over the plain below "like a star

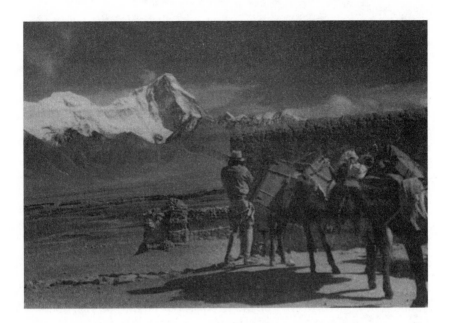

Figure 8.1 Bernard photographing Chomolhari (PAHM)

sapphire on the hand of a Hindu Goddess" all the way until they reached the dak bungalow at Phari. Having paid their respects to the Phari fort commander (Dzongpön) and sent off letters, telegrams, and several rolls of film to Calcutta for developing, they rested briefly and were off again the next day.

By now the quiet plodding of the small group across the south Tibetan plains had proved ample inspiration for Theos as he sat astride his pony bound for Gyantse. Anxious for the opportunity to photograph Chomolhari, Theos was disappointed to see the mountain that had appear so vividly the day before now shrouded by clouds. It was the anger of the local gods, the villagers told him, at the presence of the British mountain climbers. Theos knew well of Chapman's hope to climb Chomolhari, and indeed had planned on meeting up with him in Phari. As he had traveled toward Gyantse, Freddy Chapman and Charles Crawford, who had preceded him by many days, had been delayed by the weather; they were just then beginning their final ascent of the mountain's peak.[16] Theos admired their attempt, for if one "could but imagine Mt. Rainier rising 27,000 feet out of an Arizona desert [one could] get the feeling one has sitting on her lap at Phari about five miles from the base at which she goes straight up like a rocket." Indeed, Theos thought, "to have all the inspirational beauty of a barren windblown waste land surrounded by rolling, light brown mounds off to the distant snow covered horizon is quite enough to awaken the dormant awe in any lost and weary soul," and it sent him "into an emotional photographic orgy." As far as the people were concerned, for Theos, the similarities between the Native American communities he had visited two years earlier and the Tibetans he was now encountering was clear:

'Tis no wonder that the Tibetan never leaves his own country, and when he does his consciousness aches until his return, for nowhere can one find a more perfect physical awakening of his inner soul, for the rare atmosphere of the altitude soon begins to make the whole system breathe and by such subtle fanning the sleeping serpent of man's dormant self slowly begins to rise and its hissings are recorded by the heart. . . . When the essence of man is in continuous repertoire with the universal flow of life, he neglects to carry on the externals beyond the necessity of his existence. This may be attributed as one of the reasons why the American Indian failed for countless hundreds of years to make any material advancement. It is only when man is robbed of his consciousness by the intricacies of materialistic societies that he tries to compensate for the deficiency by the embankment of material complexities, never realizing what it is that is driving him and what he should be looking for.

This loss was the pathology that Theos saw as driving Euro-American culture as a whole. Rather than striving to reawaken that more primal religious sense, he felt that as "Westerners"

we battle on, generation after generation, trying to set up a system that will provide for that which man lost when society commenced to be an unsurmountable machine. It matters not in what way we are able to improve the external conditions of men, his purpose will never be fulfilled, for the effort is all in the wrong direction. Temporary relief may be the outcome, but the fester of dissatisfaction will only manifest itself in another channel. He who has spent his energy in the struggle will have passed through this short cycle with the least possible amount of discontentment, thanks to the ego of man, but those who follow will only be helped in that they have a more unwieldy machine to keep the increasing multitudes at work. The day will come when the whole thing

will collapse, for man is slowly weakening his own capacities, and therefore the future will no longer have the drive to continue the struggle.

Like it or not, he thought, "the West" would be forced to confront its own
inadequacies as a society and eventually return to a more natural, har-
monious religious state. But such progress would not happen of its own
accord: "if only one would come who could guide man back into the right
channel of life, for then any society would work that would provide for the
distribution of the necessities of keeping up a physical existence."

Lost in a whirlwind of such thoughts, Theos soon found himself lost in
a much different whirlwind, as the late spring blizzard that was buffeting
Chapman and Crawford on the peak of Chomolhari became only barely less
than a blinding snowstorm on the plain of Du-na, and Theos and Tharchin
were forced to take shelter in one of the makeshift rest stops set up along
the way for tiffin.[17] The Du-na dak bungalow that became their refuge
from the snow was little more than a "four wall dung enclosure . . . whose
ceiling was nothing but the carcasses of dried animals, the only food they
had." Nonetheless, invigorating themselves with hot water and instant cof-
fee while they waited out the storm, Theos and Tharchin put the time to
good use strategizing for Gyantse, with Theos guiding Tharchin through
his plans—"the various tasks" clearly outlined for Tharchin "to take up
immediately" upon their arrival. The following few days blurred together
as they passed various landmarks, from small bungalows to the lake at
Dochen. While Chomolhari passed farther and farther into the distance
behind them, they posed for photos and staged scenes for filming—Theos
sending Tharchin on ahead so as to be able to film him overtaking the pack
train between Dochen and Kala—and soon the last leg of the journey was
upon them.

The final day's ride had been a quiet one, broken only by the sound
of the footsteps of Theos's donkey beneath him echoing off the canyon
walls and the distant tinkling bells on the harnesses of yak trains ornately
decorated and transporting more and more wool south toward India. After
passing the famous Buddha carved in red sandstone from the cliffs outside
of Kangma, ten days after setting out from Gangtok, on Sunday, May 23,
they passed the two small stupas below the ancient Nanying Monastery at
the canyon mouth and finally approached Gyantse. The sight of the fort in
the distance brought an uneasy excitement for Theos, as he reflected that
"at times I can hardly believe that I am here, if so why and how come."

Although Theos had achieved this first stage of his trip, whether or not permission to visit Lhasa would be forthcoming depended entirely on his actions—and more realistically, on Tharchin's actions—over the coming days and weeks. Theos consoled himself with the knowledge that eventually an invitation would come, even if a few years later, when he would "be still more prepared to make the best out of such an opportunity." Come what may, Theos was determined not to waste any opportunity that might present itself in the meantime. He was not jealous of those who had gone to Lhasa, as much as he lamented their wasted adventures.

> The thing that hurts most of all is what little those who come are able to take away. It is nothing but a great adventure into the great unknown. Being a forbidden spot on earth, people seem to think it enough if they merely walk over the ground; and so we have to continue on waiting for someone to lose sight of the adventure long enough to let us in on the treasures that have been stored away by the faith of ages.

Even photographically, Theos was determined to make his record as different as possible from everyone else's. It was fine to document what one was *seeing*, but far more important, he felt, was to photographically convey what one was *feeling*.

Early the next morning, Theos was dressed and on the ground before the sun had even risen. After more unpacking and some breakfast, he and Tharchin went to pay a visit to the Acting British Trade Agent in Gyantse, Captain Gordon Cable,[18] who, quite annoyingly, made clear that he already knew far more about Theos's activities and plans up to that point than perhaps even Theos did, and informed them further that neither Theos nor Tharchin should so much as leave their bungalow without first informing him of their actions and intentions. "Is there any place where the petty traits of human character will not exert themselves and man find a way to make himself supreme?" Theos thought. On a similar courtesy visit to Cable's counterpart, the Tibetan Trade Agent in Gyantse, who conveniently happened to be the abbot of the local monastery, a somewhat more amicable accord was achieved—and plans set into motion. Just the same, Theos knew, he would have to tread carefully around the British.

As luck would have it, the next day, May 25, would be the fifteenth day of the fourth Tibetan month, known as "Saga Dawa"—the annual celebration of the birth, enlightenment, and "final nirvāṇa" of the Buddha—and there would be considerable festivities. Informed by Tharchin that Theos was a devout (and rich) Buddhist on pilgrimage from America, the abbot suggested that it would only be appropriate to include Theos in the coming days' activities and offered to incorporate a "long life ceremony" on his behalf, with a thousand-butter-lamp offering. Tharchin informed the abbot that Theos, for his own part, would be honored to serve as patron for the celebratory events and graciously accepted the honor of being allowed to feed the entire monastery, some fifteen hundred monks.

Theos knew that this was his opportunity to put to use the information he had gleaned from William McGovern's book. McGovern had succeeded in avoiding detection by adopting a series of mannerisms that enabled him to pass as a Tibetan to the casual observer, although he failed when closely scrutinized. Nonetheless, when confronted with a situation that could potentially expose his identity, McGovern's approach was to try to respond as any Tibetan would. Whereas this was a clever attempt at disguise on McGovern's part, Theos realized that he could deploy the same strategy to precisely the opposite end—to invite scrutiny and put forth a very public image.

Arriving early the next morning, Theos found that the entire monastery had turned out, assembled in the courtyard before the main temple and seated in row after row on long carpets. Guided through the kitchen and upstairs to the small audience chamber, Theos and Tharchin were greeted by the abbot in his full regalia before being seated on cushions nearby and served tea and sweets; all the while, the cavernous space of the hall below reverberated with the deep chants of the monks. Returning downstairs with the abbot, Theos was led on a tour of the monastery complex commencing with a tribute to the late Dalai Lama, represented by the chair he once sat on, displayed on the grounds before the main temple. Walking forward with a white silk *khata* in hand, Theos prostrated before the chair, then offered the silk scarf, draping it across the seat. The impact of this small gesture on those who witnessed it was far greater than anything that he could have imagined, for never had any resident of Gyantse witnessed a white man—certainly not any of the British they had met—pay any sign of respect to their religion or spiritual leaders the way Theos had just done. Before the day was over, the entire populace of Gyantse had heard of the public profession of faith and respect and was fully convinced of his sincerity.

For his own part, Theos was indeed sincerely moved when, upon entering the main assembly hall, he was struck by the vision that awaited him:

There were three thousand candles in this dimly lighted sanctuary, and your wildest imagination will never be able to picture the impressiveness of these hundreds of twinkling lights which were placed in a row of two completely around the room. The walls were decorated with handpaintings of the deities, displaying master craftsmanship on the part of their Lama artists. The Buddha was of the most impressive size, all studded with precious stones. The sixteen bodhisattvas which are usually painted on the walls were represented here in giant figures adding immensely to the impressiveness of the environment which would instill religious devotion in any soul—even the most hardened heathen would want to bow or do something. That is the feeling that it gives you, that you must do something, you know not what and you know not why, but a something deep within is moved that perhaps you never realized existed before.

No less impressive to Theos was the sheer quantity of gold, semiprecious, and precious gems that seemed to adorn every stupa, statue, and shrine within the hall, and it boggled his mind to "fathom the wealth" stored away inside the monastery. Having disbelieved the accounts he had read, thinking that "the authors borrowed considerably from their imaginations," he was convinced when he saw the temple with his own eyes that those accounts must only have scratched the surface concerning "the untold wealth that has been amassed" by the monasteries.

Theos was duly impressed by all that he saw that day, and reflected on the fact that he had not seen any account, or even mention, of such sights in any of the books that he had read. "To date, there are no records of any white man ever entering such chambers of the great monasteries at Lhasa. Even Waddell, Sir Charles Bell, and David MacDonald, who perhaps have enjoyed the most intimate relationship with the Tibetans, of any European, fail to relate any such experience of opportunity." He concluded, therefore, that he must be the first to have seen such things, and further suspected that he could claim this status as "the first" in many achievements, if his luck held out. "To be invited to the world center of these teachings would be the first time the barrier has been broken. People have stolen their way in, fought their way in, and got in under various pretenses, but no one yet has been invited to make a pilgrimage to Lhasa and had the heart of their teachings open to him." With this in mind, Theos continued to "carefully lay a diplomatic foundation."

Tharchin as well was doing his part. No sooner had the day's events transpired than Tharchin wrote up a short account, highlighting Theos's generosity, and sent it down to Kalimpong for publication in the next issue of *The Mirror*, knowing full well that it would be read in Lhasa in a matter of weeks—conveniently, just about the time that their petition to visit would be received. The simple, one-line article read:

AN AUSPICIOUS SAGA DAWA

Fourth Lunar month, fifteenth day: At the Pal-khor-chö-de Temple in Gyantse, an American Sahib named Bernard along with 1,000 [butter lamp] offerings, presented both tea and monetary offerings to each member of the assembled monastic community, and in this way, humbly venerated and paid his respects [to them].[19]

With that short piece of "news," Theos's campaign was well under way.

The centerpiece of the next day's events at the monastery was the ritual dances, which Theos was invited by the abbot to attend and film and photograph to his heart's content. He had been advised in Gangtok by Gould that he "would probably not be able to attend," and reflected with some amusement that if the British authorities "only knew the depths to which I have penetrated, they would run me out of the country immediately for various political reasons." Nonetheless, Theos felt quite safe in attending the festivities since he doubted Cable would give much thought to the Tibetans' opinion. After dining with him the night before, Theos concluded that Cable had little more than contempt for the Tibetans—"he does hate them—in typical English fashion." Nonetheless, Theos made a point of casually informing Cable that the "Tibetan Trade Agent" had given his permission to attend the dances. Cable then, per protocol, informed Theos that in that case, he would collect him at the bungalow the next morning and accompany him to the monastery.

Arriving early, Theos and Cable were left to their own devices, as the abbot was otherwise engaged in overseeing the many affairs of the day, the pair wandered about in the main hall, with the altar fully stocked and illuminated with butter lamps and molded and painted butter sculptures. Having been given permission to photograph what he liked, Theos began his attempts to document the various temples, though hampered by the presence of Cable, who, his disdain for the Tibetans being well known by

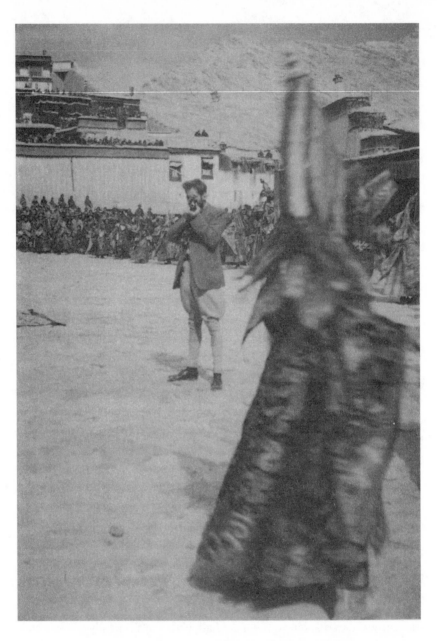

Figure 8.2 Bernard filming the dance on Saga Dawa at Gyantse (PAHM)

the monks, was not allowed access to some areas—a fact that Theos knew well enough to diplomatically avoid.

> With the officer about it was a bit difficult to go too far, for he is not accepted in the same light as I have been, yet I had to see to it that he had the feeling that all was open to him, but after my tour of yesterday it was obvious how much they permit the outsider to see even though he comes with all the official prestige of England. However, it is my experience that prestige without personality does not get one beyond the rules and regulations that govern all political courtesies.

Nonetheless, Cable could easily scuttle Theos's plans with the slightest word, so he remained careful in their interactions.

Initially "thrilled" as he had approached the monastery that morning, seeing the sky clear with the horizon forming "a perfect background of turbulent clouds," upon exiting the temples after a few hours, Theos was saddened to see that the distant clouds had disappeared and the sun had been blotted out by a heavy dust storm. Cinematographically, this was less than ideal:

> I had come prepared to take the entire dance in color for I wanted to preserve the splendor of their costumes, but the weather cheated me out of the opportunity. As a result, I had brought little Pan film; so I was more or less compelled to go ahead and try to record something in color which I did at a fiendish pace, for such chances come so seldom, I felt it wise to get all that was possible, for I can always cut but I will never be able to add once the procession has passed. But it hurt me every time I started the machine going, for all looked so drab and hopeless; but what to do— grin and bear it under the hope that something might be forthcoming.

Resolving to carry a sufficient stock of black-and-white Pan film with him from then on, Theos, joined by Tharchin, set about documenting the dances in still and 16-mm color film, lamenting that when he was able to preview the films for the first time, six or seven months later, he might be disappointed at having "to show such inferior work after the endless precautions that have been taken."

While Theos kept Cable occupied at the monastery throughout the morning, Tharchin—far from disinterested in the day's coming events—had taken the opportunity to meet with the Gyantse fort commander (Dzong-pön), a young man in his late twenties who had risen to his rank through a fortuitous marriage with the daughter of a noble family. Dorje Wangyal—known as Chokte[20] to most—was a friendly, well-educated man for whom a government post offered a convenient means of supporting himself in his religious practice. He had heard, before Tharchin had even arrived at the fort, of Theos's display of respect the day before, and being duly impressed, he was favorably disposed to help Theos in what ways he could. Hearing that Tsarong Lhacham's daughter and son-in-law, Mary and Jigme Taring, had arrived in Gyantse as well, Tharchin sent a courier to their house, re-questing a meeting for the following day since Theos had missed the op-portunity to meet them in Kalimpong. Although he was making progress with the various Tibetan officials he was encountering, Theos felt that his "greatest difficulties are going to be with the British Official" and remained fearful of the British authorities, thinking that "it will be impossible for me to overcome the petty jealousies that exist amongst them to win them over in the limited time that is remaining." It was all the more painful since every-one told him that even if he won over the Tibetan government, they would still defer to the British, "who will undoubtedly dissuade them to grant me the requested permission." Consequently, he concluded, the British Trade Agent, Hugh Richardson, in Lhasa, would have to be wooed as well.

The next day, beginning—as he did when possible—by writing a letter to Viola, Theos told her about his ongoing "diary" of activities replete with "a few personal reflections that are stimulated by this environment and ex-periences" and jokingly informed her, "you now have a real Tibetan Lama" though "his feelings of love are unaltered." The rest of the morning, with Tharchin by his side, he devoted to logistical activities, from exchanging Indian rupees for Tibetan silver to strategizing about the contents of vari-ous letters they knew would need to be written to the Lhasa government.

Having received word the night before that Mary and Jigme would call on him in the morning and would like to invite him for the dinner that eve-ning, Theos summoned up all that he could remember about them based on the entries in the British Mission diaries that he had read in Gangtok a scant two weeks earlier. Jigme was a prince of Sikkim, the eldest son of Taring Raja—the putative king, who had stepped down from the throne in order to lead a more simple life[21]—and Rinchen Dolma ("Mary") was the daughter of a minister of the Tibetan cabinet. Both had been edu-cated in English schools in Darjeeling and after their marriage,[22] with their knowledge of English, assumed roles in administering their families' fortunes. Although a few years younger than Theos, Jigme was the commander-general of all the military forces of Tibet, a role he had assumed at the age of twenty-one when his father-in-law, the great Tsarong Shapé, fell from favor with the Tibetan government. Thoroughly impressed by the man, Theos remarked,

> He possesses a very shrewd mind and a keen imagination, anxious to expand the outlook of his country. With such personalities as this in the government Tibet will not remain isolated for more than one more generation at the outside, for the younger generation with the tolerance of the present will be able to carry out the manifold desires of the younger set today who are being hampered by the archaic traditions of the past, held to by the older ones who must be continually favored.

After a long conversation, Jigme suggested to Theos that they meet again to discuss "some of the possibilities" that Theos could see for Tibet. Delighted to assume the role of a political advisor, Theos agreed, pointing out the obvious lack of encouragement that Jigme could expect from the British in India, who were far more concerned with maintaining Tibet as a "buffer nation" than with benefiting Tibet or the Tibetans. Consequently, Theos actually had some useful insights to offer:

> They know nothing about their metal resources, but from all external conditions, there must be metal to be found, for there are large areas of metaliferous rock; so a few skilled mining engineers are needed. They fear industry because they do not have coal or petrol. Well, they are constantly digging mastodons and what have you out of the Gobi Desert and the geologists tell us that this country is all very young, having been raised up only a few million years ago; so it is not at all unlikely that they might accidentally strike oil or something if the proper examinations were made. With little additional cost the cost of transportation over these endless plains could be reduced by the development of a few roads so as to permit the loads to be carried by bullock carts instead of on burro back. This would handle many times their present exports. It is true that it would throw the present people out of a living; but that power could be easily diverted into some other channel that would be more constructive. They only have a little over 3,000,000 people to deal

with, and there is hardly any tract in the world as large as this that will not accommodate that many souls. If properly organized, they could utilize all excess labor in some sort of industry for if they just put the beggar to work they would be able to compete with Japan for the low cost of labor. And so one could go on and on.

With such insights and recommendations, Theos ingratiated himself with the Tarings. Feeling he had secured their friendship, he knew only one man remained in Gyantse who could help him further, the Gyantse Dzongpön, Chokte. And with Tharchin's help, Theos had already secured a meeting with him over dinner in a few days' time.

Following the dinner with Mary, Jigme, and Taring Raja—and all the attendant complications, since "there are more or less three different families in this one family, so there was a bit of etiquette that had to be solved with regard to the proper presenting of the scarves . . . after which a good time was had by all, once I had been told that it was unnecessary that I observe the little formality—which of course is a part of the formality"— Theos was delighted to discover that Jigme had taken up photography as a hobby. With this common interest, Theos and Jigme decided to indulge themselves taking portraits and group photos of the party, going so far as to dress Theos up in full Tibetan official's garb with Jigme's hat and signature of rank, his long *sok-jil* earring, with Tharchin doing his best to document it all using Theos's spare camera.

Although the ensuing days were filled with more events—horse racing, archery competitions, and the like—Theos set his sights on meeting with the Dzongpön, Chokte. They had already met once before, when earlier in the spring Chokte had gone on pilgrimage to Bodh Gaya, returning to Tibet via Calcutta and Kalimpong. Now, however, they would meet in a much more formal situation. Still, given this familiarity between them and Tharchin's friendship with him, they felt they could be more forthright about their plans and had a frank conversation about their desire to reach Lhasa. "He is a very devout Buddhist," Theos observed, and consequently, was eager to help another Buddhist—as Theos had publicly demonstrated himself to be—on his own pilgrimage.

We stated our plans and he told us exactly what should be done, and if all was carried out it was his prediction that there would be no doubt as to the permission being granted. He, himself, is very much in favor of my being allowed to visit their holy center, and he volunteered a personal letter to the Regent, along with mine, recommending a favorable consideration.

Although Theos and Tharchin were aware of Chokte's influence with Reting Rinpoche, unbeknownst to both, if anyone could have secured the Regent's support it was Chokte, who had an intimate relationship with the man.[23] Nonetheless, as powerful as Reting Rinpoche was at the time, Theos and Tharchin knew that winning him over would not be enough—the entire cabinet would have to give their approval. The time this would take was on Theos's mind—a concern he conveyed to Chokte, being convinced that he would have to return to Kalimpong before such approval came, which then naturally would necessitate an immediate return to Gyantse. Chokte, however, suggested that he not worry about such things and instead enjoy his time in Gyantse, to which end he invited him to a picnic the very next day.

The festivities and contests of the previous day concluded, Theos and Tharchin commenced a "whirlwind of teas and parties" beginning at 8 a.m. at the picnic tent of an aristocratic family before joining Chokte and his many friends at his residence for his midday party.

> Yesterday I had been inside this house, but this time we were escorted into a small courtyard at the end of which was his tent, and this was grandeur personified, for it was like the palace itself. The Captain and myself being the only two Europeans in the country at the time had to uphold our races along with about fifteen of them, but with their graciousness and hospitality, it is one of the easiest things in the world to do. No sooner than we arrived, sweets and tea was served and this was kept replenished until a little after twelve when the dinner was brought on which took us until after three to eat it, for at no time were there less than fifteen dishes on the tables and none of them remained for long. I failed to count the number but from the few times that I did check up, there must have been far over fifty courses, because I did note down over thirty and then I stopped.[24]

As for the guests themselves,

> The girls were done up in their "Sunday best" and the men in those enviable silk brocades. Never have I been in such a group where all the

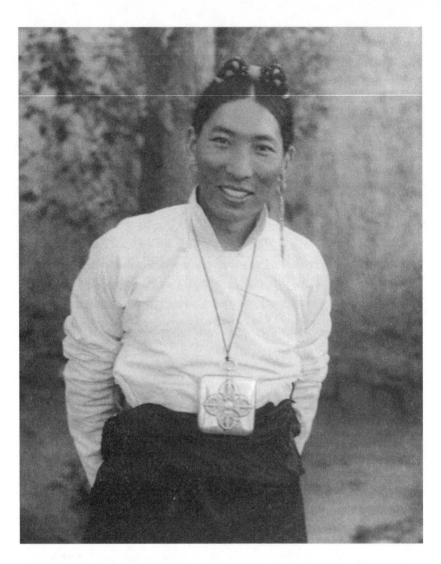

Figure 8.3 Chokte, the Western Fort Commander at Gyantse (PAHM)

personalities present were so overwhelmingly charming. To have twenty in a tent this size for seven hours, and then only leaving because they feel that they have to, is about as high a compliment to the Tibetan character and their charm as a host, as could ever be asked. The Nepali agent was there along with the head of the Commissary Department for the India troops stationed at the fort; with them and the Taring family we had a jolly lot.

Tibet, Tantrikas, and the Hero of Chaksam Ferry

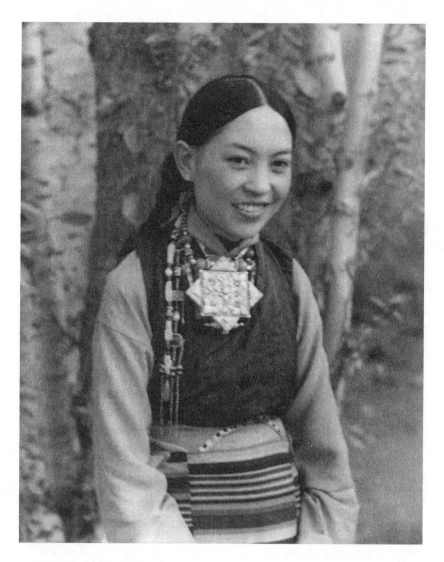

Figure 8.4 Namkye Tsedrön, Chokte's wife (PAHM)

Theos himself—unlike Cable, who was fulfilling his political obligations—was happy to socialize with the entire ensemble, and with one in particular.

Like so many before and after him, Theos was smitten by the beauty of Chokte's wife, Namkye Tsedrön,[25] as well as her personality—she was a woman whose "sparkling thoughts" could "stimulate a keen conversational evening":

Never could one find a more charming face to gaze upon than the spar-kling bright black eyes that light up the smiling countenance of the Jongpon's wife. We often think of the beauty of the Japanese women as capturing the prize for the East; it is fortunate that they do not have to compete with this type. The amazing part of it all is that their skin is as fair as my own, bordered with this glistening black hair done up in two long braids tied together at the bottom by the pink tassels which are woven in the hair.

As the afternoon drew to a close with games and entertainment from Japanese and Chinese phonograph records, Theos felt confident that he had conducted himself quite well, earning the friendship of the assembled guests without sacrificing documentation of the event, as Tharchin had been saddled with the duty of photographing and filming the gathering throughout the day. Ready to bid them all farewell, Theos was shocked to learn that rather than departing, everyone else was preparing to return to the picnic tent to commence the evening meal! Quietly discussing the situation, he and Cable decided to politely excuse themselves, and having paid their respects, rode back to town.

Thinking he would have the evening to himself, Theos was somewhat disconcerted that Cable then wanted to talk. Knowing how important it would be to stay on Cable's good side, Theos agreed, which meant staying for a proper British dinner. Cable, it seems, was intrigued by Theos's pho-tographic equipment, and in particular, his "duplicating apparatus" for the Leica.[26] Taking advantage of this enthusiasm, Theos took the opportunity to quiz him about all the people they had just met. "From him," Theos wrote,

I was able to get some of the historical background of who these various people were, and where they came from, and what they were doing; and in the end I find that it is all the same as any social climber in our own world. Some poor boy who has been able to get a break in life, and is now out to retrieve the old family fortune—and in these particular instances they are succeeding—for they are today about the highest collection of individuals to be found in Tibet. They at least represent the most power-ful families of the country.

Nonetheless, Theos could see how precarious his own situation was. He had earned Cable's friendship, though at the price of having to play a sporting game of polo the next day and then join a discussion of world politics. For Theos, the perilous state of Tibet was all too obvious, and given the possibilities of another world war,

It is almost heart rending when one hears about how Tibet is trying to keep in preparedness with their antiquated equipment. They think that it is impossible for another nation to ever attack them because of their high barriers of snow and ice. Little do they realize that within a few hours a complete army could be brought up here from India, for it is just a few hundred miles in a straight line, and the entire country is a landing field. There might be a few minor casualties, but in all events they could land. As for modern means of warfare, they know nothing, not even those in charge of their forces. The country is so poor that they cannot even afford to fire off a few shots now and then to test their equipment let alone try to train an army; so what chance have they? As it stands, their ignorance of such facts lets them rest in their idleness. The British sit quietly by and let them do what they want, for it helps to make them think that they are a force. . . . But luckily enough they do not understand this means of existence, for their life is chiefly one of meditations with a small group trying to bring about a change which will take many years, for it is impossible to change the nature of the animal overnight.

Indeed, the motivations behind Tibetan society were far closer to his heart than the aims of his English-speaking brethren, who diverted themselves with games of polo, cricket, and the like. "This sort of thing always cuts deep," he remarked, "when they say that they have to carry on in this manner to help while away the time, for my greatest difficulty is trying to find time enough to get done the little that has been planned." Indeed, Theos thought, "if I could have my own way and reach my goal, I would never waste such vital time on the back of a horse; but now it has turned out to be one of the necessities of my job, because without their good will it would be impossible for me to go to Lhasa."

Just the same, Theos knew that his time would have to be divided between his studies—which he vowed to do every morning even if it meant waking up at 4—and various social obligations, both in Tibet and at home. Determined to support the "deep interest" that Tibet held for "all outsiders who are not fortunate enough to visit these parts," Theos spent one morning alone addressing more than a hundred postcards to friends and family back home, and especially took great pains to write a lengthy letter to the youngest of his half-brothers, Marvene, offering him some advice from the experiences of his own life. However, the greatest difficulty wasn't writing his letters but "being able to get enough Tibetan stamps for it is history for them to ever have such a thriving business; so a special order has to be sent to Lhasa to have them printed."[27] Theos spent the next few days running back and forth from his residence to the home of the Dzongpön "for his consultation on each move," as well as in repeated games of polo with Captain Cable and even a hunt for gazelle—a highly problematic venture, given Theos's publicly professed Buddhism.[28]

For the local population of Gyantse, Theos was a bit of a curiosity and the object of much fascination, which garnered him repeated visits by monks and the townsfolk alike. On one occasion, afternoon tea with some monks from the local monastery, Theos was able to entertain them with his camera equipment. Taking turns photographing each other, the monks, having no end of fun as well, went so far as to take off some of their robes and dress Theos up as a monk, then insisted on taking several pictures together with him.

But all of these activities were "robbing [him] of precious time," and to facilitate things as efficiently as possible, Theos resolved to send Tharchin on to Lhasa alone to plead his case in person, for "with Tharchin going in to present the story which I have built up for him, it was the feeling of everyone concerned that permission could hardly be refused; so our hopes were high." Remaining in constant contact with Lhasa via telegraph and letter, Theos and Tharchin learned that their gifts sent from Kalimpong had never arrived. Disheartened, they knew their attempts to woo the authorities without accompanying gifts would be "the worst breach of Tibetan etiquette." Immediately they dispatched a letter to Lhasa to learn what sort of gifts Cutting had sent to the officials there and more importantly, what the reaction had been. Sending telegrams to Calcutta, Theos ordered more gifts for delivery to Gyantse while he and Tharchin made a new plan. Thinking that he would soon have to return to India alone, Theos vowed to travel as slowly as possible while Tharchin went to Lhasa in the hope that he could cable Theos en route to return. Luckily, they soon received word that their gift packages *had* arrived, but were stuck in the post office right there in Gyantse, awaiting the return of the Tibetan Trade Agent, who had left on a trip of indeterminate length. Securing permission to retrieve the packages themselves, Theos and Tharchin resumed working on drafting the letter to accompany the gifts and requested a meeting with their friend the Dzongpön again.

Working up their proposal, Theos and Tharchin put forth what they thought would be a convincing petition. Reviewing their letter, however, Chokte felt that it was inadequate for the task at hand, and he rewrote the letters of petition and had them copied onto good Tibetan paper by a professional scribe for Tharchin to deliver. Beside himself with excitement, Theos felt assured that he would get permission to proceed to Lhasa.

> You should hear the letter that he has written to each of the officials as well as to them as a group. He has taken a few of my ideas and spread them out in the "King's English of Tibet." The letters themselves would almost win my goal. As he says, the Tibetan is a very queer sort of person and there are certain things that he is sure to think of, and by attaching his emotional reactions with the proper Tibetan proverbs, he is left with only one decision; so he has poured out the best that he has in him, all in my favor, because he is so happy to find that I am such a firm believer in their teachings.

Feeling that their plans were well afoot, Theos turned to the subject of religion with Chokte and his beautiful young wife, who followed the teachings of the Nyingma sect that traced itself back to Padmasambhava in the eighth century. Discussing his own fondness for the teachings of the great Guru Rinpoche, "they brought out endless volumes and commenced to tell me no end of the teachings in these sacred books." Showing Theos the very seven-book set by the fourteenth-century scholar Long-chen-pa that he had been told about in Yatung weeks earlier, they informed him that the books "more or less contain all of Padma Sambhava's teachings, but they are to be found nowhere in Tibet today except in Kham, and there are only a few sets left." Even for Chokte, a high-ranking government official, acquiring the books had been difficult, and only after several years of searching for them had he been able to secure his own set. Nonetheless, feeling a shared bond of religious commitment with Theos, Chokte "promised to let me have them if I am unable to find another during my visit in Tibet," and understanding the heartfelt offer being made, felt "rather fortunate in this opportunity."

Beyond even these matters, Theos found that he was able to relax and socialize with Chokte and Namkye who together, he felt, embodied the ideal relationship—something he made a point of letting Viola know in a not too subtle manner:

> Once these details had all been attended to, we turned off on to the subject of religion. He and his wife commenced telling me about various religious books. She is just about as keen a little woman as one wants to talk to let alone look at for she is as beautiful as a woman can be, without being of your own kind, which of course is the best.[29] After having spent endless hours in trying to read these manuscripts in Tibetan, and then to see her race over the lines faster than you could go if they were in English, makes you a bit envious. She is well versed on all the teachings of Buddhism, as well as familiar with all the literature, for apparently they both do a great deal of studying together. This is something that you admire in the Tibetan in contrast to the Indian; that his wife is his every day companion in all that he does.[30] She is always with him, and if you think that you are likely to have a private conversation with him, you are wrong, for she is always there and has very valuable suggestions to offer. She has that perfect charm of being able to let him run everything, do everything, but serve as an unintruding companion . . . as in our own society you will find that behind the scenes the reason for the man's success is because of the wife that he has.

In all honesty, however, Theos did think that theirs was an ideal arrangement. The Buddhist texts always spoke of two necessary prerequisites for religious practice: the leisure time that wealth and privilege could afford and the good fortune to be able to utilize it with proper instruction. While Chokte and Theos had both of these—or so Theos hoped—Chokte had something more: a companion with whom he was of a single mind and single purpose in their religious life.[31] As much as Theos tried to convince Viola that they had precisely such a relationship as well, still he had his doubts about the level of commitment from her side.

Nonetheless, feeling flushed with success with Chokte's letters of support to both the Kashag and Reting Rinpoche, Theos immediately sent a wire to Calcutta requesting "more films to come immediately, because so many pictures have been taken en route and about this section, that there is not enough to photograph this sacred center of the world satisfactorily with what is left." Indeed, he thought,

If this invitation is granted, it will be the first time in the history of the country that one has ever been invited to make a pilgrimage to this holy center and it will almost mean that things will be opened to me that others have never been permitted to see; so I am very anxious that it all turn out. Because of my studies, I am placing everything on the religious angle, because when all is said and done, I am more anxious to peer into their hidden beliefs than I am to looking [sic] at the barren streets of Lhasa which I have already seen several times over in photographs taken by this recent mission and in the endless books that are available on this section of the world. But nowhere is it possible to find out anything about what goes on behind these walls and thereby keep this social structure together century after century. It will undoubtedly be one of the most revealing experiences of a lifetime so far as the understanding of foreign thoughts is concerned.

Thus, with the letters written and Tharchin's departure for Lhasa scheduled for the next day, Theos reflected that "there will be nothing for me to do but sit and hope until his wire is received telling me to make haste for Kalimpong or Lhasa." Although everyone reassured him that his plans would succeed, "it all sounds so good that I am afraid, for I hardly know of anything ever working out that smoothly for me." Sure enough, just before Tharchin's departure for Lhasa, Theos received word from Kodak in Bombay that they were out of Kodachrome film, "which means that there are only about two rolls of this film in all of India." Nonetheless, deciding to hedge his bets on reaching Lhasa, Theos made the decision to send both still and motion picture cameras along with Tharchin in the hope that even if he was denied permission to go himself, at least Tharchin could obtain some still photos and color film footage of the city. Thus, along with some rolls of film, Theos gave Tharchin his "wish-list" of photos, as well as texts and specific questions he hoped to have answered. The motivation was "not to obtain a more comprehensive knowledge of Buddhism, but to know more about the living principles of Tantra which in my estimation offers the most complete explanation of a way of life." Through these studies, he felt, "it is possible to have an answer for every phenomenon known to man. It gives a reason for all the conditions of man, from the low to the high. Above all, it gives you a theory of life, which enables you to understand anything that may ever come to pass."

Somewhat disconcerting for Theos was the fact that with Tharchin gone, "my one and only means of speaking a little English will be gone, for I will be left here with the boys who do not know a word of English, and the one Tibetan that I know of that does speak English lives about seven miles away." Not to be disheartened, Theos resolved "to come forward and see how I can make things happen in a strange land with a new language," since "one in all, it is rather an opportunity because it forces me to use this other means of communication which I am trying to develop." Still somewhat apprehensive about speaking Tibetan himself, he wrote, "I will have to be on my toes, because they do not offer you any charity [since] they all feel that you should speak their language as well as they do." Just the same, Theos could always rely on Tharchin, who took care of as much as he could before leaving:

Due to the fact that I am going to be left absolutely alone and will have to function the best I can with the little Tibetan that I have, we have tried to see to it that all complicated affairs are settled before his departure for I can hardly be expected to enter a Tibetan diplomatic circle as yet even though I may be able to join up with a bunch of muleteers. From the standpoint of learning this language? I am rather looking forward to the experience, for it will force the issue. While Tharchin says everything first in Tibetan, and when I do not understand he repeats in Tibetan, I finally break him down to a few English words which he condescendingly gives me so that I may make the sense of the full statement. This is hardly enough, for I always listen with the subconscious feeling that in the long run I can get the answer in English. Then even when I understand him perfectly, I find that my reaction is always to answer in English while now I will have to answer in Tibetan, for they cannot understand a word of English; which means that I will have to alter my nature of thinking.

Before leaving, Tharchin paid one last visit to Chokte to have the professionally scribed letters signed and sealed by him, and to discuss Theos in his absence. From his dealings with the British and visits to India, Chokte was understandably suspicious of Theos and his interests, for "it all sounded too good for him to believe when coming from a European," but Tharchin reassured him that Theos was, in fact, quite sincere in his actions and intentions. With that, Chokte reaffirmed his willingness to help

Theos reach Lhasa. As a final gesture, he called on Theos and Tharchin just before the latter's departure, bringing along his set of the *Seven Treasuries* of Long-chen-pa—the condensation of the Nyingma teachings[32] attributed to Padmasambhava.

> Now he offers to give them to me in order that I may be able to spread their teachings in America. He has spent a lot of effort in making sure of my true feelings in this matter, and is now confident and wants me to have them, for he feels that he will do a good turn for the world if he makes it possible for these books to be used for such a purpose as mine. . . .
>
> But still more touching is the gift that he brought with him. He had told me on my visit of a Thangka which he had that had been blessed, first by one of the head Lamas of this sect many generations past and has remained in his family ever since. I had been told by others of this possession which he had, and that if I could but have it, I would be sure of success in my purpose to spread their teachings. Of course, it seemed ridiculous to ever think of being able to possess this venerated object of faith, but now that he was sure of my feelings in these matters, he had brought it to me after the necessary ceremony at his monastery by the head Lama.[33]

By this gift of a Padmasambhava *thangka*, "from everything [that] has gone into it through acts of friendship and the sacrificing necessary to pass it on," Theos was touched and overwhelmed, and accepted it possibly "with greater feeling than with which it was given." It was Chokte's hope that the rest of Theos's life would be spent "laying the foundation for the spreading of these teachings," so he had visited a lama to have it consecrated for transferral to Theos. Theos related to Viola that with this ceremony he had received "authority from the Kargyupa sect to carry on its teachings in our country" and confessed that "it is exactly what I hope that I will eventually be able to do," for which Viola congratulated him on "becoming a Lama." Truly appreciative of their trust in him, Theos invited Chokte and Namkye to visit him and Viola in America, which they promised to do once direct flights from India were established.

After several logistical delays and false starts, Tharchin finally began the three-day trip to Lhasa on the sixth of June, certain that he would be able to present Theos's case to all the important parties within days of his arrival and promising to wire Gyantse as soon as a decision had been reached. Alone for the first time in a while, Theos returned to his usual routine of letter writing and sorting, identifying, and mounting the contact prints he had begun to receive from Calcutta. With few distractions beyond Captain Cable, Theos had time to contemplate the agenda for his life that seemed to be unfolding before him, recording it all in his diary. "If Tibet has done nothing else for me," he wrote, "it has captivated my imagination [and] filled me with ideas on a material outlet for my all consuming purpose."

As he was writing to Viola again, a long letter from her arrived, written almost three weeks earlier, addressed to him care of Kalimpong, since she couldn't muster the nerve "to address an envelope 'Gyantse, Tibet.'" Giving him news of her life and responding to his earlier letters, she particularly advised him that he "mustn't just pipe dream," and that if he was serious about his planned activities, he should take concrete steps to make them a reality. He had informed her earlier that he would type his letters to her despite, he knew, how much she preferred to receive letters handwritten in order to feel closer to him. Stressed out from her internship, Viola told Theos that she found it just as hectic as being married to him and, as if she didn't have enough to do, "where in the world," she wrote, "did you ever get the notion that I preferred your writing by pen instead of typewriter—Perish the thought! never would I willing take on those god-awful hen tracks of yours that I have to puzzle over to extract the meaning that often tantalizes me for hours—when I could have nice typewritten keys instead. No—no—a thousand times no!" Taken slightly aback, Theos simply responded, "So you don't mind the typewriter—well Yaks and what have you have been bringing it along for you," and besides, he apologetically wrote, as far as interning being like their marriage, "that is hardly fair," and he promised her so much leisure time upon his return that she would be bored.

But Theos was struggling with his own tendency to boredom, stranded in Gyantse, though it was more like apprehensiveness. Within days of Tharchin's departure, he had settled into a routine of morning meditation, playing polo with Cable—followed by "our usual discussion of what-nots about nothings that is so in keeping with unimaginative sociability necessary to while away the useful hours of a life time by purposeless consciences," language study and writing in his diary, followed by the seemingly endless barrage of visitors checking up on him in an effort to keep him company in Tharchin's absence, which occasionally proved fruitful.[34] But for Theos, "the rich part of the day" was "the quiet morning after four and before eight" when he could remain in that postsleep calm and allow his mind to reveal what he perceived as its innate wisdom to his conscious self:

For today I merely passed the time away in order to re-enter my meditative hour whose silence holds an indescribable enthrallment or something. No longer do I have to plan on thinking of anything—all that is necessary is to put myself in the presence of the early morning quietude of nature and let myself become receptive to what takes place within. Often the mind has not yet recovered from its sleepiness, and is not anxious to think; but soon something starts to move deep within, and shortly I find myself all [in] concentration on something that I am not yet aware of, when suddenly I find the mind wrestling with an idea, trying to find the most shapely form for its expression; and it is never satisfied until the thought will pour out as smooth as water from a vessel. Once it is out, it is through, and is likely to wander to any extreme if it is not recalled from within, and it is during this intervening period when a union is trying to be established between the subtleties of the subconscious and the agent for external expression. (In fact, it is so much like fishing that I hesitate to point out the analogy), that I receive my strongest emotional awe that is supposed to be so closely related to the mystical experience, and as with that experience I have no conscious control over it. All happens like a flash and is gone again, but I have found that during this prolonged discipline that it comes more quickly as well as oftener, remaining for a longer period. However I most note that the experience gained by a contact with this unconscious reservoir is by far richer when the mind is removed from it which is the experience had in establishing this union through Yoga, for there the first principle is to banish the mind, but now that I am anxious to record the feelings that comprehend various problems in life, I let this awareness of growing understanding and insight formalize itself through the mind. Today I am not so much interested in whether these answers are right or wrong as I am in building up this capacity to attach the problem of knowledge through this intuitive channel to be the true path for truth . . . never have I been able to establish such a definite relation between my inner world of feeling and the mind.

From these meditations, Theos was beginning to develop his own understanding of what it meant to be enlightened and gain what he saw as the capacities necessary to lead others in the religious life as a teacher:

I have been able to become conscious of the subconscious; so now I continue on just to keep the channel from closing up on me, until I can take the next step, and some day I hope to be able to use all of this. It is not contended that there are no other ways to this end, but for one who knows nothing about this should they follow any of these other methods, they never become aware of what was happening, and thereby are unable to use it and suffer when the stream is cut off which is often the case. This explains a great deal of the unhappiness experienced on the retirement from a very busy and successful career—the stream has been cut off and those people find that they are hardly ever able to re-establish it again. Now this other method which I uphold, enables one to carry on in the same manner as everyone else, yet at all times be conscious of what is taking place and thereby be able to get considerably more out of such worldly activities, and as a result contribute more, but at all times conscious of what is taking place, never letting the stream be cut off. On retirement from any such life, he is able to continue his inner growth, for this is what it is. In other words, through this time-worn method, one is able to see the outcome of all external activity and thereby know how to choose. He knows why some people are happy and others are not, and how it can be corrected if the patient is able to submit to the treatment which is often not the case. Then too, when he finds one exceedingly happy, he knows the nature of that happiness, because he knows why it exists, and once he can examine its source of stimulus, he can predicate many things concerning its future. In other words it permits the individual to approach life with a great understanding, and so be able to penetrate beyond the fiction of all worldly forms, and the most lasting solace to be found in this life is understanding, for it is not so difficult to adjust to misfortune, pain, discomfort, sorrow, and grief if we but understand it.

As the days rolled by, Theos found that his isolation from Tharchin was having the desired effect on his language skills; he was "getting along fine with the chaps even though there is no one around to interpret." Indeed, "so far I have been able to explain everything that has come up and there has been nothing that I have not been able to understand." Just the same, Theos preferred his time alone to the seemingly endless social affairs made deadly dull by the presence of Captain Cable:

My personal reaction is that I am so disgusted with such doings that I do not give a dam [sic] what sort of a nit-wit I may be able to rate; I would rather be silent and dumb than gay and brilliant at such soul-killing affairs. It just about drives me insane—and what to do—you can't leave, and they will not let you sit and watch, or sleep. Here we are a group from all the corners of the earth, with nothing to talk about, except regret that there is not a pack of cards around so that we will not have to play checkers. In the heart of Tibet—one of the most interesting places on earth, with one of the most up and coming personalities of the country, and still nothing to talk about because our friend knows all there is to know about Tibet from his previous year's experience up here. Then too, it must always be remembered that an Englishman knows all there is to know, and especially so when the family has been able to stagnate for six or seven hundred years of recorded disintegration. . . . Jigme is a very interesting personality and speaks English as well as myself. Is there not enough left in humankind to warrant a little effort spent in the direction of extraction? From all outward appearances, the answer is no. . . . It would be easier to climb Everest than to go through one of these ordeals daily, but they like them. . . .

I must admit that my reflections on the English race as revealed by this sort of a specimen, was not very complimentary to them or me. These people know all the answers in the world, and silently plant themselves in such remote corners and bide their time while waiting to talk over the control of the "animals" which surround them. There is only one culture in the world that is right, and that is this good-for-nothing disintegrating English race. Everything else is archaic and unworthy of any consideration. I do not believe that any group of people on earth hold such a national EGO as does this race. They even like to think of us as a bunch of upstarts that do not know what is happening. . . . Thank god there is no way to mar the beauty of the country. If you can just get to [a] window and gaze for a few minutes into space, watching the dance of the late evening shadows, all will quickly settle within and you will be yourself again.

Day after day—as much as he hated it—Theos persisted in his social obligations, even sending a polite and respectful letter to Hugh Richardson requesting a small extension to his Tibet permit, to allow him to finish his studies and avoid a rushed departure since, from his brief correspondence with the agent a week earlier, he had gotten the impression that unlike Cable, Richardson "seems like a real human being."

For several days, Theos was able to maintain his composure, his life punctuated by small encouragements and successes in the form of telegrams and messages: Tharchin had arrived in Lhasa, Chapman had successfully reached the peak of Chomolhari, three others had attempted to cross into Tibet illegally only to be stopped and escorted out,[35] and most significantly of all, Cable was about to leave Gyantse. While Theos was happy for Chapman, who had "climbed the highest peak yet reached by man," as his "only ambition was to get married and settle down, not knowing," Theos remarked somewhat sarcastically, "that he can get married without settling down." Likewise, although happy at Tharchin's news, he was more than amused by the scrambling he witnessed on the part of the British authorities to deal with unauthorized intruders to Tibet. In the most recent case of a Swedish woman apprehended near Yatung, "it has never bean known to have Indian troops arrest a white woman" for "apparently, they never had a provision in their book of rules for a woman who might intrude; so what to do." Remarking on the event at length, Theos observed,

When someone tries to break through . . . on the face of the matter it all looks very simple, but the undercurrents are strong. It is not so much that they care, but each official must protect his face. He must see to it that all is handled in a judicious manner. They are not looking for ways to offer service, but it is promotion that they are thinking about, and one of the things that they like about this spot is that they are given considerable prestige and have nothing to do, but always come out with some sort of a promotion. In the event that something goes wrong and they are called upon to act, it may turn out that they will make a mistake, so they are scared to death. You should see them run for cover in their mad effort to duck responsibility, one person gives an order, and he turns it over to the next in command with instructions, so that if anything does not work out as planned, he will not be to blame; and so it goes on until

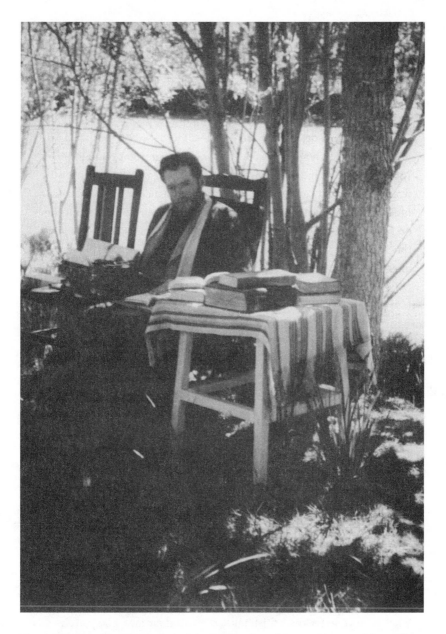

Figure 8.5 Bernard writing and studying in Gyantse while awaiting word from Lhasa
(PAHM)

it winds up in the hands of some incompetent babu who doesn't know what it is all about; so everything goes wrong, but no one cares for the rest are so protected so that they cannot lose, and the poor babu has nothing that he can lose; so it is impossible to find a better system of shakers. And in the meantime, the poor girl sits around in jail wondering what is going to happen, not knowing that wires, cables, and phone calls are being made, all over the world—almost—so that she can have a pleasant journey home. It makes you want to run right out and holler, "Come and catch me, I am on my way to Lhasa," for all the higher ups would delight in it because they would have a chance of going to Lhasa in order to catch you, and they are all so afraid of their positions that they do not dare cause you any inconvenience; so if you should get hungry, the safest thing to do is to get caught; and then all will be cared for in a most elegant fashion.

More than anything else, he was overjoyed at Cable's impending departure for the leisure time it would afford him. Unfortunately, things would get worse before they got better: with the arrival of Colonel Leslie Weir and his wife, cricket and tennis were added to the list of Theos's social obligations, not to mention a general increase in the amount of English conversation in the town since Weir's wife "complains of being unable to sleep or eat, but from the sound of things, the altitude has no effect on her voice-box." Moreover, in a matter of days, the only Tibetan attached to the British Mission in Lhasa, Rai Bahadur Norbu Dondrup, would be passing through Gyantse en route to Lhasa to relieve Hugh Richardson as British Trade Agent.

All the morning, and late last night, mules kept coming, bringing the effects of Norbu who will be with us tomorrow on his way to Lhasa to relieve Mr. Richardson who will return to Gangtok via Shigatse. From here on into Lhasa there are no accommodations; so one must provide his own, and this is what consisted of his advance transport—tents and what have you—for the British must keep up their face, and you should see the caravan the high officials and wealthy landlords take when they make a move—almost a small city in itself; so Norbu is trying to uphold the prestige of the English. In keeping with the custom of the country, there will be multitudes out to meet him tomorrow at the fourth mile. When another is coming, it is the practice to always go meet them so that they can accompany them for the last few miles, and likewise when one leaves, a farewell party always takes place down the line a few miles. Once you travel for days over these vast plains you understand the meaning of this bit of respect. He being a Tibetan who has been elevated to this position in the British Foreign Political, his own countrymen think a great deal of him; so he is honored on both sides wherever he goes, which of course is the thing that the English want, and that is why he has been chosen for the job—not because of any deep affection. He is pleasant enough to meet, for he speaks English fairly well, but his character is that of the typical yes-man always trying to figure what is the right answer and willing to play on all sides of the fence until he is forced to choose, which of course he manages never to do, and for this reason he is more or less unable to do anything really constructive, but sort of acts as political-social go-between to promote friendly diplomatic relationship. At all times you know that he is not your friend, but you wonder whose friend he is, for you can see that he is no more interested in the other fellow than he is in you; but it is all a question of which of the two will bring the most to Norbu, so that leaves me out; but I have a frank American way of handling all such diplomatic eels.

It was not the difficulty of the situation that bothered Theos so much as the annoyance of dealing with condescension, posturing, and hypocrisy. "Why," he exclaimed, should he "have to tolerate it all in Gyantse, for we find it around every corner at home?" However, he would persevere, since "this is a very vital part of the game, for if I did not stand in to the extent of being able to be a guest from sun up until bedtime, it would be hopeless for me to even think of getting anywhere in the country."

Waiting for all and sundry to leave Gyantse—Norbu for Shigatse and everyone else for Yatung—Theos accepted an invitation to lunch at the Taring estate, some ten miles outside of the city. When he spoke with Mary Taring about his apprehension over not having received any word from Lhasa, she advised him to send a cable to the Kashag, requesting that they give his application "their earliest attention," and to contact her sister, Tsarong Lhacham. When he returned to his bungalow that afternoon, however, he was met by a telegram from none other than the Regent himself. His request to visit Lhasa had been accepted:

LHASA

BERNARD, GYANTSE

RECD YOUR LETTER HOPE YOU RECD WIRE FROM KASHAG THAT YOU
ARE MUCH RELIGIONSHIP MAY VISIT LHASA AS YOUR DESIRE WIRE IF
YOU NEED DWELLING HERE = REGENT

He had done it. He had succeeded. Theos was beside himself with excitement. That telegram, he thought, "I will never forget as long as I live."

Within days, word had spread and congratulatory telegrams began arriving—from Gould in Gangtok, and Frank Perry in Kalimpong. Having finessed the situation, Theos felt that he was aware enough of the intricacies of Tibetan politics to "create a loophole so that I can bring others with me on my next visit—which may mean that there will be a pilgrimage of American Buddhists to Tibet within a few years."

Theos now had a busy schedule ahead. In addition to having to mount and label over a thousand recently arrived contact prints, in Tharchin's absence he had to see to all of his logistical concerns personally, from ordering more film and gifts from India to arranging for stores for the trip to Lhasa. In addition, Theos was thoroughly absorbed in his intellectual preparation for Lhasa. Even though he had "a fairly complete library" with him "on all the externals which I have read," he still needed to review it all again "in more minute detail so as not to miss anything." Unfortunately, insofar as religion was concerned, his only resource was L. Austin Waddell's *Lamaism*, a book recognized as embarrassingly biased and inaccurate even in Theos's day. Instead, he knew he would have to start more or less from scratch in his study of the religion.

Theos had been repeatedly told that the essential teachings of the Long-chen-pa tradition were crucial for understanding Tibetan tantric Buddhism, and when it came to the specifics of Tibetan Buddhist doctrines, there was no substitute for the living tradition. As with all these texts, he wrote, "the surface amounts to nothing more than a lot of emotional poetry that says absolutely nothing, but once one has the key to the analogy that is being given, there is little difficulty in understanding its hidden depths, and this is only possible to obtain from the individuals themselves." The broader implications of the tradition were interesting to Theos, for "they do not necessarily write these things in this hidden form to make them obscure, but it is [their] impression that this is the best form for the mind to handle them, for if they are written in a more abstract manner, it will be impossible for anyone but the most learned to comprehend them and in the last analysis, they are anxious to teach others." Nonetheless, he wrote,

> My whole purpose is to penetrate to the bottom of their religious teachings, for therein lies the driving power of the past and the waning framework of today . . . It is not going to be what one sees that will give these answers, but it is going to be the insight gained from the external experience—it is essential to peer beyond in order to sound bottom—as it is with the hidden mineral wealth of the world—one does not see this precious metal but he discovers the dike and knowing the country, he can predict 999 times out of a 1000 what mineral wealth will be found there [when] exploration work is carried on, and so it is with the hidden elements of life—first you learn to understand the character and then you examine the facts in the light of this knowledge and you can be fairly certain of your predictions even tho the people themselves do not know what is coming for the most of them as with the rest of us in the world, do not even know ourselves.

This level of understanding was essential, Theos felt, since "It takes a great deal more [than] a mere grasp of all the factual material involved in this highly complicated system of ritual. The truth is simple enough, and this can only be understood thru the feelings."

It was a conviction that he would express over and over again. This challenge, to gain what Theos thought would be a *real* understanding of the Tibetan people, was something he felt had not been accomplished by any Western writer thus far. Despite the detail in their accounts, "the difficulty with all these descriptions is the fact that they deal only with the majestic external beauty of the Potala and the narrow winding streets of Lhasa which when all [is] said and done does not give you much to go on so far as an understanding of the people." Indeed, Theos thought, the material produced by members of the British Mission thus far seemed concerned with relating the difficulties of "the Mission" itself, rather than gaining any real insight into the Tibetan people, their religion, and way of life. The typical British civil servant, he thought, "could be next to this culture for ten thousand years" and still remain "rotting in his own ignorance and never think to ask a question—but make dam [sic] sure that everyone that he passes salams [sic] him . . . I find that I hate the English and their stagnated traditions."

However, sitting in Gyantse and having read the British Mission reports, Theos could also see that more immediate concerns would affect his desires for study and hopes for the future, for political and social change on the Tibetan plateau was inevitable.

No place in the world does there exist a race of people as untouched as the Tibetans—why is this so with four world potentates trying their best to conquer them; however, on the other hand, a breakdown is coming. Thru what avenues will it proceed, and why must it come? Is all of the past to be discarded? Is there anything to be salvaged?

The answer to these questions, even Theos could not say, despite his other "insights."

Although Hugh Richardson had offered Theos accommodation at Deki Lingka, the British Mission headquarters, west of Lhasa, which would afford him the opportunity to discuss such political issues with the Mission staff. Theos politely (and strategically) declined, suppressing his urge to tell them that he thought them too "satisfied, egotistical, bigoted, conceited, prepossessing and anything else that you can add" to be of any real use to him in his studies. Unbeknownst to the British Mission, Theos had already arranged for his own accommodations and would be the guest of one of the most powerful and influential families in Tibet, and instead would reside in the house of Lord and Lady Tsarong.

Only the day before he intended to leave did the official telegram from the Tibetan Cabinet arrive:

BERNARD OF AMERICA
    GYANTSE
    RECEIVED YOUR LETTER WHICH WE SENT UP TO THE REGENT AND PRIME MINISTER STOP
    AS YOU PROBABLY KNOW TIBET BEING A PURELY RELIGIOUS COUNTRY THERE IS GREAT RESTRICTION ON FOREIGNERS ENTERING THE COUNTRY BUT UNDERSTANDING THAT YOU HAVE A GREAT RESPECT FOR OUR RELIGION AND HAVE HOPES OF SPREADING THE RELIGION IN AMERICA ON YOUR RETURN WE HAVE DECIDED AS A SPECIAL CASE TO ALLOW YOU TO COME TO LHASA BY THE MAIN ROAD FOR A THREE WEEKS VISIT STOP
                                                            KASHAG

With this final piece in place, Theos paid one last visit to the Tibetan Trade Agent, Rai Sahib Wangdi, to pay his bill for accommodations at the dak bungalow, and to the recently arrived Eastern Dzongpön to request letters of transport to Lhasa, which would instruct the local village headmen to provide him with pack animals and sundry necessities. These final details out of the way, Theos was ready to depart. Although the typical trip from Gyantse to Lhasa required ten stops over ten days, Theos was too anxious to pander to the financial protocols of each way station and hoped to make double stages, arriving in Lhasa after only five days. Of course, in Tibet as in India, nothing ever goes as planned.

As he waited in the bungalow the night before departure, his transit letters had still not arrived from the Dzongpön. After several more envoys making inquiries, the letters arrived, but accompanied by a message from the local village headman that he could not provide pack animals for at least two more days—a delay that Theos had no intention of tolerating. Instead, Theos met with the headman, and it was finally agreed that transport would arrive at 6 a.m. the next day.

Hoping that he had sorted that situation out, Theos took the opportunity to send telegrams to Lhasa with his revised schedule, only to learn that the Lhasa telegraph operator had gone home early and simply unplugged the telegraph line (as they were wont to do). Resigned to his messages going out the next morning, he found his attempts to have any telegrams sent to him at Gyantse forwarded to Lhasa blocked as well. Such was not done, Theos was informed, but they *could* transcribe the messages and send them on via postal carrier to Lhasa. "Hell they might just as well not be sent!" Theos thought, and trying to contain his rage attempted to negotiate other solutions to the problem, before finally just giving up and deciding to deal with it later. "The only thing narrower in this world than the thoughts of an Indian Babu is that of another under him, and no matter how high you ascend into the kingdom of Babudom—they are all dumb!"

Returning to the bungalow, Theos discovered that the mail had arrived, bringing a letter from Viola. On the verge of being "about to sail out into another sea of the great unknown," he found it both a happy contact with home and a reminder of all the mundane concerns she faced daily that made her life so radically different from his. Reminding him that with the right emphasis, their trip could be tax deductible, Viola suggested that he maintain "a sort of monthly itemization of expenses" and save his receipts. This would be easily justifiable if they could succeed in setting up a Tibetan wool importing business, and she informed Theos of what she had found out about the business in America. In other news, she informed him, his father had arrived in New York, and though she had seen him briefly, he had not visited his brother in Nyack, and was now "reorienting himself" back in Los Angeles. Asking him to keep in mind different strategies for self-promotion—something Theos needed little reminder about—Viola informed him that their friend Herbert had a new system for making large-format photographic enlargements, so he should earmark some photos for this purpose, and as an example, included with her letter a newspaper clipping from the *New York Times Magazine* on the search for the fourteenth Dalai Lama in Tibet, written by Sir Charles Bell and illustrated with photographs by Nicholas Roerich.[36]

Even though the mail went from Kalimpong to Phari every day, it was transported from Phari to Gyantse only twice a week. Anticipating of the next day's departure, Theos was too excited to sleep and so took the opportunity to write to both Viola and DeVries. To Viola, Theos wrote of his activities up to that point, taking the time to quote the "Historical Document from the Representatives of the Lord Buddha on Earth"—his telegram from the Kashag—and couldn't help gloating a little in response to Viola's earlier concerns.

it might be your reaction to think that I am crazier than ever before; however if you do, do not hesitate to tell me so, because that is the most important thing in life so far as I am concerned . . . it is that uncontrollable little bug that keeps pushing my way around like this—and now Lhasa—to the moon next I suppose. Aside from all these things, what do you think of the whole affair—have I been out of my head to work this all out and then make it happen by myself. You do not have to say much, because the truth of the matter is that I pretty well know how you feel about [it], otherwise there would not have been those long, long, long continual letters exchanged between you and Welch—nor would you have suggested that I get Lindbergh to fly in; so you see, you really have given me your answer months ago.

Nonetheless, Theos reminded her, "Please do not get mad and do not talk, because when all is said and done, it doesn't amount to three whoops in hell . . . and always know that there is a Lama who loves you and it is growing deeper and deeper with each added experience." Feeling vindicated by his success despite Viola's worries, Theos remained convinced of the validity of his course of action.

Writing to DeVries, Theos adopted a decidedly different tone, not feeling any need to justify himself in her eyes. "My Dear DeVries," he wrote,

> I have no idea how much you know about the inaccessibility of Lhasa which is one of the most Sacred Cities of the world to which virtually no one is permitted to go, and never in history has there been a record of an invitation being extended to one to come there for the purpose of a religious pilgrimage . . . All this being true, it makes me feel that I must have tapped something deep that such a privilege has been extended to me . . .
>
> [L]et us plan now on some long quiet uninterrupted hours when I can relate these endless activities which will reveal an insight to be found in no books, in fact, it is impossible to put them into name and form . . . Everything only furnishes more food for thought, and so I am excepting [sic] this privilege with a greater receptive consciousness then [sic] has ever been before. . . .
>
> From now on I will be far removed from any regular mail service; so please forgive if you do not hear until I contact Western Civilization again.
>
> Lots of Love,
> Theos

This was precisely the sort of letter DeVries would have expected, for unlike her soon-to-be ex-husband, Pierre, she was convinced already that Theos was naturally spiritual.

Finally ready for sleep, Theos decided not to leave anything to chance and gave instructions to be awakened at 3:30 a.m. Roused as instructed, Theos immediately sent one of his "boys" over to the muleteer's house to ensure that the mules arrived by 6. With some effort they began to arrive at 5:30, and when they were finally loaded and sent off at 7, Theos turned his attention to the telegraph office one more time. For the better part of two hours, telegrams were sent north to Lhasa and south to Darjeeling and Calcutta. Finally convinced that his messages had gone out and none was waiting to be delivered, he returned to the bungalow, and together with his assistants, headed off down the road to Lhasa.

After a little more than a half an hour, Theos began to get the impression that something was not quite right. Querying his companions, he discovered that none them actually knew how to get to Lhasa; they had been following his lead down whatever random path Theos had chosen going out of town. Turning back to Gyantse, they decided that the simplest course of action would be to follow the telegraph line. So, once again, they were off.

Back in landscape that seemed familiar, Theos finally began to find some mental rest. The road ahead was very reminiscent of the packed dirt trails he had spent so much time traversing as a young boy in Arizona. The high canyon walls of rock and earth rising sharply for hundreds of feet on either side lent the scenery a certain comforting feeling and gave the sense that his presence there was purely natural. Of course the rushing water at the bottom of the canyon offered the only incongruity; where dry riverbeds of sand and scrub greeted the traveler through Arizona, here the perpetually snow-capped peaks kept the rivers lush and flowing, winding their way to India and the oceans beyond. With the occasion monastery or hermitage dotting the mountains in the distance, the idyllic vision spread out before him laid his otherwise preoccupied mind to rest as they traveled throughout the day.

The days that followed offered Theos unending anecdotes to fill his journals with. From the rest stops where the staff cleaned and shined the tables by spitting on them to the glint of the glaciers approaching the pass at Karo-la, sparkling for miles around, the whole valley seemed teeming with life and beauty. Small, gopherlike animals darted between the feet of his pony and scores of small sparrows swooped from side to side as they passed through narrow gorges. Indeed, the wildlife filling the land seemed almost tame.

Despite the weariness of travel, Theos remained determined to record "the details of the day," realizing that they would be likely to be lost if he did not set them down. It was not always easy, however, since Theos's typewriter was traveling with the pack animals, and he would often have to wait for them to arrive to add to his diary.

The middle of the second day, Theos and his party spied a lone figure approaching in the distance. Theos eventually recognized the man: it was Norphel, his syce, whom Tharchin had taken along to Lhasa, headed back to escort Theos the rest of the way. While the two men were overjoyed at their reunion and the success of Theos's petition, of greater import was the content of Tharchin's letter to Theos that Norphel had been carrying. Beyond detailing his activities that had led to the success of his envoy, Tharchin wrote that he had been busy laying the foundation for Theos's arrival; in addition to talking about Theos with everyone he met in Lhasa, Tharchin had "friends at Drepung and Sera and told [them] about you and all the monks are waiting for you."

For three more days, Theos and his party pushed on, passing the stops of his preordained itinerary, pausing for a meal or a night's rest—longer if fresh transport was needed—documenting every stage of the journey with a photo or two. When they reached the ferry point at Chaksam, their pack animals were loaded onto "a large wooden ferry" while they made the crossing in small yakhide boats beneath iron chains dangling overhead—the remnants of an old suspension bridge dating from the fifteenth century. Stopping at last just past Chu-shur for the night, they found Theos's efforts to rush the trip had paid off: it was June 23, and the next day he would arrive in Lhasa.

Although Theos had succeeded in pushing the entire party seventy miles in one day, it was not without consequences: the next morning the party awoke to discover that one of the ponies had gone lame. With nothing to be done and only two fresh ponies available, Norphel stepped forward and offered to walk the last fifty miles to Lhasa. With no other option, Theos agreed, and he and Hla-re set off, leaving Norphel to walk, falling farther and farther behind as the day progressed.

Norphel, however, was far from resourceless, and several hours later as Theos and Hla-re approached the Lhasa valley, the sound of galloping and yelling startled them from behind. Having negotiated with local residents along the way, Norphel had secured his own pony and was racing to catch up. Eager to show Theos the best vantage point for his first glimpse of Lhasa, Norphel led the party to a small hill. From this outcrop eight miles out of the city the crowning architectural achievement of Tibetan civilization, the Potala Palace, could be seen. Each day, as the sun broke over the mountains, from all around the Lhasa valley, the golden roofs of the Potala shone like a brilliant beacon in all directions to lead pilgrims toward their destination. This, at least, was the effect it had on Theos, making him and his party all the more anxious to reach the city.

After negotiating a rocky ridge, we entered upon a broad highway, which still further widened into a twelve-lane thoroughfare, overcrowded with yaks and donkeys, and us on our royal horses riding in between them. It was but a short distance before we came around the bend which sheltered the great monastery of Drepung, the largest in the world, holding in the neighborhood of 10,000 monks. It was a startling sight: white masonry studded over with the black spots, which indicated the endless series of chambers, gloomy cells of meditation. . . . I had seen endless pictures of this sanctuary, yet it was wholly unlike such preliminary impressions. The truth is, no film could possibly convey its majesty. There is a sense of immaculateness about it which eludes the camera, so faithful in capturing external forms.

As they passed the monastery and drew closer to the city gates, they found an official government escort waiting for them. No sooner had they made their greeting than Theos spotted "Tharchin racing thru a cloud of dust" coming to meet them. It was a happy reunion for all, and Theos was overjoyed to see Tharchin again, for he knew that without Tharchin's assistance he would never have made it so far. In addition to bringing the small movie camera with which to film Theos's arrival—"he never forgets anything," Theos thought—Tharchin also brought fresh horses, courtesy of Lord Tsarong, upon which they could pass through the western gate into the city. Passing by the Potala and on through the small enclave of buildings that formed the city, they headed just south of the central temple of the Jokhang to the Tsarong estate. Although Lord Tsarong had been scheduled to survey bridge construction that day, Tharchin informed Theos that upon hearing of his pending arrival Tsarong had postponed his plans in order to properly greet his guest.

Arriving at the front of the main house, Tharchin was ready with two white silk *khatas* for Theos to present to Lord Tsarong and his wife, Tsarong Lhacham. Too embarrassed to use his broken, low colloquial Tibetan, Theos offered his *khatas* in silence rather than risk offense with nonhonorific speech, before being led into his quarters, his home for the coming months. A model of modern comfort and civility, the Tsarongs' home was exquisitely decorated with both Tibetan and European furniture and a wealth of modern amenities imported from all around the world, and even an orchard of apple trees, whose seeds had been imported from America. "The house itself," Tsarong's son recounted,

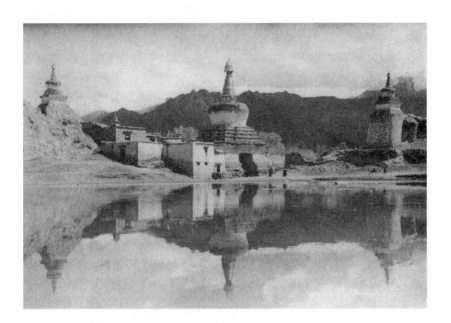

Figure 8.6 The Western Gate into Lhasa (PAHM)

was a two-storied, rectangular building containing thirty-six rooms of different sizes. Concrete steps in front of the house led to a big hall. The hall had beautiful carvings on the wooden beams and pillars, and exquisite drawings and paintings on the walls. Doors from this hall led to the eastern and western suites, and an inner door led to a staircase going up to the second floor of the mansion. This main hall was large and spacious, measuring thirty feet by thirty feet. . . . Four large store rooms lay behind the main suites and hall on the ground floor. The upper floor contained a similar hall, which was set aside as the main family chapel, known to everyone in the house as the Choegyal Khang. This name, meaning "The House of the Religious Kings" was given because images of three religious kings of Tibet were enshrined there.[37] . . . The walls of the Choegyal Khang were lined with scriptures and *thangkas* (religious paintings), and a large altar in the center of the room was full of offerings, butter lamps, and incense which burned continuously throughout the day and night. All family ceremonies and prayer gatherings took place in this room. A corridor from the staircase led to the east and west wings. Each suite contained a spacious living room, a bedroom, a private prayer room, a bathroom, a large storeroom, and an office. One of the living rooms set aside for our guests was pillarless, and iron beams were substituted for wooden ones, which was much of a novelty to our relatives and friends at that time. A library containing many foreign books, a guest suite, and a banquet hall were situated behind the family rooms. ... The house was, on the whole, well planned and spacious, including modern windows with glass panes, which were much talked about in Lhasa, as houses in Tibet did not have glass windows at that time.[38]

As impressive as all this was to Theos, most impressive of all was Lord Tsarong himself. Although he was a man of small stature, his bearing and very presence conveyed far more.

Born in 1888, the Tibetan year of the Earth Mouse, Dasang Damdul spent his early childhood in Lhasa under the care of an aunt. Sent for tutoring to one of the many private schools in Lhasa,[39] he came to the notice of the Thirteenth Dalai Lama through his teacher, Khangnyi Jinpa, a steward of the summer palace. Always a keen observer, "the Great Thirteenth" noticed that the young boy in the steward's charge was exceptionally intelligent and had him transferred to his personal staff.

Called "Chensel" by His Holiness,[40] in time Dasang Damdul became one of the Great Thirteenth's most closely trusted advisors, accompanying him both as a political consultant and as commander of his personal escort. When Francis Younghusband and the British army invaded Tibet and advanced on Lhasa, the Great Thirteenth fled north and east toward Mongolia and China, taking Khangnyi Jinpa and Dasang Damdul along as part of his entourage. Over the course of their five years of self-imposed exile from Tibet, His Holiness gave religious teachings throughout Mongolia and China,[41] while Dasang Damdul learned to speak Mongolian and received Russian military training courtesy of Tzar Nicholas II's envoy in Mongolia, Agwan Dorjiev. Following their meeting with the Chinese Empress Dowager in 1908 and the subsequent deaths of the Chinese Emperor and Empress, it was decided that the time to return to Tibet had come: reports were beginning to arrive of military aggression by petty Chinese warlords in the borderlands.

By the time the party returned to Tibet in 1909, reports of Chinese looting and murder on the Tibetan–Chinese border were increasing, and shortly after the Tibetan New Year in spring 1910, Chinese forces arrived in Lhasa itself at the order of Chao Erh-feng—"the butcher Chao," as he was known—randomly shooting residents of the city on sight. Once again the

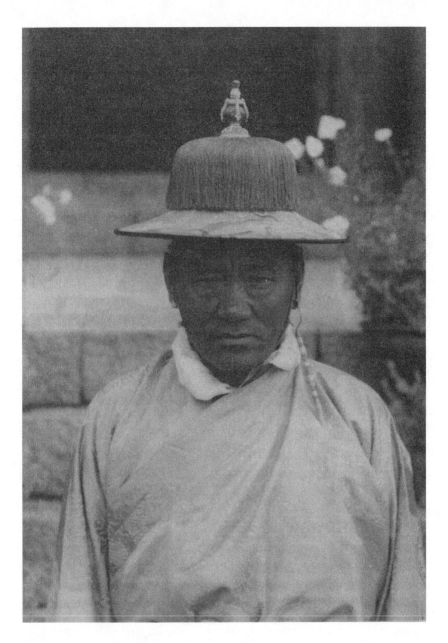

Figure 8.7 Lord Tsarong, Dasang Damdul (PAHM)

Great Thirteenth assembled his entourage for a flight from his homeland. Anticipating the worst, they left that very night, crossing the Kyi-chu River at the Ramagang Ferry south of the summer palace, and making their way south and west toward Sikkim and British India. Directing operations from Chamdo, receiving his lieutenant's report on this, Chao Erh-feng was enraged and offered a reward to the man who would bring him "the head of the Dalai Lama."[42] Dasang Damdul and his men followed the escape route taken by the Great Thirteenth's entourage—as did the Chinese force pursuing both of their parties—and at Chaksam Ferry four miles outside of Lhasa, decided to make a stand.

With only sixty-seven men to serve as the rear guard for His Holiness, Dasang Damdul was seriously outnumbered by the pursuing force of close to three hundred Chinese troops. Crossing the river and pulling their boats to shore, he and his men took up positions on the far ridge and waited for the Chinese troops to arrive. Shortly after dawn the Chinese had assembled on the far shore of Chaksam and seeing the ferryboats secured, had begun building their own rafts by ransacking nearby houses. Remaining in hiding, Dasang Damdul waited until the Chinese troops began their crossing on makeshift rafts and wooden beams, and then, firing the first shot himself, he and his men opened fire. Before the smoke had cleared his small Tibetan guard had felled more than half of the Chinese force. Having successfully engineered his first battle at the age of twenty-one, for his actions in defense of the life of the Thirteenth Dalai Lama, Dasang Damdul would come to be known as the "Hero of Chaksam Ferry." Out of ammunition and feeling that they had bought the Great Thirteenth's entourage as much time as they could, Dasang Damdul dispersed his men, and taking two servants with him, headed south to join His Holiness in exile.

It was the young David Macdonald, stationed as British Trade Agent at Yatung, who personally met the Thirteenth Dalai Lama upon his arrival at the border town[43] and secured his safe transport southward across the border.[44] Although Macdonald then waited for Dasang Damdul, word of whose imminent arrival had been sent from Phari, by the time he reached Yatung, fresh Chinese forces were already at the border, with the promise of a reward for his head as well. Disguised by Macdonald as a postal carrier, despite suffering from exhaustion, Dasang Damdul succeeded in crossing through the ranks of the Chinese guards while they lay in their cots smoking opium. Safely reaching Kalimpong, Dasang Damdul rejoined His Holiness's party. David Macdonald would later turn down a knighthood for saving their lives, though he accepted their friendship unconditionally and remained close to the Great Thirteenth and Dasang Damdul's family over the decades that followed.

For more than a year, Dasang Damdul stayed in the entourage of the Thirteenth Dalai Lama as he traveled in India[45] and consulted with the British authorities, receiving more military training, this time by the British in Darjeeling. By 1911 it was decided that the time had come to retake Tibet from her Chinese occupiers; charging him with leading the effort, the Great Thirteenth conferred upon Dasang Damdul the title of Commander General and sent him back to Tibet. Proceeding north from Sikkim toward the Ghampa Dzong (fort), and gathering men and arms along the way, the new commander first retook the fort at Shigatse before moving on to Nadong and then to Lhasa, bringing several Chinese soldiers who had come over to the Tibetans' side.[46] Meeting with loyal factions in Lhasa who had remained in communication with the Great Thirteenth—members of the newly formed War Department of the National Assembly (the *Tsongdu*[47])—Dasang Damdul strategized about the best way to take the Chinese garrisons. For many days the fighting went on, often hand-to-hand in the streets, led by Dasang Damdul himself. In the end nearly all the Chinese troops had been defeated with only a few holdouts remaining. Cut off from their supply lines by the recent Chinese revolution and the fall of the Ch'ing dynasty, the last Chinese holdouts quickly lost morale and eventually surrendered to the commander's forces.[48]

Adding humiliation to their defeat, the captured Chinese soldiers were stripped of their weapons—except for the officers, at Dasang Damdul's instruction—and, prohibited by the Tibetan government from returning to China by traveling east across Tibet, instead were forced to go south to India and thence to China by boat. Although Dasang Damdul secured permission for some soldiers to stay in the city, where they ran Chinese restaurants and the like, most settled in Calcutta, populating that city's Chinatown district and making a life for themselves in the Indian subcontinent.

With the Thirteenth Dalai Lama and his aids en route back to Lhasa, members of the Tibetan aristocracy who had aided the commander held a secret meeting of the national assembly in which it was decided to arrest all the government officials appointed by the former Chinese military administration. Although actually appointed by the Thirteenth Dalai Lama, the head of the House of Tsarong, Kalön Wangchuk Gyalpo, was included on the list by his political enemies, and before the Great Thirteenth could return to Lhasa, he and his eldest son had been murdered. Forced to deal with the ongoing political intrigues in his government, the Thirteenth Dalai Lama lamented the desolation of the House of Tsarong and to maintain its lineage, recommended that the Commander General, Dasang Damdul, be married into the family and take over as head of the household.

Given the title of lord (Dzasak) and later promoted to cabinet minister (Shapé),[49] Lord Dasang Damdul Tsarong—Tsarong Shapé, as he came to be known—would spearhead the Great Thirteenth's modernization initiatives over the next twenty years. Charged with modernizing Tibet's defenses and social infrastructure, he began a campaign of construction, importation, and training designed to meet the needs of the Tibetan nation facing imminent external threats. Inviting S. W. Laden La—who had served as liaison officer to both the Panchen Lama in 1905 and the Dalai Lama in 1910 in India—up to Lhasa from Darjeeling, Tsarong had him reform the Lhasa police force (personally serving as Lhasa's Chief of Police for several years) while Tsarong reformulated the Tibetan military along the lines of the British model. A contingent of four students was sent to England for technical training, and a new mint for producing standardized, machine-made Tibetan currency was established, which Tsarong personally oversaw. Importing generators from India, Tsarong electrified the streets of Lhasa, installing street lighting and telegraph lines and even constructing a makeshift movie theater in one of the local parks (lingka).

By the early 1920s all of the Great Thirteenth's initiatives were well under way, but they were expensive, while the financial base of the Tibetan government remained weak,[50] and Tibet still faced major challenges in modernizing its infrastructure. Although progress was being made, some problems seemed unavoidable. In 1925, an outbreak of smallpox decimated the population of Lhasa, and years later, visitors reported that one could still smell the stench of death on the outskirts of the city, where the bodies of the dead had been burned.[51] Seeing that much more remained to be done, on his own initiative, Tsarong explored the possibility of mining some of Tibet's natural resources, gold and other ores, as a means of funding the new measures, but reactions were strongly negative in many quarters and Tsarong was forced to abandon the idea. Instead, members of the aristocracy put forth another option.

Ten years earlier, during the immediate aftermath of the overthrow of the Chinese occupation, the Ninth Panchen Lama, having always had close ties with Chinese patrons—a fact that greatly contributed to the wealth of Tashilhunpo Monastery in Shigatse—understandably had become nervous about the events unfolding in Lhasa, since on several occasions he had met and had amicable relations with the Chinese occupation administration. Laden La had been allowed to serve as mediator between the Panchen Lama and the reinstated Lhasa government, but the détente was an uneasy one and a decade later, relations began to break down again. Arguing that the Panchen Lama and his Shigatse administration had never been properly punished for their collaboration with the Chinese ten years earlier, factions in the Lhasa government decided that heavy taxation on his Shigatse estates would be an appropriate means of both punishment and funding the new modernization measures. Thus, when additional taxes were proposed for the aristocratic families in Lhasa, a 25 percent tax on all the estates of the Panchen Lama was put forward. Refusing to pay the new taxes and fearing for his life, in 1923 the Ninth Panchen Lama fled Tibet for Mongolia and China.

Even with some of the advantages that the Great Thirteenth's progressive measures had brought to Tibet, not everyone was happy with the new course, or with the men he entrusted to implement the changes—least of all with the young and energetic Lord Tsarong and the apparently increasing power of the military.[52] While his opponents spread rumors that Tsarong was positioning himself for a military takeover of the government, it was Tsarong's attempts to enforce strict military protocols in the new Tibetan army, in particular, having two men shot for murder—in contravention of the Tibetan government's prohibition against capital punishment—that ultimately undermined his efforts. It was the excuse his opponents needed to point to his presumption of autonomy from the country's central authorities.

As a result, on his way home from a visit to India for military procurements, Tsarong was informed by messenger that he had been relieved of duty as commander of the Tibetan military. A few years later, in 1929, as more ambitious elements within the Tibetan aristocracy led by the Finance Minister, Tsipön Lungshar,[53] strove to consolidate their power and influence in the Tibetan government, Tsarong was targeted as a potential threat to their plans and even stripped of his position as cabinet minister; later he would be offered the post again but would decline it.

In the midst of these intrigues, the Great Thirteenth could see the dangers for the future of a free and independent Tibet. Although traditionally, the Dalai Lama gave a teaching every year as part of his regular New

Year's activities, in 1933, His Holiness the Thirteenth deviated from the past pattern of speaking strictly on religious matters. Instead of a prayer or dedication, this time he issued a proclamation—a warning—that would be repeated and read far and wide, carried in Tharchin's *Mirror* newspaper, and even translated into English:

All of you, both Sangha and lay people alike, should do all that you can to help preserve the unique spiritual heritage of our country. In turn, the stability of this heritage depends upon the strength and wellbeing of our unique form of government. If our government remains strong, our heritage can be maintained without degeneration. Whether or not this can be achieved depends very much upon the strength and integrity of the individual people working in the various government positions. The present international atmosphere is not very good for us. A number of our neighbors are building strong armies and seem to be motivated by hostile and aggressive attitudes. Their actions do not encourage confidence in a peaceful future. We have come up with a strategy whereby we can avoid being invaded and taken over.

Unfortunately we seem to be of a situation internally wherein everyone working in the government is motivated solely by self-interests. Monks and lay officials alike, both high and low, everyone with any government position seems to be concerned more with personal gain than how to contribute to the wellbeing of the country. Falsity, flattery and deceptiveness seem to have become integral features of political life . . . if we just continue with the present trend for chasing self-interests alone and competing with one another for who can set the worst example, the future can only bring disaster. This is being unkind to both oneself and others. It is self-deception, and is a great weakness bringing harm on both immediate and long-term levels. . . .

It is perhaps not right for me to confidently stick out my neck and speak to you as I have above. But I thought that if I were to say these things to you there may be some amongst you who would listen. I have set out these ideas as reminders and as material for reflection. The decisions concerning them are up to you. I really hope that you don't make the wrong choices.[54]

By December 1933, as it became clear to the Great Thirteenth that little was changing to secure the safety of Tibet, many say that he took matters into his own hands. Dismissing the abbot of the medical college, Khenrap Norbu, as his personal physician, a few weeks later the Great Thirteenth became ill and with little warning, suddenly died. As word spread of his death, different factions braced themselves for the ensuing political struggle. To the east, the Paṇchen Lama mobilized a Chinese army and prepared to return to Tibet to head a new interim government, but few people in positions of power would have welcomed such an obvious subversion of Tibetan autonomy. Sending supplies to reinforce the Tibetan army at the Chinese border, the cabinet and national assembly instructed commanders in eastern Tibet to keep the Paṇchen Lama from bringing a Chinese army— and the Chinese government—with him to Lhasa. With Chinese influence thus held at bay, others had their own plans.

It had been close to three hundred years since a king had controlled the destiny of Tibet. When the Fifth Dalai Lama—"the Great Fifth"—summoned the warlords of Mongolia in the late seventeenth century to crush an imperial army bent on overthrowing him and the growing strength of the great monastic universities of the Lhasa valley, Tibet became united under his rule, and the world witnessed the closest mankind ever came to realizing Plato's dream of a benevolent philosopher-king. But not everyone thought so, least of all Tsipön Lungshar, who, having accompanied the four boys sent to England for Western education twenty years earlier, admired the British system of governance, but moreover saw in England a role model for the peaceful transition from a monarchy to a civil government. Hoping to engineer a similar overthrow of Tibet's monastic government, by the time of the death of the Great Thirteenth, Lungshar and other members of the aristocracy had been plotting for some time.

In this atmosphere of political intrigue, two men in particular vied for power in the struggle for a nominally secular future Tibetan government. One was Lungshar, a personal friend of the late Thirteenth Dalai Lama and one of the four *shapés* who dominated the cabinet. It was he who had engineered Tsarong's downfall and positioned himself to take over the military. His political scheming in recent years had made him powerful and his lavish treatment of the monasteries and military had given him a strong base of support, but he was disliked and distrusted by the other members of the aristocracy. The other figure in the forefront of political machinations was Kapshöpa,[55] an early recruit to the inner circle of conspirators who had earned the favor of the cabinet by dint of his amiable nature but who, unbeknownst to all, had higher ambitions.

Working together at first, they gathered a group of friends and founded their own political organization, the Unification Party. Holding clandestine meetings, they recruited more and more followers and one by one, their opponents fell through their political conniving. By May 1934, the government seemed ripe for takeover and Lungshar made his play for power. But Kapshöpa had struck first. Moving the Unification Party meetings into public view, Lungshar had become overconfident. He boldly put forth his proposal for a new government and a new constitution that would turn Tibet into a republic. Assured that he would win over the hearts and minds of the cabinet and lead Tibet into a new era, he overplayed his hand, for the cabinet and national assembly had already been tipped off to his motives. Just days earlier, Kapshöpa had warned high-ranking leaders in the government that Lungshar was plotting their assassination and at the same time, led monastery officials to believe that the establishment of a republic would spell the end of Buddhism in Tibet in their lifetimes.

When Lungshar walked into a cabinet meeting days later, rather than receiving the affirmation he expected, he found himself in the middle of an inquisition. Kapshöpa, although there to testify against him, in the process indicted himself as well. What could have been a true political revolution turned into a fearsome backlash. Before the dust had settled, a half dozen nobles were stripped of their lands and titles and sent into exile. Lungshar himself received the harshest punishment of all: his eyes were to be gouged out and he was to be imprisoned in the dungeons of the Potala Palace, condemned to spend the rest of his days in darkness and squalor.[56]

Tsarong had weathered all of these turbulent events at a safe distance—in Western Tibet at the time of the Great Thirteenth's passing—and thereby escaped retribution. Despite his demotion and the loss of the Thirteenth Dalai Lama as his personal friend and protector, Tsarong's fame and reputation as a just and truly "noble" man only seemed to increase, leading Ernst Schäfer to declare *him* the "uncrowned king of Tibet."

Still a powerful man at age fifty, Lord Tsarong had an air of personal fortitude that was not lost on his young foreign guest. Lord Tsarong was "as charming a personality that one could ever hope to spend an hour [with]," and as time went on, Theos's esteem for the man would only increase, for Theos could see that "he continues his education of the outside world, already being miles ahead of any other Tibetan in all of Tibet." With the threats of the modern world constantly at Tibet's borders, Theos felt there would be hope for the Tibetans "if they had another hundred like him."

Led to his suite of rooms on the ground floor of the Tsarong home, Theos was impressed by the luxury of it all:

> The low cushions upon which one does all of his work, etc. were cover[ed] with their lovely Tibetan rugs of oriental design. The wall likewise carried out the pattern of the room with a beautiful border painted in red, green, yellow, and blue. And so this was to [be] my home in Lhasa—never could I dream of such comforts, for I also had a separate bedroom, and store room for my boxes, as well as a toilet with modern thimble, towel rack, and portable bathtub—in fact, it was all much better than many places I had been in India.

Along with a Western-style desk for his convenience, Theos had everything he would need for the coming days.

When he joined Lord Tsarong and his wife for tiffin, through Tharchin as translator, Tsarong had many questions for Theos.

> He was anxious to know what I felt could be done for his country and what possibilities there were etc. etc. so the most of the afternoon was spent in going over these details which he was eager to hear about, but as he said at the end it is a self-satisfied religious country so what to do—let them continue on, for they are all happy as they are, and new things might cause trouble, for it will necessarily bring them to the place were they will have to negotiate with the rest of the world using India and China as markets for exporting and importing; and this will get them involved; so they will continue to remain isolated from the rest of the world.

After several hours, not content to spend his first day in Lhasa indoors, Theos insisted on going out to the telegraph office and the British Mission, ostensibly to visit the British Political Officer, to whom he was obliged to announce his presence in Lhasa, although the Tsarongs insisted that both were "out" for the day and unreachable. Eventually locating the office, Theos did indeed find the British telegraph operators out, but was able to work out the details of sending and receiving telegrams from Lhasa before visiting Deki Lingka, home to the British Mission.

Meeting the Political Officer, Hugh Richardson, and Reginald Fox, the telegraph operator—who, having heard of Theos's arrival, took his presence as an excuse to leave a day-long Tibetan party—Theos sat down with them for what would be a long talk. Of Richardson and Fox, Theos's first impressions were not far from his expectations.

[Richardson] was a most understanding chap. Rather young—in his thirties, very slender with the typical Oxford Droll and overflowing with their brilliancy, not knowing much about anything—but should never be able to detect this because of all that they do know. His partner, Mr. Fox, who is the wireless man, is a nice heavy set chap, making the impression of a "very nice boy" at the beginning, when afterwards I discovered that he was only an over fed devote [sic] Catholic. They were both keen about cameras; so for hours we went into such details, they bringing out endless pictures for me to see. Knowing my interest in Buddhism, the conversation drifted to many of their teachings with our intelligentsia always pointing out an error that the mind may have. Long ago, I learned to never argue once I know my personality—and never hope to instruct—for they do not want the embarrassment of learning from you—but will straighten things out privately, if you do not touch the pride and only plant the seed for them to nourish alone; so we talked and I listened.

Their teatime talk having turned into dinner, which then ran late into the night, Theos rode his horse back to the Tsarong estate "at a full gallop in the moonlight under the Potala." Upon arriving at his temporary home, he was startled to find the entire courtyard of Tsarong's estate lit up with electric lights, which made it feel "very comfortable." Paying his respects with a final cup of tea, he retired for the night.

Waking early the next morning, Theos sat down to plan his agenda for Lhasa, since he was determined to "do that which has never been done before by a European so far as it is possible to find out from present records." Soon, however, it was time for breakfast—the Tsarongs having insisted that Theos take all of his meals with them. Both a blessing for the opportunity it offered and a trial as a challenge to his language abilities, Theos was happy and apprehensive at the same time. While he felt more than comfortable stammering out what low Tibetan was at his command when speaking with servants, he was at a great disadvantage when speaking with the

Tibetan nobility. Determined to force Theos to improve his Tibetan, Tsarong Lhacham suggested that Tharchin take his meals in a separate room—to keep Theos from relying on him as translator—and promised him long tutorial conversations throughout the day while her husband was otherwise occupied.

At the top of Theos's list of things to discuss with Lord Tsarong was the acquisition of a Kangyur and Tengyur. Although the new Lhasa Kangyur was a good fallback option, Tsarong informed Theos, the better Kangyur-Tengyur pairs were to be had from Narthang (near Shigatse to the west) and Derge (in Eastern Tibet). The former was printed from carved wooden blocks that had deteriorated with use and age—realistically, all the prints were good for by then was as decorative editions or for mixing into mortar for *stūpa* construction—but the Derge blocks had been cast in iron and offered the best quality reproductions. Tsarong himself had only obtained his copies by sending his own paper and ink to the printing house in Eastern Tibet. Indeed, Tsarong thought it would not be difficult for Theos to obtain permission to leave Tibet via China, passing through Derge, instead of returning south to India, and thereby obtain a copy for himself.

Finishing breakfast, Tsarong prepared to inspect the new Trisam bridge southwest of the city, having postponed the trip from the previous day, though he agreed to first look over Theos's presents for the officials with whom he would soon be meeting. Everything Theos had bought had arrived intact, but he was dismayed to learn that although his present for the Regent, Reting Rinpoche, was suitable, it was customary to give him *two* presents. Retreating to a room in his house, Tsarong returned moments later with one of the many museum-quality artworks adorning his home, giving it to Theos to use as the second gift.

Although Theos had hoped to find time to study, soon it was time for lunch, and at the midday meal, he and Tsarong Lhacham were shortly joined by the first Tibetan official to call on him, Khenrap Kunsang Mondong, one of the magistrates of Zhöl (the administrative complex at the foot of the Potala Palace), arriving with gifts on behalf of the Kashag: "a half a dozen sacks of flour and about fifteen dozen eggs, a large sack of butter (50 lbs or so) and a large tray of vegetables." One of the four boys sent to England along with Lungshar twenty years earlier, Mondong spoke impeccable English, and together they discussed "all sorts of things—of course always planting seeds"—with Theos convinced that he was quickly gaining proficiency in "this game of winning diplomatic points in idle conversation."

Finally excusing himself to attend to the logistics of his stay, Theos visited the telegraph office again, where he found telegrams from Viola, his mother-in-law, and his brother-in-law, congratulating him on reaching Lhasa. That same day, Theos received his first batch of letters via the British Mission, including one from Viola sent weeks earlier, congratulating him on becoming "the First American Student of Tibetan Buddhism." Informing him that the Kangyur shipped from Calcutta had arrived safely in New York and was stored in her mother's house in Nyack, she took the opportunity to tell him all about *her* life over the past few weeks, including starting her internship in the psychiatry ward at Jersey Medical, as well as the reactions to their resignation from the CCC.[57]

The next morning came early for Theos, as the realities of his day-to-day time commitments became increasingly clear. He had been given permission for only a three-week visit to Lhasa, and he would need almost every second of every day to accomplish everything on his agenda. Consequently, Theos would have to spend hours each morning prior to breakfast in order to fix his plans for the day, write his diary, make an effort at language study, and document his photographs.

Having heard that the Regent would be returning to his monastic estate in a few days, Theos put meeting with him at the top of his list of activities for the first day. It would be a very sensitive and important meeting, for

I may come back to these parts if I am able to establish a strong enough contact—which I am trying to do in my silent little way—the future is always with us, and knowing the uncertainties that lie ahead it is always safe to arrange as many possible avenues as opportunity will permit so that regardless what happens, there will be some way around—and the more I contact people the more I find that the world moves according to the form and not the feelings—give anyone the word in the right way and the world is yours for the asking—it is not what you ask but the way in which you ask for it; so we are learning the proper methods according to their psychology.

A young and relatively inexperienced man, Reting Rinpoche had been appointed the Regent of Tibet following the death of the Thirteenth Dalai

Lama, partly on the basis of the favor shown to him by the Great Thirteenth on his visit to Reting in 1933, shortly before his death.

At that time he gave the young Reting his own divination manuscript and dice, supposedly telling him, "I have been using these and they have proved good and if you use them it will prove useful for you too." Reting's supporters argued that this was a sign that the late Dalai Lama wanted him to become regent. Reting was also famous in his own right for having performed several miracles as a child.[58]

Arriving at Reting's residence in Lhasa, constructed with the most modern amenities, Theos was impressed by its grandeur. "He has recently built a new palace here," he wrote, "with a flowering garden all around—all very formal but with its green lawns broken by their luxuriant growth of flowers, it affords a real inspiration for anyone and the way his room is fixed the garden forms up the decoration of the entire wall on one side which is all glass and a one way visible Chinese screen affording him his privacy." With every degree of formality that Theos was expecting and more, he waited in the antechamber to Reting's audience room with Tharchin by his side. Given a butter offering, a small Buddha statue, and a manuscript, Theos and Tharchin were led into the audience room where, along with a *khata*, Theos presented his offerings to the Regent and received his blessings. Striking in appearance, Reting Rinpoche was "a very thin delicate spiritual sort of a personality with a very sensitive nature." The formal aspect of their meeting having passed, with Tharchin acting as translator, their conversation began in earnest.

I was seated just a foot or so in front of him and we had a long conversation over the Buddhistic religion and my plans for spreading it in America with him offering to do all that he could to further my mission and wishing to pass on thru me the necessary sacred object blessed with his own hands after the bestowal of the power of [it] on me to carry forth this divine instruction.

Indeed, the impression Reting conveyed to Theos was that he was

the type that one really likes to associate [with] if they turn out to have a good mental foundation to coordinate their deeper nature. There was no doubt about him being a truly spiritual individual but at the same time very keen, for his mind was sharp and grasping, as well as filled with ideas. Along with it all there was a reasonable sense of humor to balance up emotional disorders as they appeared, for in the course of time I had him laughing as a part of the relief of the situation.

Curious about Theos's unusual presence and interest in Tibetan Buddhism, Reting asked many questions and offered his opinions as well.

He was most eager to learn of all that I wanted to do and how come I have such a deep interest which seemed all the more amazing, he attributing it to a past life in this part of the world as a spiritual teacher or leader—they can only explain things within the scope of their own understanding. He advised me to make a list of all the things that I was anxious to secure and he would see to it that everything possible would be done about it—so now I feel confident about securing my copy of the Tengyur. It will probably be given to me with his blessing, but that is handled all right, for it is also the custom that I pay my tribute to their shrine which cost the equivalent; when all is settled and we have poured forth the emotions of our soul, the check books balance just a little in their favor, but since this is the way of getting things, it must be followed, for it is hard enough to have the privilege of making such an offer in order to have such books or what have you. In our conversation, all the seeds of the future were planted and also for my return etc. He is now anxious to watch my work and help me if necessary by giving my personal disciples his personal blessings; so that means that I will probably be granted the privilege of returning to this land and bringing friends with me by the mere asking—and as it stands today, I am the first American who has ever seen him.

His audience with Reting concluded, Theos's next stop was the home of Yapshi Langdün Küng, the Lönchen[59] (Prime Minister) and nephew of the Great Thirteenth. At age thirty-four, Langdün Küng, like Reting, was considered young for such a post. He had been described as "a rather stiff and uncommunicative young official,"[60] an impression that Theos came away with as well, feeling that "it is difficult to say how much ground I gained, but seeds were laid so that will come out with something more than I have already obtained." And so, returning to the Tsarong estate, Theos spent the afternoon reading his mail, as more and more gifts of food arrived at the house from various officials and aristocratic families.

For his third day in Lhasa, Theos was scheduled to meet the officials next in rank below the Regent and Lönchen, the four cabinet ministers who formed the Kashag. First on this list was the most senior member of the Kashag, described by the British Mission as "very conservative and not very intelligent"[61]—the minister who had most strongly opposed Theos's presence in Lhasa and had lectured Tharchin on both of his prior visits about "the evils of allowing people to enter their precious land." The conversation that took place that morning, not surprisingly, merely transpired in Theos's presence and remained entirely between Tharchin and the minister, Lang-chung-nga Shapé, Pemba Dhondup.[62] Since Theos had wisely discussed his aspirations with him in advance, it was up to Tharchin to convince the minister to support him. Watching Tharchin display his utmost honed humility before the minister, "poor old Tharchin," Theos thought,

> is going to have himself sucked away before he leaves here in his effort to demonstrate his humble respects to all who rule; however it is the custom, and it is mighty fortunate that he has the manner down pat, for it does have its effect, but I feel sorry for the poor chap, for he cannot speak above a whisper and must draw every other breath and wait to be forced into a seat on the floor and should they say anything at all encouraging, he has to bob-up and down like a floating ball along with the usual sucks, gasps, thank yous, and what have you, but he does it so graceful, that I feel it is pretty much natural with him, but I find that he never fails to use his head in conversation; he is always there to see an avenue thru which I can shove one of my aims which—have loaded him full & long before we leave. In fact, all vacant time is spent in preparing him for anything that might turn up; so that he is so filled that it just cannot slip by unnoticed.

Feeling that they had gained some ground in pleading their case, Theos and Tharchin ate a quick lunch at the Tsarong home before going out again to visit another cabinet minister. If the encounter with Lang-chun-nga Shapé had been trying, the meeting with the Kalön Lama, the one monastic cabinet minister, fell at the opposite extreme.

Kalön Lama, Trekang Shapé, Thupten Shakya[63] was the product of an aristocratic family with a long history of ecclesiastical service to government dating back to the days of the Fifth Dalai Lama. His uncle was at one time the personal physician to the Great Thirteenth, and having accompanied them both to India in 1909, Trekang Shapé had risen through the ranks of the government upon his return.[64] As the sole monastic representative in the Tibetan cabinet, he had been Theos's most enthusiastic supporter when his petition had been laid before the Kashag. Arriving at his residence at the Potala Palace, Theos was immediately embraced by the Kalön Lama and received an overwhelming welcome.

> He came to the stairway with open arms to greet me and I have not yet felt such a warmth of friendship come over me on the meeting of a personality as I did with this individual wrapped in the Lama blanket lined with golden silk. He is an elderly man as are all of the Shapés and a bit stooped, perhaps from worship and study and an air of real friendship about. In fact when he put his arm around me and beckoned that I enter ahead of him, I looked forward to a conversation that would take years to forget . . . and I did enjoy being with him and we stayed a bit longer then [sic] usual.

Feeling the warmth not only of his personality but also of his home, and feeling that it was a good opportunity to have some of his questions answered, Theos attempted to move their ongoing conversation to more philosophical topics, but the lama casually brushed them aside, always returning to pleasantries. Instead of responding to leading questions, he suggested that they take advantage of their presence to make a tour of the Potala Palace. So eventually Theos and Tharchin excused themselves from the Lama's presence and walked from his office toward the massive stairs that led to the entrance to the palace.

Reassured by Tharchin that the meeting had gone well—it was not the lama's nature "to talk much, so everything was all right," Tharchin explained—so "one should never be offended if you cannot get a Tibetan to talk about anything other then [sic] your trip etc., for he does not feel that he should talk to you until he knows you, but once the relationship of friendliness has been established, he is then privileged to talk as he feels . . . [and] it is an unbroken rule that they will all talk about their religion in the sense of extolling it, but as for discussion [of] its teachings, you are likely to be a little disappointed," which Theos was.

As they entered the Potala Palace through the eastern entrance, Tharchin paused to read the large declaration on the wall—signed with the handprints of the Fifth Dalai Lama—before they heard that the temple of the tombs of the previous Dalai Lamas would soon be closing for the day. Hurrying through the halls, they quickly made their way to the see the gold-plated *stūpa* of the Fifth Dalai Lama, "over three stories high entirely covered with . . . a layer of pure gold—not gold leaf—but slabs thicker than a good piece of cardboard . . . with all other decorations of the finest gems to be had on earth—jade, turquoise, ruby, coral, making up the lot." The immense wealth was truly impressive, prompting Theos to reflect that "the transformation in this country would be amazing if the wealth of these shrines was sprinkled over the land to develop its natural resources."

Leaving the Potala and descending to the Zhöl complex, Tharchin led Theos to the Zhöl Publishing House (Parkhang) to show him the wooden printing blocks of his own recently purchased Lhasa Kangyur. But lest Theos think all was well in Tibet, Tharchin made a point of taking him to visit the prison, also housed at the foot of the Potala in Zhöl.

In talking with one chap we found out that he had stole a couple of charm boxes about five years ago and he had no idea when he would be released—what happens is that the government forgets who they have put in and how long they should stay—once in—always in, until the government can gain a little virtue by releasing someone on an auspicious occasion at which time you might be lucky—but never any certainty. As we were about to leave we heard sounds coming up from a trap door in the corner and we listened to the faint echo that came up from this dark dungeon below where the crying soul was going through his ritual that he might gain happiness in the next life. It turned out to be a friend of Tharchin's who was at one time a very powerful person and exceedingly learned, and having been left on the losing side of the government he had his eyes poked out and thrown in this cellar for life—I have forgotten how long he has been here, but his case is famous.

Described by Tharchin, it was not the last time that Lungshar's story would be impressed upon Theos.

The next day Theos was obliged to visit the remaining two *shapés*, Tethong Shapé and Bonshö Shapé,[65] before seeing Hugh Richardson at the

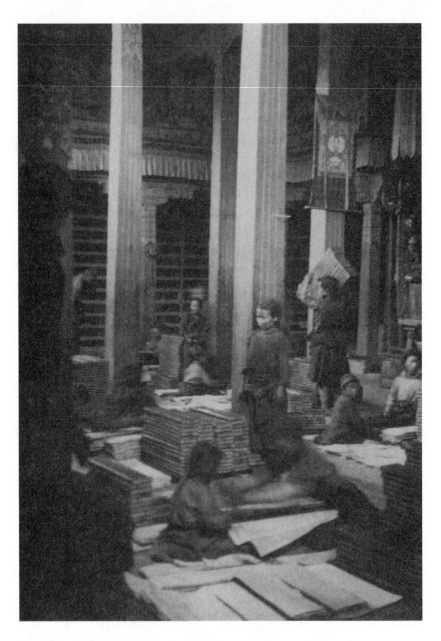

Figure 8.8 Zhöl Publishing House (PAHM)

British Mission again. But before they could leave in the morning, Theos and Tharchin were visited by the son of a high-ranking official, whom Theos learned had provided the actual entrée to Reting when Tharchin initially presented Theos's petition weeks earlier—"because of his intimate contact with the Regent."

Both Bönshö and Tethong were amiable enough, but it was with Tethong Shapé, one of Tsarong's friends, that Theos felt he could be most honest and forthright. Expressing his wish to remain in Lhasa for longer than the three weeks then allotted to him and his further desire to visit Shigatse, he openly and sincerely asked the *shapé* for his trusted advice.

From there, Theos and Tharchin proceeded to the "Holy of Holies," the Jokhang Temple at the heart of the city. Built in the seventh century to house one of the two Buddha statues brought to Tibet by the king's wives, the Jokhang was the central point of veneration, at the front of a monastic assembly hall surrounded by various smaller shrines. As they made their way into the temple complex, Theos was somewhat disappointed by what he saw, however.

Aside from the entrance, there is virtually no light to be had within the enclosed passageways. There is a large hall that goes completely around the inner room and down the centre of this lane, which is decorated on both sides with religious murals, is a row of pray barrels; so you first circumnavigate the inner shrine and store up treasures in heaven by revolving these wheels after which you enter the dark inner passage way guided by a burning bowl of butter for a torch held at your feet by the monk escort. Likewise does this inner hall go completely around its central Buddha (the present one). Off of this inner tunnel are small cells enshrining the sacred deities under the protection of a meshed screen of steel, which covers the four foot door which gives added protection to the sacred chambers. The only light within them is that of the burning butter lamps which makes them like hot ovens of sanctity. All the deities of their pantheon are to be found as well as the guardians of the religion. . . . None of the images were particularly impressive, for all were so filthy and hidden in such a thick gloom that one could have no inspirational appreciation. The majority of the images were of much coarse[r] workmanship then [sic] any I had yet seen so there was nothing of any particular interest but the jewels with which all were inlaid. The thing that caught your attention first among the shrines was the smell of mice and when your eyes accommated [*sic*] themselves to the light, you could see thousands of these rodents running all over the images eating on their robes of silk. One room was filled with the implements used to protect the place—matchlock guns, spears, helmets and breastwork of the fourteenth century and as with all the sacred places, several monks beating drums and carrying on the never ending ritual while they sat amongst the teeming swarms of mice. And so we left this dungeon of worship and strengthened our soul by a fresh breath of air in the eternal sunlight.

Returning to the Tsarong estate late for the midday meal, Theos felt somewhat awkward about his tardiness, despite having warned the household in advance. "In fact," he remarked, "they insist that I come and go as tho it were my own home with my own servants, but with it all, one cannot help but feel as tho he is imposing and especially when you are of a different race. Never have I ever felt more welcome in a strange house; so it shows there are some admirable traits in this land."

Finding that Lord Tsarong was out for the day and only Lady Tsarong at home, Theos

was left to dine alone with the Lhacham. It was a strange feeling at first, I did not know whether to risk going upstairs. The outcome was a perfect mystery, but there was nothing to do, but go; so up I trotted and had a marvelous meal with jolly conversation as surprising as it might be—truly I was more astounded then [*sic*] anyone else; however it was interesting to listen to her tell Tharchin about everything that we had talked about on his return and how easy it was for her to understand. After discussing items at hand, for some reason or other we drifted to the American Indian so I commenced telling her about the jewelry of the Navajo ladies who seem to have a similar taste as those of Tibet. She was interested as well as amazed to find that there were others who had as keen an appreciation for tourquoise as do the Tibetans. And so I lived thru my first experience of dining with a Tibetan of the higher classes who was unable to speak any English and we had to do something; so if there was comprehension of thought, we must have been talking.

With only a few moments' rest after his extended lunch, Theos briefly reviewed his notes before hurrying off again—this time for tea and dinner with the Political Officer (P.O.) at the British Mission at Deki Lingka.

Richardson was a friendly enough man, and he and Theos seemed to get along well with a certain comfortable ease, but Theos had to remind himself not to be deluded by friendship and forget their differing purposes in being in Lhasa. At every juncture, Tharchin had warned him, he was being tested, whether by a curious minister to see if his behavior accorded with Tibetan Buddhist customs (evidence of his knowledge from a prior life, as the rumors had it) or by the British officers to see if he was there to interfere with their plans. "The P.O. is here to uphold their own rights, where I am trying to learn the inside details of esoteric Buddhism and if I do not handle these [gestures] correctly, I am out before I ever start—for I should have remembered all of them from my past life etc. etc., so [these] are the things with which one has to contend."

And so, adopting his usual good-mannered friendliness, Theos sat down with Richardson for an extended chat, acceding to his opinions on Tibet and the world, as Richardson had just returned from a visit to Ganden Monastic University, east of Lhasa. More fodder for bonding over their common perspective arrived in the midst of their talk, in the form of telegrams requesting permission to visit.

While I was there, three telegrams came in asking for permission to visit Lhasa. One from a party now at Phari, and one of the others from Tucci who said that he was leaving Gangtok. He had published several articles in the *Statesman* to the effect that he is the greatest living scholar on Tibetan Buddhism and that the Tibetan Government is going to give him permission to spend five months in U province and considerable time in Shigatse as well as have a long talk with Richardson over these matters— and what a laugh we had out of some of it. So far he has not even applied to the Tibetan Government, but he is on his way to Gyantse regardless— he is being so confident—and he is filled with just enough hot air to win out since money is no object, having the entire Italian treasury behind him—and there is nothing that the Tibetan listens to more; so we will see . . . And so we discussed the follies of the world's great Tibetan experts— It is amazing what people can do when it comes to Tibet.

Laughing at Tucci's bravado,[66] Richardson told Theos how lucky he was to be there, since even their mutual acquaintance, Gordon Bowles from Harvard, had been denied permission to visit Tibet when he had applied for a visa for himself and his wife. Expressing his appreciation for everything the

British authorities had done to help him thus far, Theos casually mentioned his further desire to go overland "from Lhasa to Derge and thence on to Peking and if this was refused was asking to stay longer in Lhasa, returning via Shigatse on my way to India." Richardson encouraged him to pursue this—through Tibetan government channels—and wished him success.

Determined to do his own part to help Theos learn to speak Tibetan, the next day, Tharchin began taking his meals alone downstairs, forcing Theos to eat with the Tsarong family upstairs without a translator. This was "like a nightmare" for Theos at first, since although he had memorized plenty of words in Kalimpong over the spring, "putting them together" remained a challenge and he still could not "make a complete sentence perfectly constructed" despite his ability to "talk with servants, making it possible to travel alone all over Tibet." Nonetheless, if Tharchin kept to his word to eat separately, Theos was convinced that "there will be little doubt about being able to speak this language" before the summer was over.

Having seen to the obligatory aspects of his arrival in Lhasa, extending his visit was paramount in Theos's mind. Over lunch with Lord Tsarong, he discussed a strategy for convincing the cabinet to extend his visa, and afterward they and Tharchin began making plans according to Tsarong's recommendations. Originally conceived as a mere ploy to get permission to remain in Tibet, Theos was now forced to confront the possibility that his request to head east toward China had worked *too* well and he would in fact be sent out of the country in a mere two weeks' time.

Either way, Tsarong told him, the opening gesture in any request to the government was religious patronage—a lesson Theos had learned well in Gyantse—and Tsarong suggested that Theos sponsor the same sort of ceremony that he himself had done years earlier. Retrieving his family's financial records, Tsarong reviewed the process and costs for Theos and Tharchin to consider. Agreeing without hesitation, Theos and Tharchin began laying out the details of their new plan. The stages were, according to Tsarong, to first, notify the Kashag of the desire to sponsor the ceremony, who would then notify the various monasteries, requesting the calculation of an auspicious day; second, draft the applications for both his proposed trip and his extended stay; and third, meet with the resident Chinese representative to settle the issue of border crossings and entry into China.

Accomplishing the first two before the morning was out, by lunchtime they had an appointment to meet with Mr. S. H. William Tsiang, the Chinese envoy to Tibet, later in the afternoon.

I found him a most pleasing sort of chap as one usually finds the Chinese. He could speak good English with a heavy Chinese accent behind a mouth full of jammed up teeth as so often [is] the case with them. While there a young Chinaman came in who has been living here for three years at the Drepong monastery taking up their course of instruction. He was very keen about Buddhistic logic so we had a very interesting conversation about its various intricacies in comparison with the Dialogues of Plato—he speaking English fluently—how these boys ever manage these languages is more then [sic] I can understand; however both of them had graduated from English run schools in China; so it was easy enough to understand this much but the rest of it. . . . In most instances it takes the Tibetan about fifteen years to complete their course of study—the most of them finishing after they are forty with a few exceptions in the early thirties, but with this chap's background he has been able to start off further down the line and thereby make greater speed, but with all he is figuring on from six to ten years. We look upon the requirements for many of our professional degrees with horror because of the time they take, but here [it] is almost a lifetime job after you are fully equipped; however he is filled with youthful enthusiasm and looks forward to all of it with joy. All he can look forward to in the future is getting back to his work—studying—and such is the way the Chinese do things—a hundred years for preparation and then settled down to a little work—never any great haste.

The young Chinese man studying at Drepung Monastic University seemed to offer the promise of Tibetan and Chinese Buddhist collaborative study and mutual respect, but appearances could be deceiving. Tharchin, having written to Sir Charles Bell several months earlier, had already reported on the activities of such "students" at Drepung. Referring to the Chinese minister who had accompanied Ngak-chen Rinpoche from Lhasa through Kalimpong the previous February, Tharchin wrote to Bell,

The high official of China who was in Lhasa since 3 or 4 years, he came with Hong Musong & stayed in Lhasa, with him there were several young men who knew English also. Some since, they were doing lot of secret service in Lhasa, though this official pretended to learn the Tibetan religion and stayed in the large monastery of Drepung. His young men were making maps and taking the temperature of Lhasa.[67]

While Theos was thus engaged discussing philosophy and requesting that a telegram be sent to Nanking for an entry visa, Tharchin was busy paying close attention for his own ends and for those to whom he owed his allegiance, the British Empire.

Just as Theos continued writing his account of his experiences in his diaries and letters home, Tharchin had been keeping his own notes on the comings and goings of various Tibetan and Chinese officials, as well as the rumors in the streets. Formally writing them up, he sent them out of Tibet via the British Mission to Sir Charles Bell. A mere two days after their meeting with the Chinese official, Tharchin wrote,

> I came up to Tibet for nine weeks leave from the Mission and accompanied with an American gentleman named Mr. Bernard. He got pass up to Gyantse for 6 weeks, but he applied to the Tibetan Govt. that he may be allowed to come to Lhasa & it was granted & he is now here. I came up two weeks ahead & he arrived here on the 24th June. . . .
>
> After paying respects I went to pay my respects to the Chinese officer who is here, as I met him when he was going to Tibet via Kalimpong & I took photo & published in my paper. He was very glad to meet me. I tried to talk with him friendly & asked many questions concerning the relationship between China & Tibet.
>
> He said me, that the Tibetan Govt. has agreed that they are under the sovereignty of China Govt.[68] So he is here, still there are few questions which are not settled, but hope to settle soon. Regarding Tashi Lama:— He told me that he is at Kikodo [Jyekundo] & will start for Tibet at the beginning of July. He will reach here in October or latest in Nov. The 300 Chinese body guard are coming with him. If the Tibetan Govt. try to stop or make trouble, the Central Govt is going to help & also he said that there are over 10,000 soldiers in the province of Kham, in Dergey, Chamdo, Bathang & Dartsedo. Also the Central Govt. ordered the officer of Ziling to send troops if any troubles rise. Also he said that he is going back on arrival of new officer, who is accompanying Tashi Lama.
>
> Then he told me that the Chinese Govt & the British Govt. are very friendly, but he was complaining Mr. Gould that when he came up to Lhasa last year, he sent his man to welcome him on the way with Khada & he thought that he will call him at first, but he never came so he also did not go to see him, so they never met each other, for which he is very sorry. . . .

They have wireless station & daily they are sending messages to Nan-king. Some English knowing Chinese young boy are studying at Drepong & trying to win over the monks.[69]

Indeed, while Chinese agents posing as monks attempted to win over Ti-betan factions, Japanese agents *also* posing as monks—Mongolian monks—were doing the very same thing. The Mongolians had offered the strongest support for Japan in the ongoing war, having been shown considerable favor during the Japanese occupation of China, with Japan even promising to establish an autonomous government for Inner Mongolia.[70] But Thar-chin's main concern was Tibet and its implications for British India. He continued,

> I had a very private talk with Tsarong Shape (at present Dzasa) & he also told me that Tibet is bending towards China. All the officers talk with me openly as they do not doubt me. Also Tsarong told me that the discipline of the Tibetan Army is very bad, it is not good as before, the old rifles are not good, but of course they hope to get new, but when the army is not good, not properly trained he fears even if good rifles, it will not get much help. He has lot of idea to improve it, but it seems that he alone can't do much, neither he has any power to act.
>
> Now I close the letter. I may get some more news & different news about the new Dalai Lama, I will let you know. Regarding political news if I have some money to spend I can get many, but which I am unable to do so, nor think wise to do so. Any how I am a loyal British subject so, I am trying to get some news & will let you have again. I may stay here one month more.[71]

Kept informed of these conversations—if not, perhaps, the only one Tharchin was telling—over the days that followed Theos tried to relax and do more sightseeing, in the various parks scattered around Lhasa, the Jokhang and Ramoche temples, and the Dalai Lama's summer palace west of the city while Tharchin and Tsarong tried to finesse plans on his behalf.

Tharchin had submitted Theos's petitions to the Kashag just before they adjourned for their twelve-day summer picnic, so there had been no time to discuss them and a successful supplication appeared to be up to Tsar-ong. Meeting with Reting Rinpoche to discuss his ongoing duties in Lhasa, Tsarong took the opportunity to convey to the Regent Theos's desire to host a garden party for the Kashag. Reting replied, however, that it was *he* who had planned on hosting a feast for Theos at his Lhasa residence upon his return in a month's time. Theos was overjoyed by the implication that Reting had already decided to extend his visa. Counseled by Tharchin not to miss an opportunity to ingratiate himself with both the British and Chinese authorities, Theos decided to invite both the British Political Officer and the Chinese representative to the party as his guests, thereby allowing them to meet unofficially and both save face by not having to be the first to call on the other.

Although actively engaged in study, research, and negotiations, Theos still found moments alone with himself—usually early in the morning or late at night when he was writing his diary—when he could reflect on his life. Above and beyond the radically different intellectual life of America that awaited him on his return, it was the lack of even the opportunity for the sort of life possible in Tibet that was most disconcerting. "I only wish that I could find the same degree of contentment and inner satisfaction at home as I have been able to contact in this section of the world," he wrote.

> Never having lived to quite the same discipline I can hardly say that it is impossible in the world of activity, but I do know that they are diametrically opposed to one another; so now how to adjust them. Never before in my life have I been able to bring up as much of the stored up energy that rests within and at the same time be conscious of it. Before it has only been a driving force for unfatigable external expression of action which soon develops into the expression of nervous energy because of the agitation rather than the driving force of that creative flow of life.

It was also in these moments of quiet that Theos discovered some of the advantages of staying at the Tsarong estate. The Tsarongs were benefactors to a number of residential houses at the surrounding monasteries— the aristocratic families each being responsible for the welfare of different "regional houses" or Kham-tsen (*khang tshan*). The Tsarong family had a close relationship with the Kham-tsen for the Tsang region of central Tibet, which meant a more or less constant stream of visitors. From the family's tutors, the learned scholars Geshe Chödrak and Geshe Kedrup from Sera University, to many other high-ranking geshes from Drepung, Sera, and Ganden, many highly educated lamas were available for Theos to have contact with.[72]

Inspired by these encounters, Theos decided that he should do his best to document the great "Three Seats of Learning" of Drepung, Sera, and Ganden for the benefit of future students, since

> it is my feeling that a strong impetus of scholarly investigation is going to be guided in this direction, for the country is not going to remain closed forever. If the Chinese take up therein again, they will permit students to come, and little by little enough good will is going to be established that even the Tibetans will allow people to enter for the purpose of study. . . . With the foundation which I am laying at the moment I feel that it is going to be possible for me to return and be permitted to bring along several of my sincere disciples who I will be sure and have well trained before leaving the States so that not one detail will be overlooked.

But this was just one more item to add to his list of things to do, and already Theos felt "there is so dam much to be done" with "never a void moment—in fact I often wish there could be one," as his exit plans were requiring more and more attention.

Not surprisingly, many of the people he talked to about traveling east to China remarked that it would be a dangerous trip, with bandits and Communist rebels in the hills. Consequently, Theos began planning for his preferred route home, via Shigatse and Sakya, hoping to even visit "the first monastery in Tibet," Samye—"only two days around the mountain" south of the city—if he could find the time. This, of course, was his biggest concern. To make matters worse—timewise, at least—Theos finally began receiving contact prints of his hundreds of photos from the previous two months in the mail from Calcutta. Should he wish to label and mount his contact prints for Lhasa as he had done for India and Gyantse, Theos realized that he was going to have to wake up by 4:30 every morning just to see to his basic necessities before dealing with each day's new activities. However, he ran out of cardstock to mount the prints on, so gave up on doing so for the Lhasa photos, deciding to attend to them "next Christmas."

Overwhelmed by the details of sponsoring a *puja* at the Jokhang and Ramoche temples in a matter of days, Theos and Tharchin relied heavily on Lord Tsarong's guidance as well as his financial strength, with Tsarong putting up the cost of the ceremony on Theos's behalf in silver bullion[73]—which included not only all the silk *khata*s and monetary offerings (six *sho* per monk[74]) but also the cost of eight hundred pounds of butter, over a thousand pounds of barley flour (*tsampa*), and the "four hundred coolies" required to carry it all into town.

While the preparations were under way for the ceremony at the Ramoche Temple, Theos utilized his time to the best of his abilities, doing his best to maintain a respectable appearance, even if his best efforts often involved innovation—such as getting a haircut and beard trim with a pair of garden shears. Splitting his time between study and planning, Theos made sure his politically savvy social function came off without a hitch. Making a point of visiting the Regent prior to his departure for Reting Monastery, accompanied by Tharchin and Tsarong, Theos reiterated his desire to remain in Tibet beyond his allotted three weeks. The Regent, rather casually over lunch, remarked that he had discussed his application with the members of the Kashag, who had "granted everything that I had requested." However, "As for going to China, they were willing to permit me to proceed, but with things so dangerous on the border at this particular time, they felt it was a very unwise move, but if it was my desire, they would not stop me and then it would give me the opportunity of securing the Tengyur from the Derge blocks."

Preparing to leave, himself, in a few days' time, as a final token of his good wishes, the Regent gave Theos not only the traditional white silk *khata* with a red silk "protection cord" but also a small Buddha statue and a copy of the recently printed, illustrated edition of the *Sūtra of the Fortunate Aeon.*[75]

Although Theos still needed the "official word" from the Kashag itself, with Reting Rinpoche's assurance, he began making plans for the next two months since there was "no doubt about being able to remain," in Tibet at the very least, to continue his studies. The new plan was to "go to Ganden to return via Samye and thence onto Shigatse to take in Tashilhunpo and Sakya." With the logistics of his extended stay more or less guaranteed, Theos and Tharchin indulged in some social events in the valley, most notably picnicking with Tsarong's family, to which Tharchin invited his mother-in-law and sister-in-law. Feeling somewhat more relaxed, Theos shed his Indian British clothes and arrived at the picnic in full Tibetan aristocratic dress. "They were most amused to find me in Tibetan dress, but really got a kick out if it. When all [is] said and done, I find that it actually puts them more at [ease than] anything else that I could do." Indeed, as the weeks passed, Theos found that this had definite advantages: "The Tibetans are very pleased over the fact that I am willing to wear their dress, for it more or less puts us on the same level of taste, and then when I try talking to them a little, they are more pleased than ever and at once all barriers seem to be discarded."

Thus enjoying themselves, Tharchin, Theos, and Lord Tsarong took photos of one another in turn, talking at length with those around them. While Tharchin socialized with his in-laws and Theos chatted with British and Tibetans alike, the rest of their lives seemed a world away. For others, however, the two men in Lhasa were simply long overdue.

Having agreed to Tharchin's six-week leave of absence from the Church of Scotland Mission in Kalimpong, the Mission director, Robert Knox, seeing no sign of him or indication that he would soon appear, lost patience with the man he'd had little regard for to begin with. More than a week earlier, Tharchin had sent a telegram to his wife instructing her to tell Knox that he was "well on his way" back; however, when Knox spoke to Frank Perry at the Himalayan Hotel a week later, he discovered that Theos and Tharchin were still in Lhasa and neither seemed to have any plans to return soon; in fact, they had sent another telegram to Tharchin's wife—to her annoyance as well—telling her that they would be staying in Tibet for two more months and inviting her to join them. Understandably upset, Knox sent a letter to Theos, demanding the return of his employee. "Mr. Bernard," he wrote,

I quite appreciate your delight at being allowed to visit Tibet and especially Lhasa and, if you had not been in touch with those who could help you more and had needed any help from me I would gladly have done all that I could for you including the provision of an interpreter. But one thing the Mission *could* not have agreed to, i.e., allowing you to take Tharchin away from his work for an indefinite period. It is no concern of ours what he does with himself during his leave. As a matter of fact, I was glad that he had the opportunity of using it agreeably and profitably by accompanying you to Gyantse or even to Lhasa but he knew the limits of his leave and that he could not commit himself to anything else beyond those limits. . . . You may remember that, on the occasion on which you mentioned the matter to me at all, I told you how limited his leave was.

Explaining that his letter to Tharchin—which Tharchin claimed not to have received—had spelled out his expectations, Knox reiterated them to Theos:

> It pointed out that Tharchin's part of the work [at the Mission] was suffering from his absence and, at the same time, recognized that he might have opportunities of doing something in Lhasa for Christ . . . if he were engaged in your work he would have time for little else. Now your wires to me and Perry confirm my belief. So, as the situation is getting more and more difficult here, I can see nothing for it but to ask you to send him back immediately. May I say that your reference to your work in Perry's wire seems to me singularly unfortunate? Does it not strike you that other peoples' work may not appear equally or more important to them? And in this case, where the work is not man's but God's, must it be put aside at the call of everyone who likes to ask?

But of course Theos had no intention of sending Tharchin back to Kalimpong, least of all to a self-important missionary for whom Theos felt nothing but contempt, any more than Tharchin felt compelled to hurry back to work for a man who had created no end of difficulties for him from the moment he arrived to take charge of the mission. So, ignoring Knox's irate missives, they returned to their tasks at hand, knowing that Tharchin would have to return to Kalimpong sooner or later, and well before Theos. But for Theos, far more important events were transpiring: preparations for the first of the ceremonies at the Jokhang Temple that he was supposedly sponsoring.

The offering was set for Thursday, July 8, a day calculated to be auspicious by the monastery's astrological staff, and preparations had been under way for several days. Requesting permission to watch and photograph the entire proceedings, from the mixing of the flour for the sculptures to the conclusion of the ceremony, Theos took extensive notes on everything that transpired. Having seen the sheer quantity of butter and flour used in the ceremonies on a daily basis—about 10,000 pounds of butter a month alone, he estimated—he was impressed that despite the "waste" of it all being "consumed by the holy flame," one thing "of heart-rendering interest is the practice after the ceremony of turning over a portion of these ingredients . . . thru the village of Lhasa, distributing it among the poor as well as a trip to the prison where some is given to those forgotten lives of error."

When the day finally arrived, Theos was "as excited about the whole affair as [he] had been over [his] first day of school" as a child. After being inspected and seen to be properly dressed by Lord and Lady Tsarong—"one would think that I was their child going off to school and they wanted to see that everything was arranged properly," Theos thought—he was sent off to the Jokhang with Tharchin, loaded down with cameras. Despite not having "the slightest idea what was going to happen," he felt ready for what he was sure would be "one of the most interesting experiences" of his life. After a long series of preliminary prayers and rituals, it was only upon the arrival of the head of the Geluk sect, the ninety-third Regent of Ganden,[76] that the day's ceremonies could truly begin. Circumambulating the temple, to the amazement of the gathered Tibetan pilgrims (who, like the residents of Gyantse, had certainly never seen any British resident do such a thing, much less in full Tibetan garb), Theos entered with Tharchin and assumed his place as patron of the ceremonies.

With the arrival of the Regent of Ganden, the assembled monks fell into their rows, and after Theos's petition for the ceremony was read, it was time to make his offerings to the abbot. Performing the obligatory three full prostrations before the Ganden Tri-pa, Theos presented the same traditional offerings given to Reting Rinpoche—the representations of the body, speech, and mind of the Buddha. Returning to his seat off to one side, Theos settled down for what would be a very long and otherwise completely incomprehensible series of rituals and "endless cups of tea," occasionally being asked to rise and walk through the assembly as a symbolic gesture of his patronage of the offerings of food, tea, and money to the monks. After three hours, Theos was excused from the ceremonies, informed that they would continue well into the evening, even as he and Tharchin distributed copper coins to the beggars outside the temple and arranged for the blessed food offerings to be distributed to the poor and the prison.

For the next week, Theos continued to socialize while Tharchin surreptitiously bought articles for him at the bazaar. Hoping to avoid protracted haggling, Tharchin was adept at negotiating purchases under the guise of his own acquisition since Suydam Cutting, in Theos's opinion, had ruined the ability of foreigners to purchase anything in Lhasa through "his generous gifts to the monasteries and exorbitant prices paid for purchases

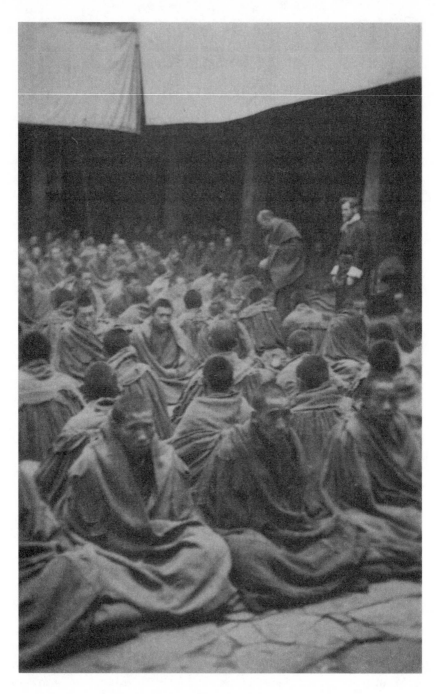

Figure 8.9 Bernard as patron at the Jokhang (PAHM)

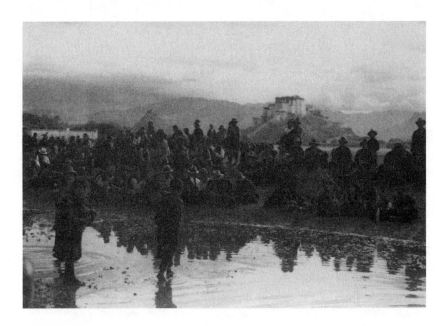

Figure 8.10 The crowd outside the Jokhang awaiting the distribution of food (PAHM)

which were exhibited in N.Y. . . . he paid such ridiculous prices for things that the Tibetan here usually throws away, so now they want to raise the price of cow dung to that of gold." Theos was not averse to paying what he had to in order to obtain the materials he was after, since "it is obvious that I am going to be equipped to buy for any museum in the country that wants to go to Tibet, but so long as we can afford it, I am going to keep all within our possession and use it all for establishing something that belongs to us."

To that end, he had Viola increase the amount of money wired to him to $1,000 a month. Tharchin, in fact, was running around Lhasa so much—looking for books, buying statues and *thangkas* from the Panchen Lama's estate,[77] and procuring various sundry items, as well as trying to negotiate for Theos's Christmas cards to be made—that he actually wore out his shoes and had to buy new ones. But far from being solely occupied with Theos's concerns, Tharchin continued to provide reconnaissance for the British Mission, the latest gossip in the streets, the perception of world affairs, or the latest details concerning the Panchen Lama and attempts to locate the Fourteenth Dalai Lama—and when he and Theos would visit

Deki Lingka on social occasions, would use the opportunity to discreetly hand over his latest letters to be sent to Sir Charles Bell in London.[78]

While Tharchin was thus engaged, Theos spent time attending Tibetan parties and picnics, where he was quizzed repeatedly about his sponsorship of the recent ritual at the Jokhang. At the British Mission, Richardson was preparing to leave for India (leaving Rai Bahadur Norbu in charge) and had a big send-off planned with all the British officers in attendance. Despite the formality of the event, the top story on everyone's list for discussion was the situation with the Panchen Lama and concerns over the Chinese, further complicated by the start of the Sino-Japanese War just days earlier (July 7, 1937).

> The Chinese . . . are trying desperately to gain control of Tibet, having been thrown out in 1911. It is interesting to note that the feeling of the Chinese is that Tibet still belongs to them and that its people are far inferior, lacking all capacities to take care of themselves which they seem to have been doing since the expulsion. So far as the Chinese are concerned there is only one supreme intelligence in the world and that is of the Chinese—everyone else is inferior; however they do make the concession that the Western world has far surpassed their wildest imagination so far as industrial advancement is concerned, but that does not necessarily mark great intelligence. It is only a matter of application of the little they have along lines which the Chinese have never given any particular thought. When they feel this way towards us, it is easy enough to figure out their concept of the Tibetan who has done nothing but preserve the Buddhist scriptures.

Indeed, given the political situation, it was hard not to see Tibet as a pawn in a larger game. To many observers, Theos included, "China has it all in mind—and Japan has China in mind with both of them looking at India behind the outpost of the British." To even the most astute observer at the time, the end result was anyone's guess.

However, unlike the British with their boredom, the Chinese with their contempt, or the Japanese with their secret strategies,[79] Theos viewed Tibet as a place wholly unlike any other, of inestimable value and fascination.

> One of the things that one learns from such an experience as living in Tibet . . . where it is essential to resort to your own imagination for any

pleasure that may be possible, is the ability to find a deeper joy out of the simple few rather than endless shallow joys out of the ostentatious infinite. This has been proved to me over and over again when I had suddenly realized that there is nothing to be had for my diversion but myself—what to do with it. . . . There are no books to be had, no shows, no modern amusements. . . . However I have had to learn to talk with the mule boys, the servants and with myself in silent reflection, and I must confess that I have failed to experience many of the moods of despondency and boredom which tend to come my way when living in the other world, and as for the rest, I find that I have found deeper joys [than] I have ever experienced before in my life and at no time has there been the sense of missing anything that I had in the past and did not have now.

They were feelings only compounded by the generosity and spirit of the Tibetans themselves that Theos experienced while attending the social gatherings of the noble families.

I must say that I have never been a stranger in a gathering of this size before where they made me feel so completely at home. In fact, I felt that I had known all of them for many years and this was one of our regular gatherings. I feel that this speaks rather well of their characters, for I cannot say the same about our people, and so my fondness for the people of Tibet continues to increase.

Still concerned about acquiring a copy of the Tengyur from Derge, Theos had noticed that Lord Tsarong had a complete set—both Kangyur and Tengyur—in his home, and that with the right emphasis, he might be able to convince his host to part with it. "I am buying up rifles and pistols from Tsarong along with an outfit of fast horses," he wrote to Viola. Even though as commander of the military in Tibet, Lord Tsarong had such things at his disposal, when Theos made his request for supplies and described his intention to shoot his way through the Chinese-Tibetan border skirmish to Derge—if he had to—in order to acquire a copy of the canon from Derge, Lord Tsarong was horrified at the suggestion. Having heard about a party of Tibetan officials recently attacked and decapitated on the Chinese border, he was sure that Theos's reckless behavior would get him killed. Expressing his concern that he might not be able to acquire a copy for himself, Theos "allowed" Lord Tsarong to convince him otherwise and to offer to "turn over" his copy of the Buddhist canon to Theos if he was unable to find another set; Tsarong would simply "order another set for himself, which will be here in three or four years."

Before Theos could make his plans for the rest of the day, however, a messenger arrived from the Gyume Tantric College. The abbot and monks who had officiated at his sponsored *puja* at the Jokhang were preparing for another ritual, this time at the Ramoche Temple. Recalling his request for teachings a week earlier, the abbot was inviting him to attend (and patronize) the Guhyasamāja Tantric Empowerment being given the very next day. Consequently, Theos and Tharchin paid a visit to the Ramoche Temple to watch (and photograph) the preparations taking place. Returning to the Tsarong estate afterward, they ran into a Bengali friend of Tharchin's who had worked for Rāhula Saṅkṛtyāyana, and whom Theos had met in Calcutta. He told them of his ongoing work with Saṅkṛtyāyana and of their mutual friend, Gedun Chöpel, who was now unemployed and living in Kalimpong.

> The chap who we met here is remaining in Tibet to keep up the contact and continue their researches as well as continue his aid in the compilation of their notes. All during last winter Rahula had with him a reputedly learned Geshe who I had met in Darjeeling with Viola. He kept this chap busy translating all thru the winter which robbed me of the opportunity of using him, for it was my desire to have him render some interpretations on things that I was translating. He is now at Kalimpong and free; so I may have the assistance of his services on my return, having already had a little before my departure for Tibet this Spring. This Bengali could speak English perfectly; so, we had a good chat on various subjects of my interest and I feel that I will perhaps get some helpful leads from time to time during other discussions when there is more time available.

Theos's more immediate concern, however, was that the last of the Indian clothes that he had been wearing nearly every day for several months were finally nearly worn out. Led by one of Lord Tsarong's servants to a local tailor, Theos had additional Tibetan-style clothes made for himself, so the next day when Theos arrived at the Ramoche Temple, he was once again dressed in aristocratic robes, to the marvel and amazement of the pilgrims, beggars, and assorted other residents of Lhasa in attendance for the blessings.

Led to the back courtyard, Theos waited while the monks assembled and the preliminary prayers and rituals were conducted, until the time was right for him to present the offerings to the abbot as patron of the day's events. Taking his seat to one side, Theos waited and watched as bells were rung, chants issued forth, and the monks of the assembly performed the rituals in full dress as the Buddha of the maṇḍala, with "a crown about two feet high, made of black velvet" with "a high border consisting of five silver sections." Without the slightest clue what was transpiring or what it meant, attending more as an observer than a participant, Theos took equal note of the manner in which the monks sipped their tea—blowing back "the froth of floating butter" before drinking—and of the hand gestures (*mudrā*) that accompanied their chants. When a break in the ceremony finally came and rice served to the monks, "attendants brought food to me and my escort which was indeed very thoughtful of them and which I enjoyed for it was way past lunch time," after which Theos and Tharchin took their leave, anticipating hours to go before the ceremony would be finished and the assembly dispersed.

Returning to their temporary Lhasa home, they found a large delivery of eggs, barley flour, and assorted gifts for Theos's use by the former cabinet minister Trimön Shapé. Planning to visit him the next day to convey his personal thanks, Lord Tsarong, hoping to expose Theos to as wide a range of religious figures as possible, decided to introduce Theos to the *shapé*'s "spiritual guide," a lama of the Kagyu sect who also followed teachings in the Nyingma tradition, and arranged for him to visit at 10 a.m. The two men—with Tharchin translating—talked at length about tantric practice and the lineage of Milarepa, and Theos was rather impressed:

If their sect develops pleasing personalities such as his, I must confess that they have something of merit, for he was like a real human being, living the same sort of life as everyone else, but at the same time providing opportunity for the spiritual side. To commence with, he has been gifted by a pleasing appearance which is left natural by his long hair as is the custom of all Tibetans. Along with his work, he has his own private home where he lives with his wife and family where he adheres to his daily discipline of study and meditation in accordance to the methods taught by his group. There was nothing sanctified about him.

He was filled with laughter, saw the joke in all things—and pointed out how foolish certain beliefs were when considered from the viewpoint of their philosophic foundations.

When relating such events to his wife, however, Theos painted a far more romantic, idealized picture:

At last I have penetrated beyond the externals of form and have made contact with one well trained in Tantric teachings. In fact I have just completed my first day of devotion demanded of young disciples. It consisted of sitting cross legged for six solid hours without a flicker and listen to all that could be imparted in that space, and I must confess that the stretch on an empty stomach left the signs of the strains; however it was all worth it, for the proper beginning has been made. He seems to be about as pleased as myself, and if I judge my reactions correctly, I am going to get a great deal of inside information that would be absolutely impossible otherwise.

For Theos's purposes, having sponsored the rituals at the Jokhang and received teachings from monks, he could claim that he was now a "lama"— at least, that was how he began to consistently, if half-jokingly, refer to himself in his letters to Viola. Just the same, Theos couldn't hide a certain amount of frustration—as well as gloat over his own cleverness—when dealing even with such an amiable figure. "This wheedling information out of esoteric priests is certainly a delicate job of silently tugging, for you more or less have to keep them talking and thru unconscious psychology induce them to talk themselves right into the thing that you are after."

Later that evening, reviewing his English-language books on Tibetan Buddhism, Theos began to think that the Kagyu sect did indeed seem to have something to offer him. Most of his information had come from Nyingma practitioners thus far, but he was open to new possibilities, while still holding to what he had been told before: that the Geluk sect was predominantly *sūtra*-based, while the Kagyu and Nyingma sects were tantric— despite the fact that the ceremonies at the Jokhang and at Ramoche had been fully tantric and entirely officiated by Geluk monks and lamas. Yet Theos simply dismissed this, believing that "wherever one finds strict adherence to external rituals and disciplines of devotion, everything that comes from that source can be discounted 99% percent."

Theos's biases against ritual and his generally anticlerical attitude were not limited to the Geluk lineage; despite his initial attraction to the Kagyu tradition based on his meeting with a lama, he found cause to vent there as well. Having paid his respects to Trimön Shapé the next day at his residence at Se-chung House, Theos and Tharchin proceeded to visit the same lama they had met the day earlier. Theos was enthusiastic about discussing the Kagyu tantric tradition, but after a lengthy conversation of generalities—while Theos covetously eyed a set of embroidered *thanka*s depicting the eight forms of Padmasambhava—the abbot told Theos that they could not discuss any further matters without his undergoing the proper ritual empowerments, and then only after the necessary preliminary practices. Annoyed at this statement, since such "rituals" were something he had no patience for nor any desire to engage in, Theos decided to flaunt some of the information he had already gleaned from his readings.

These boys talk on forever and then whenever they find that there [*sic*] wind is about to give out, they say the rest is esoteric and that it will be necessary for you to take the vows before the next step can be revealed to you. These steps do not come easy, for first of all, one's preparation is that of making 100,000 devotional prostrations to be followed by doing a *bum* (100,000) of various sets of mantras, and then making various sorts of offerings—exactly the same sort of racket to be found in India—except that they make it a *bum* here while it is a *lac* there. You should see their sails flop when you come out with a few of the anticipated answers on some of these things which they are unable to reveal—the air is hot and they start talking about something else mighty quick—and it is all more disgusting then [*sic*] it could ever be made to sound; however it is necessary to run the gamet [*sic*] of just such racketeering in order to find your way to the back of the stage where all the real work of life is carried on unknown of to those in front of life's glittering curtain of maya, and so we went home with our notes.

Dismissing the man as "nothing more than the regular religious racketeer of forgotten history" for his refusal to break his vows,[80] Theos nonetheless thought there might be something of value in the Kagyu lineage—if he could find someone who would talk with him.

As word of the previous day's event at the Ramoche Temple spread, even the British Mission learned of Theos's activities. The mission's wireless operator, Reginald Fox, took a particular interest and made a point of talking with Theos, unaware of the stories Theos had heard about him before their first meeting. Having lived in India for seventeen years, Fox had developed "a flourishing tolerance" for Indian religion, despite being a devout Catholic.

> The rumour has spread around like wildfire that I am a Buddhist making a pilgrimage to Lhasa, and so it has come to the ears of their forces; so he was rather anxious that I talk over some of their contentions. There is little that can be said in a couple of hours; however we did try to review in outline form some of the principles which are involved in the philosophic aspects of the Buddhist teachings.[81]

Far from participating in local rituals and social activities, the staff of the British Mission in Lhasa made a point of sticking to their own activities: organizing rugby games, holding "movie night" at the mission with Charlie Chaplin and Rin-Tin-Tin films, or simply drinking and dancing. Their behavior was just as incredulous to Theos as his seemed to be to them.

> What leaves me speechless is the reason for the necessity of such things. I find that they are doing this every night and now they are building a tennis court, having just erected the badminton court so they can have one game in the morning and the other [in the] evening with dancing in the night, all because they want to find some way to pass the time and give them something to do. How in the world any sort of normal intelligence can come to a place like Tibet and Lhasa of all places and have the problem of finding something to do. There is enough work available here to keep an army busy twenty-four hours a day for a lifetime and then have only scratched the surface and these aspiring souls have to figure out ways of introducing European games.

Theos felt that clearly "some people do not think much of their intellect when they consider such diversion as the best means of using it." Even the various rock carvings and artistic works scattered around Lhasa, such as the wall of images at the base of Chakpori, the mountain supporting the medical college, held "considerable interest" for him, "but apparently they

are all too crude for the sophisticated Richardson with his Oxford training." Indeed, Theos marveled that "it certainly doesn't take much to spoil
people in this world, for in no time, they are unwilling to give any credit to
anything but the very best which they can virtually never find."

Such considerations aside, Theos did observe that the British made a
point of putting on "a first class entertainment," and while they were not
entirely devoid of ideas—"one of the chaps is planning to write a book on
Lhasa . . . because of the inspiration awakened in a soccer game . . . another
wants to learn the language—and now after six months he is still holding the firm determination of definitely starting one of these days"—their
motivation seemed weak at best, and "such is the typical picture of all outposts of the British Empire."

Thus, the days that Theos spent in Lhasa were a mixture of frustration
and pacific beauty, in which "everything tended to induce an undisturb-
able inner peace and made you want to linger a while." It was a feeling
that the very land reinforced in the people, and it was something he found
particularly lacking "in the great centers of today where all has become
so mechanical and matter of fact," so much so that in America "we even
commence to despise our fellow man as he likewise dislikes you and shuts
himself up in that chilled shell of reserve." The simplicity of a moonlit pony
ride across Lhasa or the sight of the Nepali and Muslim residents of the city
playing a baseball game for their own fun and the entertainment of the
residents filled Theos with a level of joy in which he was "almost ready to
commence to love the beggars and rationalize in their favor." Of course, he
maintained, this was simply the effect of being unencumbered, as distant
from the Western lifestyle as Tibet was from New York. But the common
bond, a common humanity, could be accessed by anyone "thru the principles and techniques of Yoga," and with "just a little discipline, it will be
possible for one to shackle themselves to the grinding cogs of our social
machinery, but at the same time, keep that inner contact" with what he
liked to call "our subconscious."

Although he had received word from the Kashag that they had no objection to his continuing his studies in Lhasa indefinitely, the issue of traveling eastward remained unresolved. Having heard from yet another Tibetan
official that even members of the Tibetan government were not safe if they
traveled toward China, Theos was becoming more and more apprehensive about his half-hearted plans to visit Derge. He could not leave Lhasa

without a set of the books, for "as soon as I have crossed the Khampa la [Pass] they will [have] forgotten all about my desire to have one." The biggest difficulty, it seemed, was that Kangyur-Tengyur sets seemed to be in high demand, in China and Japan, Russia, Italy, and France. It was an odd thing to Theos. "Maybe," he speculated, "the religion is going to spread."

> With the world turning toward the mental side of life rather than towards the emotional side as in past days, it is not unlikely that these tenets would be acceptable, for they were written to be fed thru the mind and not the heart, and with Christianity holding nothing but love, it is difficult to turn mental all of a sudden in order to hold its own.

Clearly the ideas contained within the Buddhist canon could have an immense effect on whatever culture decided to adopt them, but the process of accessing the information would always be a challenge. Ideally, Theos thought,

> what I would like to do would be to select a staff of Lamas and secretaries and commence the job of translating the complete set so that those who follow in the future and become intrigued by the mystery of these characters will be able to read the thing thru in English and decide afterwards if they want to devote a life to expounding its philosophical teachings or all of its other innumerable aspects.

In the worst case, he would have to do the job himself with the help of a knowledgeable Tibetan "in about ten years," by which time he hoped "to have a little hold on the language." Since Geshe Sherap Gyatso was translating the Kangyur and Tengyur into Chinese, if he could do likewise into English, then "it will not be long before China can forget all about where they came from, and I hope that someday it will be the same for America." Indeed, with any luck, he told his wife, "a thousand years from now, America may be filled with a lot of aspiring hermits—won't that be something to rise out of the world's greatest industrial kingdom."

The next day, commencing a survey of the three great monastic universities of the Lhasa valley, Theos and Tharchin left early to reach Drepung just before sunrise, in time to photograph the early morning assembly at the monastery. As a "bearded Tibetan dressed foreigner," Theos observed with some amusement the "great commotion" his presence caused as he and

Tharchin walked through the monastery toward the main assembly hall. Photographing what he could and eating more *tsampa*[82] than he thought possible, Theos made offerings of food, tea, and money to the entire monastery, after which he and Tharchin toured the complex. From the copy of the red-inked, single-sheet Kangyur replete with carved sandalwood covers with inlaid Chinese ivory[83] to the various shrines of the four colleges, Theos and Tharchin saw it all, and walked around the circumambulation path before proceeding to Nechung Monastery nearby. Received by the abbot, they were once again fed rice and tea while Theos inquired about the monastery and its activities before the obligatory photos and their return to the Tsarong estate.

For several days in a row, Lord Tsarong had been called to the Kashag to discuss the ongoing, seemingly unresolvable situation with the Chinese. Theos's acquisition of a copy of the Derge Tengyur seemed to be one issue that Tsarong himself *could* resolve. Since each of his six estates held a copy, Lord Tsarong "has come forward and offer[ed] to sell another set which he has at one of his other six homes." With this and the acquisition of his other books, Theos was feeling more and more confident that he might succeed in "establishing a Tibetan library in America of some repute as far as our country is concerned" for with "the ardent rush from scholars of other countries on the literature of Tibet," Theos felt that getting hold of such books would only become more difficult. With any luck, he hoped, he was doing something right, and his "feelings about the future [were] a bit of judicious foresight rather then [*sic*] emotional folly."

Theos and Tharchin continued making offerings across the Lhasa valley. Having made an offering of a thousand butter lamps to the *stūpa* of the late Dalai Lama and fed the 175 monks of Namgyal Monastery, they made their next stop a tour of the Norbu Lingka, the summer palace of the Dalai Lama, courtesy of the Prime Minister, Lönchen Yapshi Langdün Küng.

After only a day's rest to study and document the previous day, Theos and Tharchin headed to the monastic university of Sera, just north of Lhasa, for another round of offerings to the monks there. As part of his sponsorship, Theos was told to mind his motivation in doing the rituals most of all:

> they tell me that the entire ritual which I am performing depends upon how much feeling I put into it, and that if I hold the right thought, that good will be forthcoming for many lives to come such as most have taken

place many lives past or I would never have wanted to come to Lhasa and perform these sacred ceremonies.

Theos, however, had his own ideas, which he equated with the perspective of "a Yogi."

> Who is to say how right they are, for the scientist of today cannot disprove it and it is tenable [in] their scheme of philosophy—and the Yogi has his own answer for all actions of a man, for he does not believe that things just happen. To him, everything is governed by a law of which we can gain understanding and thereby grow to know the meaning behind all unfathomable answers, and so I hold my secret belief.

As he had done days before at Drepung, Theos repeated the ceremony of offering food, tea, and money to the entire monastery of Sera, with all the customary activities. To his delight, however, rather than pausing during the ceremony for a simple meal, the abbots adjourned to a nearby hall where a canopy had been erected to shield them from the rain (and later, the sun) for an extended lunch with Theos, Tharchin, and various other select attendees. Having the heads of the three colleges of Sera and the abbot of the entire monastery nicely arrayed before him, Theos took each of their portraits for posterity. Following the meal, Theos and Tharchin were given a tour of the monastery, both its main assembly halls as well as the inner shrines, which Theos believed to be a special concession made to him, since "anyone can visit their main temples . . . but even for those, no amount of money will buy a pass beyond the massive doors, protecting their sacred shrines of the inner religion—the way is that of brotherhood— at which time all doors are thrown open and there is no escaping the duty of visiting each one and listening to the stories of how this one spoke and that one grew toe nails or finger nails or sweated." Eventually they were led around the circumambulation path, which afforded them a considerable photographic panorama of the entire locale with Lhasa and the Potala in the distance, on which they "used up an endless amount of film, trying to preserve the memory of that inspiring point of vantage" before returning to the city for the evening.

With only two days to prepare for their big trip to the last of the three great universities, Ganden, located in the mountains to the east, Theos and

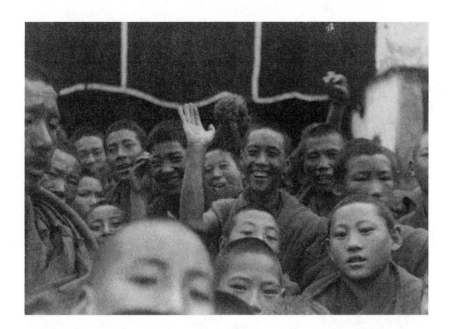

Figure 8.11 "Will the greed of capitalism smother the happiness that has been enjoyed for centuries?" Monks in front of the main assembly hall at Sera (PAHM)

Tharchin borrowed more money from Lord Tsarong to cover the many expenses that the trip would entail. Provisions for the journey of several days as well as offerings to the abbots and monks all had to be assembled and carefully packed; transport and guides had to be hired, and so on and so on. Leaving Lhasa on the morning of July 29, Theos realized he had spent more than the first month of his visit to Lhasa just sponsoring ceremonies and practicing his spoken Tibetan when and where he could.

Long before sunrise, Theos and Tharchin were dressed and seated astride ponies in the courtyard of the Tsarong estate. They could make out the dark, foreboding clouds of the Indian monsoons finally making their way north over the Himalayan Mountains toward Lhasa. Their transport loaded and ready, Theos and Tharchin departed for Ganden with their three standard servants (who accompanied them everywhere), additional men assigned to them by Lord Tsarong, their syces, muleteers, and an official government-assigned guide, planning to make the bulk of the thirty-mile ride in a day—crossing the Kyi-chu river in yakhide boats and changing transports several times. From that point it would take them only a couple of hours for the ascent up the valley to the mountaintop monastery the next morning.

Established in 1409 by the lineage founder himself, Ganden Monastic University was the seat of the head of the Geluk sect, the Ganden Tri-pa, whom Theos had already met. As they approached the monastery, they were instructed by the perimeter guard to remove the bells from their pack animals so as not to disturb the Ganden Tri-pa, who was in residence. Slightly annoyed by this obligatory show of respect, Theos complied nonetheless, taking solace in the idea that he might be able to meet with the abbot on a social level and despite his "emotional disgust," reminded himself that he was "here to learn and not criticise."

As the monastery finally came into full view, the impressive sight made an impact on Theos:

> There is little doubt about this being the ideal monastery tucked about in a hidden corner in the back bend of one of the high ridges which projects out into the valley. It was really a thrill and stimulated something inside that no other sight could bring about, providing you had ever held any ideals on what a perfect monastery should be like so far as its physical structure. Here it was among the gathering clouds of the heavens and completely hidden to everyone passing up and down the valley. It would only be a chance in a million that anyone would ever discover it, providing there was no knowledge of its existence. . . . This is truly a religious country—there is no denying of the facts; however almost any mortal dwelling in a like locality would be unable to think of anything else, for the country awakens all the religious awe any soul might possess.

Having been granted permission to spend the night at the monastery prior to the next day's offering ceremony, Theos reflected that he was "going to have the experience of living like a Tibetan Lama for a complete cycle of time and thereby hoped to contact the consciousness which goes with their form of sedentary life of devotion" and from his twenty-four-hour stay in the monastery, reach "the inner contact of the environment which I am trying to capture with my inner feelings so that I can carry away a life long understanding of the inner life of a Tibetan monk."

Of course, the day-to-day realities of life in a monastery were precisely the opposite of his romanticized expectations. "You have just about as much privacy here as you do in a hospital," he wrote, and within minutes of his arrival already "felt it a bit trying on the nerves to live in this manner," although he hoped that it was just the monks' curiosity about him as a Westerner "with a bearded face, wearing Tibetan clothes, talking to my own servants in their language with an occasional remark to them, and living in complete Tibetan fashion."[84] Nonetheless, the day had been a long one, made longer by an extended and detailed tour of the monastery circumambulation path, during which his guide pointed out the significance of "every dam rock on the hill that had a strange fissure" and the stories of the founder, Tsong-kha-pa—including about his body, interred nearby, which Theos was told (to his disbelief) continued to grow hair and fingernails that required maintenance from time to time[85]—before he was finally allowed to rest for the night.

Commencing the next day's offering ceremony, Theos went through the now familiar procedure of acting as a patron of the monastery. He presented the standard ritual offerings to the Ganden Tri-pa, as he had done three weeks earlier at the Jokhang. This time, however, the Regent took a little longer to give Theos his blessings, which Theos had not been expecting.

> We went thru a short ritual of devotion during which the warm glow of spiritual contact was felt—this being the warm hands of those who sat on the altar of life—it is a strange feeling to contact that feeling in one's ritual before such a shrine, for it was too dark to make out the live forms. We could see these holy mounds, but they might have been stone figures so far as one could tell, until the warmth of their hands and head was felt—anyone too deeply wrapped up in the emotion of the occasion would probably come away with some mighty weird tales. Having passed thru the experience with sufficient feeling to let that part of imagination take the lead, I can fully understand the reason.[86]

For Theos, this felt emotional impact was nothing more than a sign of true spiritual attainment: the ability to produce a profound emotional reaction in others. Of the rest of the inhabitants of the monasteries in Tibet, Theos had a very low opinion. They were simply part of an institution that "has developed into a social mechanism to provide for those unable to cope with the demands of life." Consequently, he thought, "the head lamas of these large monasteries are one of two personality [types]—political racketeers or a true spiritual master which is the case with [Tri] Rinpoche, but these are few and far between."

After a last brief tour through the buildings, Theos and Tharchin paid a final visit to the abbot, which included "the performance of a private ritual,"[87] before leaving to return to Lhasa. On their way down the mountain, Theos and Tharchin had a long talk during which they "had a great time reviewing a lot of the nonsense which we had just witnessed," but since it was an aspect of Tibetan life that they had ostensibly come to study, they "took it in that light."

> From all appearances someone is going to have to come along one of these days and clean out the house of religion for all the peoples of the world, for all the standing religions of the world today are beginning to wane, and this only shows that man is changing—for good or for worse he is on the move, but the traditional forms of history try to remain the same. However eventually we will out grow this shell of ages, to such an extent that we will not even be able to keep a little of it on our wings of progress—and then there will be a mad dash for freedom; however a leader will come and give expression to the universal truths of life in light of modern understanding. Today we are just unable to see how anything that was taught to the people of mythological times has anything to do with us who seem to know so much, but no more capable of coping with the inner mysteries of life then [sic] those of olden times. We are battling with the same problems of love, hate, graft, greed, jealousy, envy, ambition for power and everything else that is forthcoming as the result of man's inner sense of inferiority, and it seems that there is no society existing that does not have these traits of human nature, finding expression thru some sort of a channel—among the most primitive to the most sophisticated they always show up.

The future of mankind—if there was to be one—Theos felt could only be assured by a new world religious leader, well versed in Buddhist philosophy, something he felt to be distinct from "religion."

> Even if the more enlightened worked out a scheme which was perfect, it would not last for long, for the inferior would [be] sure to wreck it, and this can be demonstrated and proved in a thousand countless ways of

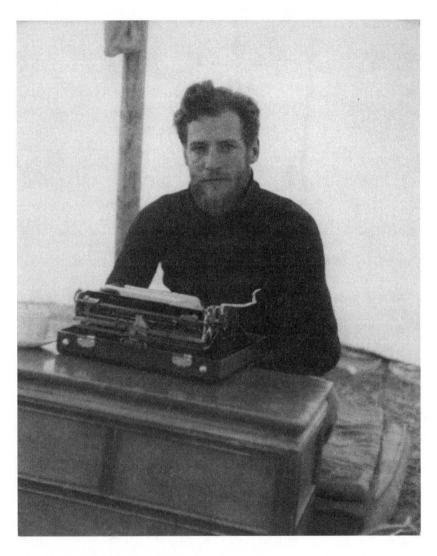

Figure 8.12 Bernard recording his thoughts (PAHM)

everyday life so we are never going to escape the need of a great leader to come and point the direction for the inner way of life—we need him more today then ever before because there are more of us who are suffering as self satisfied as a few of us tend to appear. The Western world today has developed into a mental world in which everything must be proven and explained according to a rational bases [*sic*]; therefore it is impossible for the traditional forms of present Christianity which only directed the way thru faith to hold or help the modern man; so one must come who is fully familiar with the problems of the present age and then say the same thing over again in the new way—in other ways he must mould truth into an airoplane [sic] rather then [sic] a donkey. And so I sit in a dark corner of Tibet wondering what is going to happen to man and what is the best means to serve as a vehicle of universal happiness . . . when one is able to penetrate thru the forms and get back to the original philosophical teaching of Buddha, he finds something worth giving a little reflection.

The way to introduce such philosophy to a materialistic Western audience, however, was precisely what Theos personally disliked: ritual.

Thru our extensive educational system we have developed a semi-thinking man who no longer can except [sic] traditional ritual which gives him no intellectual satisfaction; however he is in just as much in need of ritual as those in the beginning, but a new scheme of pomp must be devised for him—which in turn will also be worn out with time when the same cycle will have to take place once again, and I fear that man will never escape from the cycles of a ritual way of life—we all like clothes, but not those worn by our grandfather.

Pausing on their way back to Lhasa, Theos and Tharchin visited the retreat hermitage just east of the city, Dra-yer-pa, arriving late at night, but in time to request the opportunity to patronize a ceremony for the next day. While the next day's ceremony went as all the others had, of far more importance to Theos was his audience with a Kagyu yogi there.

They had a hermit and we were given the permission to visit him. He is one of those reputed chaps who has been living in a cave of a good many years. . . . His room was naturally very small with a large image of the thousand hands and thousand eyes of Chenresi; with several smaller images of the same deity. Then there were several thangkas, one of the thousand Buddhas, another which showed the line from Marpa down thru Milarepa and his disciples. This individual was one who was reputed to hold the Wang or "Authority" from this direct line . . . however there is no way to deny him and if someone must, it might just as well be him so we conceded all points. His entire life was spent in his small square box, just large enough for him to sit cross legged comfortably—if it is possible to be comfortable. He takes but one helping of barley flour and little milk a day and never does he lie down. This makes his tenth year in this one spot, having put in twelve years at another holy cave and now after a few more years here, he plans to go to the section where Milarepa spent his life in a cave and I take it this will finish up his time in this life, for today he is 65 years of age, but looks about forty—what the men of our country would do to hold on as he. There is not a gray hair to be found in his head or beard, and his skin still has all of its vigor as does his voice and thoughts. On a small shelf behind him, he had four large volumes wrapped up in some Indian Printed material. To the right of him in front of the small window which affords him one ray of light for the purpose of reading, were several smaller volumes. To the left of him within arms reach were various articles to be used in his ritual, and so from his position he had access to the entire room without having to move from his box. The entrance was directly in front and just over the right corner of the door coming in was a small piece of paper with the symbol "HUM" written in fair size letters—this was for the purpose of certain concentration practices. He was far from being emaciated; however he was pleasing thin in accordance with good health for such a life. His long thin fingers accentuated by his uncut nails hold your interest every time he brought them into action when speaking. Of course, I was all interest, for this was the sort of chap that I had been waiting to meet in Tibet and the reason that I have been willing to go thru with much of the external forms that have been necessary; so I was all questions, but it was impossible to say much, for he would not reveal any teachings to anyone, and in no case before such a crowd even tho several were monks from the monastery; however in our questioning and discussions, he was able to gather a little different approach than had ever come his way again, for I was able to reveal enough to give him those hidden answers so far as others who were untrained were concerned, and with this he said that he would give me some of my desired information if I would return, which meant that I was to come alone or with my interpreter; so we continued our tour in the fog, taking in all of their shrines hidden away beyond the dark tunnels into their small caves.

Tibet, Tantrikas, and the Hero of Chaksam Ferry

Attending the ceremony being held at his request, Theos was anxious to leave and return to the yogi's cave.

Once this was over, I returned to the cave of our hermit after paying my personal respects to the head abbot from Lhasa. . . . Our hermit was waiting, and after arriving, he had us lock the door and I commence[d] the repetition of my devotionals in the expression of the desires of my heart, and then he settled down to the business of repeating endless mantras so that the atmosphere might be purified or what have you. This took some time for there was considerable throwing of wheat seeds and passing of holy water and holy butter along with precious pea balls of blessed tsampa—so I had my divine nourishment before it was all over. During the whole ceremony I had to remain cross legged before my holy master of this divine line of saints on earth. However I was in for whatever went with the process of getting what I wanted, for I had found out that this chap had covered enough literature to be of some value to me, and I also knew that if I could win my way to him in the form of a disciple or what have you that it would give me an opportunity of securing books that would be impossible otherwise, for I have been trying ever since my arrival in Lhasa to secure certain material on this subject and find that it is absolutely impossible for those who have it will not part with it and in no event will they impart any of its knowledge and prayers to the outside; so it was up to me to work my way in, regardless what it might necessitate in the form of humility. In fact on my arrival, I virtually crawled to him as is customary when making a request from a learned master of divine wisdom, and in this position I placed one end of my *kata* on his low table and strung the rest out across the room which is the manner followed when making a request. . . . On my offering he immediately responded for me to be comfortable and then we commenced to work in the manner which I have just stated, he had several books which he used to commence the service from which he mumbled with a ringing voice in the typical Tibetan rhythm which one can never forget nor can he ever repeat. At various intervals thru out his reading, he placed various sacred objects on my head as well as throwing the other articles about which I have mentioned. Before commencing however, he placed over his left shoulder and under his right arm a cloth band on which three lines were sewn in reddish thread which represented the three centres of the body where the *lung* [energy] travels—Sushumna,

Ida and Pingala. This was according to the Tibetan beliefs—which is little different than the Indian, in that they have the right nose connected with the right side in contrast to the Indian with its crossing over. At the various centres were woven the mantra which went [with] it and which was repeated as the entrance was made. And with this, he passed on the authority of the direct line of Milarepa to carry on his teaching and spread them to those who were worthy. Then commenced the instruction on their various practices of meditation, concentration, breathing and the union of the two spiritual poles within. All was as I had been taught in India except here they used the burning of incense to mark the length each breath should be—just a means of adapting to the element of time—about six inches marked one breath and they teach that one must do it at least twenty one times.... Now when speaking with regard to these centre[s] he had a chart which he used and explained its meaning from a small handwritten book which gave this ritual in a very brief form, the illuminations having to come from him with these as a guide. The entire process took virtually all of the afternoon, but now I am prepared to go to work before the last step of ascending into heaven or something—however I appreciated the opportunity and that I was able to instill enough confidence on virtually a glance to gain this entrance which has never been done before by one from my country. He then permitted to take these brief books so that I could have a copy of them made for my further use when instructing others; so in all I did gather a wealth of material, for I know that it is impossible to get otherwise, for all of this sort of thing is written by hand and not printed from public blocks.

The amazement of the Dra-yer-pa monks at Theos's being granted an audience with the yogi, as well as the empowerment to practice "Heat Yoga,"[88] and being allowed to borrow his books only added to Theos's sense of accomplishment. Flushed with success, he returned to Lhasa and arranged to have the manuscript copied.

Over the next few weeks, Theos continued to acquire books and take more photographs of Lhasa and its people. He also made a point of enjoying the time he had earned: indulging Reginald Fox with the occasional game of badminton, socializing with the newly arrived Dr. Morgan and Lord Tsarong, keeping abreast of the ongoing Sino-Japanese War[89] exploring the city and the surrounding area, attending, describing, and photographing ritual dance performances, and socializing with aristocratic families. Feeling relaxed, he began to take notice of more and more around him, including young Tibetan women, from the daughters of nobles to the poorest peasant girls and even the occasional teenage nun.⁹⁰

From that point on, however, Theos's activities all began to revolve around logistics. Attending to the Kangyur and Tengyur, he got a geshe "to check all the volumes"—Theos following along with the help of the recently published index to the canon published in Japan, which Tsarong had a copy of—and had them properly wrapped and sewn in yak hide "so as not to get wet on their long trip on mule back to Kalimpong." Thinking about ways to capitalize on his experiences in Tibet, Theos saw "so many possibilities on the horizon of capitalistic hope," given the fascination with Tibet that existed in the rest of the world. Since he had copper mining rights in Arizona, Theos could imagine a whole new industry in copper Buddhist images, for "the markets of China, Japan, Burma, Ceylon and parts of India to say nothing of those of Mongolia, parts of Siberia, Sinkyang, northern Turkestan etc. are not to be looked at lightly, for being Buddhist they will all take a small image as quickly as our country will buy a Bible . . . when you contact religion, you are in one of the softest rackets on earth and it seems to be the same all over the face of the globe without any exceptions." Lecturing and teaching, in fact, seemed a natural occupation to pursue, and it would offer him open-ended employment since, he said rather cryptically, "I won't be killed for some years yet."

Likewise, giving thought to his eventual return to Tibet, Theos envisioned first writing a few books—a process well under way in his diaries, which by early August amounted to well over 150,000 words. Knowing of the interest in Tibet and based on the fame he would achieve, Theos felt he could easily charge would-be explorers $10,000 each for the privilege of accompanying him on a return trip. His only competition, besides the British Mission staff,⁹¹ was Tucci, who was still stuck in Gyantse and "trying desperately to come on to Lhasa," even offering Rai Bahadur Norbu "an Italian Title" if he could use his influence as British Trade Agent to get him there.

Coincidentally, a telegram sent to Captain Cable in Gyantse by Theos, boasting of his success in Lhasa and the wealth of photographs obtained, was accidentally delivered to Tucci instead, which sent the Italian scholar into a rage, thinking that Theos—"a nobody"—was taunting him. Insulted by this, Tucci "got on his high horse . . . but the British . . . took him down in a hurry." Consequently, the British Mission staff informed Theos, Tucci had decided instead to document Gyantse in excruciating detail and was "taking pictures of Gyantse just as fast as he can click a camera" with the intention of publishing a book. Not to be outdone, Theos resolved to "beat him at his own game" and write a book that would make T. E. Lawrence's *Seven Pillars of Wisdom* look like "a short story in comparison."

Already planning for their return trip to India, Tharchin began securing sufficient quantities of silk for wrapping the books and yak hides for packaging,[92] commissioning special printings of Tibetan stamps for Theos's hundreds of Christmas cards, and engaging carpenters to build boxes to hold it all. Time was of the essence, for although Theos could (and planned to) remain in Tibet, Tharchin knew that he would have to return to Kalimpong soon, having already stretched his employer's patience beyond the breaking point; he had received yet another letter from Knox threatening to evict Tharchin's wife and family from their home (owned by the mission) if he did not return immediately. Consoling him, Theos told Tharchin that although he personally "could shoot" every Christian missionary for such behavior, "the quicker Knox kicked him out, the quicker he [could go] to work for me like a real human being and not a Babu," for Tharchin, in Theos's opinion, was "certainly more deserving of far more [than] a contemptible Christian mission will ever pay him." Recognizing that he had created the problem for Tharchin himself, Theos took on the responsibility of solving it for him as well, wiring Knox to tell him how important it was for Tharchin to remain in Tibet with him, for the benefit of "those of the outside world who are going to want the results of this opportunity which has never before been had by a foreigner." He did not have to wait long for a reply. In addition to threatening one more time to evict Tharchin's wife and family, Knox informed Tharchin in a separate telegram that he had cut off his pay the moment his six-week leave had expired, and he was to return immediately. Theos was not happy. "I decided right then and there to myself," he wrote, "that the moment that he went off his pay role he went on fulltime on mine, providing Tharchin wanted to take on the new work as a fulltime job which has the possibilities of a long dreamed of piece of life work for him." In any event, Theos declared,

He is not returning to Kalimpong until I have finished by job and if Knox wants him for a few months while I return to America and make final arrangements, and if Knox is not agreeable, Tharchin will continue right on with me paying him anything that any Christian beggar has to offer for his begging assistance. . . . I even hate that aspect of Tharchin, for he is no better then the rest of them when he gets off on one of these avenues; however being a Tibetan even tho under Christian influence which was only commenced in the beginning because of the foresight of a parent to make an easier and better living for his family, he still holds his hidden beliefs in certain teachings of Buddhism . . . in fact, one of the most lamentable phenomena of present day human existence is a belief in any sort of religion—regardless what name it comes under—it is all the same—ignorance of the lowest order; however with this sort of an attitude it is easy enough to guess what my actions would be on the receipt of a telegram telling me to "send Tharchin at once"—I'll send him straight to hell first, for I know that he will wind up there sooner or later if he follows the other course, and fast traveling in any direction is always more fun; so irregardless of where one is going, he might as well enjoy the excitement and exhilaration of a little speed, and so Tharchin stays with me.

In the midst of this unfolding melodrama, thousands more contact prints were arriving from Calcutta, and Theos was swamped with the task of organizing them. To make matters worse, the task was complicated by the fact that, having "kept Tharchin supplied with camera and film," he was accumulating pictures twice as fast as he normally would, and the resulting contact prints were "a mess." Although Tharchin was experienced in the use of a camera, he was "not familiar with modern ideas on the subject of the photographic art," and most of his photos were "not worthy of publication." When he was shown Lord Tsarong's photograph albums, Theos endeavored to make a list of everything notable that Tsarong had photographed in order to try to photograph it himself. To compensate for Tharchin's photos, Theos decided he would have to redouble his efforts to "take a picture with a 'feeling' behind it," revisiting the Norbu Lingka, the Jokhang, and Potala Palace, as well as climbing Chakpori hill to take pictures from the vantage of the medical college.

Throughout it all, the books "continued to pour in"—including, Theos claimed, a Tibetan translation of the *Caraka Saṃhita*,[93] which excited him immensely since it offered a means by which Tibetan and Sanskrit medical vocabularies could be bridged. Nonetheless, he found the days that followed "more or less devoid of any imagination" since although he had hoped to spend more time photographing Lhasa, the monsoon rains from India had finally come, and most days were overcast, if not actually rainy.

Resigning himself to studying and watching the tailors sew wrappings for his books, by the end of the summer, Theos was spending "hours upon end of constant drill in order to get a few of the fundamentals [of literary Tibetan] before it is time to leave this section of the world when it will be impossible to carry on the studies for some time." Yet he was still struggling with the written script, for while the simple block-print-style Tibetan lettering was easy to master, it was only ever used in printing books; no one ever wrote in it. Everyone used the cursive form, and because all of Tharchin's and the geshe's notations were written in that script, Theos felt "that it is essential that I learn to read it." But it was not easily self-taught. To help his guest, Lord Tsarong made a point of trying to keep Theos busy, and hopefully learning as well; helping him with the script and with his pronunciation of written words.

The highlight of these weeks for Theos was the occasional mail delivery from India—whose timely arrival had suffered of late with the departure of Richardson and Gould and the discipline they brought to the British Mission staff. "It is truly a gratifying feeling to receive messages of encouragement from old friends who have almost past [sic] from your memory because of the indifference we hold towards one another in our busy world of affairs." From the letters he received from time to time over the summer, he could see that much of the drama of his distant life in America had continued unabated, and it often left him "virtually dumbfounded."

Glen wrote to Theos that he had had a "long talk" with Evans-Wentz, who was "anxious that I come on to Oxford where he believes that he can give me a great deal of help." From his mother, he learned of the latest news concerning his brothers and her own life, including her pending divorce. He remarked to Viola that his mother was suffering this fate because of her unorthodox religious beliefs; in response, Viola told Theos he had nothing to worry about in that regard, reaffirming that "tho our lives are funny, I am sure that they are sound" and that she had confidence in him and what he was doing: "you—with your capacity for ecstasy, are fulfilling yourself."

For Viola, the day-to-day events in her life centered around her internship at the medical center and her plans for her "psychiatry apprenticeship" in the fall—assuming she could get accepted to a program—although her connection to P.A. and the CCC had already cost her one position. The focus of her personal life remained her friends from the club, and in particular, the ongoing strife between her one-time guru, P.A., and his soon-to-be ex-wife and Viola's closest friend, DeVries. She reminded Theos to take care of himself "in these different moments of breath-taking living" and "be happy in the knowledge of our love," and while being touched that he was thinking of her and their "Christmas card" for the coming year, Viola still cautioned him with her concerns. "It also scares me a little for you," she wrote, "in the sense that you are existing on such a peak of experience right now that it will be difficult not to let everything afterwards seem rather anticlimactic." She encouraged him to keep writing to her since "it helps tremendously" to prevent "a too widening gap that would be very hard to span" when they would be together again.

Although appreciative of Viola's letters to him, Theos concluded that while "it is interesting to read of the activities which fill every hour of their lives, for on the most part they all seem to be so busy that there is hardly time for an extra breath," and yet, he continued, "I must confess that it is that sort of activity that I want to duck, for I feel that it is the strongest poison of our civilization to the imaginations of man." Nonetheless, there would be no escaping it anytime soon, and Theos knew that he would need to continue to function in the world, and at the very least, have a fixed address and a plan for the future. Viola suggested that he write from Lhasa to a number of organizations, from the New York World's Fair—which was planning a "Hall of Religions" exhibit—to the Lotos Club and The Explorers Club in New York applying for membership, since his acceptance to the latter would at least provide him with a mailing address.

Deciding that her advice was sound and that he should not neglect his contacts back in America, Theos wrote to all of the organizations, including The Explorers Club—feeling assured of membership since hearing, to both his and Tharchin's delight, that Tucci had been denied permission to visit Lhasa. He further mused about reading Tucci's future rendition of his failure in this regard.[94]

As the weeks passed, the time of Theos's departure loomed near. Suydam Cutting arrived in Lhasa and, unable to stay with Lord Tsarong as he had wished, he and his wife decamped at a small house at Sara Lingka arranged for them by the Tibetan government. As a reflection of Tibetan-style hospitality, Theos ventured out of the city to meet them. Although they would cross paths from time to time over the next week and a half, Theos was actually quite determined to keep an eye on his rival "in order to see that he does not uncover anything that I have failed to pick up which would be a disgrace on my part," and took exceptional joy in Cutting's repeated

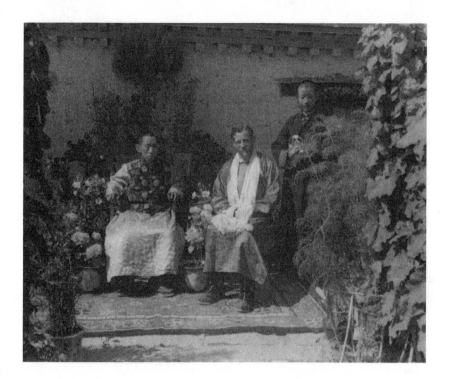

Figure 8.13 Bernard with the Regent, Reting Rinpoche (PAHM)

amazement at seeing Theos talk with his Tibetan servants without the aid of a translator.

Yet with each summer day, there seemed to come another photographic opportunity, from festival dances[95] to the chance to film a "sky burial," in which dead bodies were to be cut up and fed to vultures. After photographing and filming this last event, Theos related the details to Viola, describing the scene in which "all along the cliff the vultures were waiting." Upon reading his letter, "so was Theos," she sarcastically remarked.

As the final pieces of Theos's plans fell into place, it was Reting Rinpoche who came to Theos's aid when he was still unable to acquire the "twenty five volume set" of medical textbooks, since every printer in Lhasa was engaged in producing the *Collected Works* of the Thirteenth Dalai Lama. With these last books obtained and a photo of Theos with the Regent to commemorate their friendship, he and Tharchin prepared for their departure from Lhasa.

Tibet, Tantrikas, and the Hero of Chaksam Ferry

By now, their plans had been settled. Theos and Tharchin would leave together, making their way to Shigatse to visit Tashilhunpo Monastery, the seat of the Panchen Lama. As Theos paid his respects by visiting Tethong Shapé and the Kalön Lama, who had both warmly welcomed him to Lhasa, they equally offered him their utmost prayers for his future successes, and while the Kalön Lama invited him to return to Tibet in the future, Tethong Shapé offered "to attend to anything on the Kham side that might come up" in the course of Theos's future studies. There then followed in rapid succession visits with Cutting, the British Mission staff, the Chinese envoy, and every merchant eager to sell him something at the last possible minute.

In his final meeting with the Regent, Reting told Theos that spreading Buddhism in America was the most important thing he could do, and that he, Reting, would like to visit America someday and could perhaps come to see him. In the meantime, in order to help Theos in his endeavors, Reting suggested that he write a letter on his behalf to President Roosevelt, if Theos would agree to deliver it personally. Unable to refuse, Theos graciously accepted the offer and, slightly stunned, return to the Tsarong estate with a letter from Reting Rinpoche to FDR—in both English and Tibetan—that read:

To His Excellency the great Mr. Roosevelt, President of America, White House, Washington, D.C.V., E.C.I.,

The bearer of this letter, a citizen of your country (kingdom), Mr. Theos Bernard, has great faith in the Buddhist religion, and is possessed of great wisdom, mild, and a good disciple.

Especially has he the greatest desire to cement the friendship between Tibet and America. It is of importance that all of you who are concerned, should have a high regard for this matter, and render such assistance as lies in your power, in order that the Buddha's doctrine may prosper exceedingly in all directions.

This letter is sent by the Regent of Tibet, the Hu-thuk-thu of Ra-dreng Monastery, from the Happy Grove of the All-Good Beautiful Palace of the Shi-de Gan-Den Sam-Ten-Ling, on the Auspicious Date, the tenth day of the eighth month of the Fire-Bull Year. (September 1937)

Stamped with his personal seal, it was an impressive, if unusual document.[96]

At a final afternoon tea with Lord and Lady Tsarong, the melancholy of his last day in Lhasa was beginning to catch up to Theos, and on their return from visiting Tharchin's mother-in-law, he happened upon one of the geshes from Drepung, who had been working at the Tsarong estate checking and labeling all of his books. "The experience that dam near wrecked me," he recounted, "was when I spotted a lama waiting at a corner a couple of miles out of town and rode up to find that it was my geshe who I had seen just a few moments ago at Tsarongs. . . . He had walked all the way out here to offer me his Kata." Though a simple gesture of fond wishes on the geshe's part, it shook Theos deeply, and for the rest of the evening he was left inexplicably "haunted" and lonely; riding back to the Tsarongs' in the moonlight, he could only wish that Viola were there to offer him comfort in her arms.

Assembling in the courtyard at four o'clock the next morning, their transport caravan would head to Gyantse while Theos and Tharchin went to Shigatse, a journey of several days. Traveling once again through the same stark, yet beautiful terrain so reminiscent of the Arizona lands of his childhood, Theos was back to his old self and took his inspiration where he could find it. Following the traditional route from Lhasa to Shigatse, they passed one more time along the shores of Tibet's largest sacred lake, Yam-drok-tso. Resting for the night at the fortress ruins of Phe-de overlooking the lake, while his hosts busied themselves with burning juniper branches in the votive censers dotting the mountain pass, Theos took the opportunity once again to write to Viola:

At the moment, I am sitting in one of the filthiest dung heaps to be found in the world and known by the Tibetans as a house. Well, the truth of the matter is that I am so dam busy and concerned about other things that the most of the time I do not fully realize my environment until I realize that it is impossible for me to move without wading in it up to my ankles . . . in no way am I trying to complain, for I can look out the window and behold one of the most beautiful lakes of the world tucked away up here to harbour the nectar of the melting Gods on the High Himalayan peaks. If I will but stop the machine for an instant, I can faintly hear the silent lapping of the quiet waters on the narrow shore—listen . . . . hear it—it is all moving and the splash is carried through the echoing canyon walls while the water finds its way to the other shore to be sent back. The sky is banked high with thunderbolts all ready to open up and wash us away—bang—there goes the thunder—and it is real thunder—after the lightening, it rumbles and roars until your whole insides commence to quiver just a wee bit—but gee, you like it—if you like nature. And such is my trip from Lhasa to Shigatse.

Arriving in Shigatse in late September, Theos and Tharchin repeated the now standard procedure of requesting the privilege of making offerings of food, tea, and money to the monks of the local monastery while waiting for permission for Theos to proceed to Sakya, all the while photographing and filming.

Since Theos was able to claim the friendship of both Ngak-chen Rinpoche and Reting Rinpoche—not to mention Lord Tsarong, whose reputation, Theos discovered, extended all the way to Shigatse—they were able to meet with the governmental officials, both the acting fort commander and the Lhasa representative overseeing the operation of the Shigatse region since the flight of the Panchen Lama. Having received permission to proceed, Theos was set. However, for the first time, he would be truly on his own. The caravan of pack mules was en route to Gyantse from Lhasa, so it was imperative that Tharchin go on ahead to meet the convoy of books, clothes, and all their sundry acquisitions from the summer. Theos would have to head to Sakya alone and negotiate his own way, accompanied by only his syce and coolies.

Arriving in Sakya with letters of introduction, Theos was received by the household of the Sakya Hierarch, given accommodations at the Phuntsok Palace, and scheduled for an audience with the man himself. As the regency of the Sakya lineage alternated between two families, the new head, the Sakya Tri-chen, was Ngawang Tutop Wangchuk,[97] and Theos was quite impressed. "Next to Tsarong," he wrote, "I have not met such a burning personality, for no sooner than I spotted him and before a word had been uttered, I felt as tho he might have been a life long friend and I truly felt a twang of affection for him which is rather exceptional on my part." As much as he was struck by the force of the Hierarch's presence, he felt an even stronger emotional reaction when he met the man's eldest daughter.

I had only arrived at my suite in the palace and was in the midst of writing down my notes, when I suddenly felt the presence of someone watching me . . . I looked up to find the most radiant face that I had ever

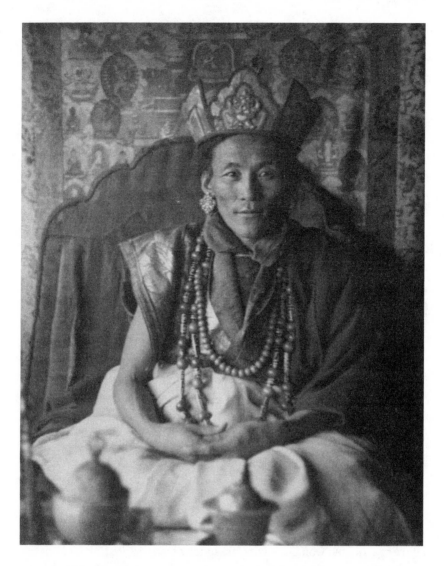

Figure 8.14 Sakya Tri-chen, Ngawang Tutop Wangchuk (PAHM)

seen watching my every action. It was like a dream—An Asiatic Princess.
I could well understand why Knights of Olden had so willingly gone to
their death in the mere hope of a chance to win the heart of such a
creature. She was as tho of another world. She did not belong to the
people of this world. Her features were sharp and well-defined as tho
chiseled by the hand of some divine sculptor. Her rich black hair formed

Tibet, Tantrikas, and the Hero of Chaksam Ferry
269

a sharp line around her face. She had everything that every girl has dreamed of since their earliest childhood. . . . Not a word was exchanged between us. I could not have spoken had it been a matter or life and death. I did not know what it was, but whatever it was, I never wanted it to end. . . . Everyday she came to my room and we would look at one another for hours at a time, never uttering a word, but living in the depths of the same consciousness. The feeling never waned, but became more intense with time. I would almost forget at times, the purpose of my mission, where I was going and from where I had come. I was lost in something that seemed eternal. . . . I was on [my] way—where I did not know—it was not home, for never in my life had I felt more [at] home. If home is where the heart is, this was home for me.

Upon being informed that the young woman was destined to be ordained as a nun since she had been formally recognized as an incarnate goddess, Theos began to speculate on the reason for his strong feelings for her.

I enquired more about my friend, and learned that she was being trained to be a nun. She was believed to be the reincarnation of a divine dietess. Her religious sect would not have prevented her from marriage, but where was the reincarnation of her divine counterpart? How would they find him? To me it was the ideal marriage, for this would have been the Union of Souls and not the marriage of bodies. In fact, she was already united with her divine counterpart, it was merely a matter of recognition of its physical manifestation.

At the end of a long summer in Tibet, Theos had finally succumbed to the allure of a Tibetan woman. Having asked for permission to film and photograph the Hierarch's entire family, for Theos, it was Tupten Wangmo who compelled him the most.

Truly one glimpse of his eldest daughter who is 15 is like striking a match. She was gowned in golden silk and wearing a shoulder cape of brilliant red which lighted up her beautiful innocent face of childhood curiosity. From a distance her black hair glistened as tho it had been polished, and at no time did she take her eyes off of me trying to take a picture . . . she has one of the few faces that I have seen in this country that radiates with intelligence and once you know her father, the reason is obvious; however this evening, I likewise met her mother whose face is marked with a strong determination, and speaks with a well disciplined mind.

It was the Hierarch himself, in the end, who was most fascinated by Theos. After hearing about Theos's activities over the past months, the Hierarch too offered to write a letter to "the King of America" on Theos's behalf. Like Reting Rinpoche, he emphasized the importance of Theos's mission:

> To the Most Illustrious King of America who is interested in all the Virtues.
>
> This letter is sent by the Hierarch of the Phun-Tshog Pho-Drang (The Perfect Palace) of Sakya, with greetings.
>
> An American gentlemen named Bernard, who has great faith in the Religion, arrived here. Rest assured that I have rendered him all the assistance that lay in my power. If a Buddhist Monastery is established in your Precious Majesty's Kingdom, there will be no pestilence, nor will there be any war or famine in your country. Perfect happiness and prosperity will prevail.
>
> Pray remember that in whatever state you may chance to be reborn, you will have long life, and fortune, power and glory beyond description will be yours.
>
> It is good to hear that the King of America sympathizes with the spread of the Buddhist Religion to other countries.
>
> As I have requested earlier in this letter, please be graciously inclined to render all the assistance that lies in your power, to help this gentleman, (Bernard) who has a pure mind.
>
> This letter is sent with a Silk Scarf of Greeting from the Phun-Tshog Pho-Drang of the Noble Sakya Monastery, on the Auspicious Date, the fifth day of the ninth month of the Fire-Bull Year. (October, 1937)

The Hierarch went further to offer that if Theos gave him a list of *thangkas* and texts he wished to obtain, he would personally have them procured and sent down to India and on to America, for having gone on pilgrimage to India himself in the past, he was well aware of conduits for shipping materials across the border. Indeed, coming to pay his respects to the Hierarch before leaving, Theos was encouraged to return to Tibet:

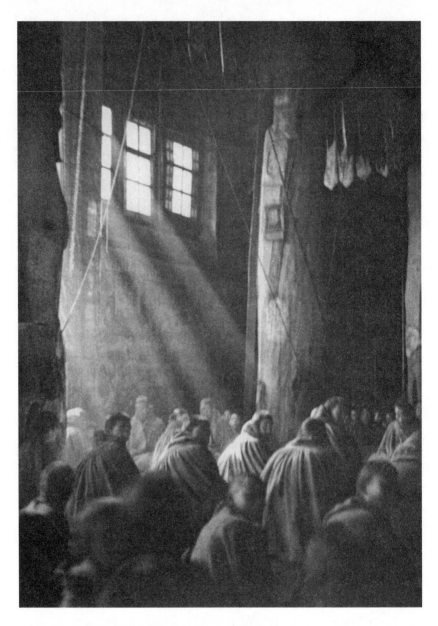

Figure 8.15 Morning assembly at Sakya Monastery (PAHM)

He received me in his large audience hall, seated on his high throne . . . and draped in that beautiful red . . . which helps to light up the dangling leaf shaped turquoise earrings and his long necklace of coral beads. . . . As before, he was radiating like an over heated radiator on a cold day and expressed many regrets that I had to leave after such a short while. He not only asked but he insisted that I return to Tibet once again, and enter thru Northern Sikkim so as to visit with him first . . . as well as permit me more time to study and go over their vast collection of literature of which I have referred. I must say that he is one individual with whom I would enjoy looking forward to another visit . . . perhaps after a rest of a couple of years I will feel a pressing urge to come and not stop to consider what the trip is going to be like—in fact, I will look forward to its difficulties and demands.

With all that he had hoped for accomplished, on October 9, 1937, Theos packed his bags one last time and began his journey south toward Sikkim and India. Following the short route suggested by the Hierarch and guided by one of his men, he passed through the seldom traveled lands and valleys—some maintained, home to one of the mythic "hidden valleys" of Tibet—due east from Sakya and south past ancient ruins and long-forgotten *stūpas* to the Sikkim border. After two days of rapid travel through barren valleys and over increasingly colder and colder snowy passes, Theos crossed the Se-bu pass, and returned from the "ethereal vistas of the Gods . . . bounded on all sides with nature's glittering necklace of ice," back to the land of men.

NINE

"The Clipper Ship of the Imagination"

The great majority of readers and hearers are the same all over the world.
I have no doubt that the people of your country are like those I have met
in China and India, and these latter were just like Tibetans. If you speak
to them of profound Truths they yawn, and, if they dare, they leave you,
but if you tell them absurd fables they are all eyes and ears. They wish
the doctrines preached to them, whether religious, philosophic, or social,
to be agreeable, to be consistent with their conceptions, to satisfy their
inclinations, in fact that they find themselves in them, and that they feel
themselves approved by them.

—ALEXANDRA DAVID-NEEL[1]

WHILE THEOS WAS WENDING his way back to India, Tharchin had been
busily at work on his behalf. Accompanying all their belongings back to
Kalimpong, Tharchin had already begun promoting Theos as the latest
great explorer of Tibet. While Viola was forwarding Theos's letters to old
professors, friends, and family in America, Tharchin was wiring reports
from Gyantse to Calcutta about their great adventure in Tibet before either of them had even returned. Based on a letter from Tharchin, the *De-
troit News*—fascinated as much by Tharchin as by Bernard—ran an article
in early October telling of their exploits. Indeed, all of Theos's friends and
family had mobilized on his behalf. In Tucson, his mother had contacted
the largest state newspaper, the *Arizona Daily Star*, forwarding his letters,
and articles began informing the public of "the Ex-U.A. Scholar" and his
adventures, with more stories to follow, in both Arizona and New York.[2]

Before Theos had reached Kalimpong, Tharchin had contacted the *Calcutta Statesman*, which ran an article on their adventures,[3] and Frank Perry
had already negotiated a UK exclusive interview with a Calcutta reporter

for London's *Daily Mail*,[4] a widely read—if not very widely respected—tabloid newspaper. His public relations campaign well under way before he had even set foot on his home soil, Theos Bernard declared to this Calcutta reporter, "I am the first White Lama—the first Westerner ever to live as priest in a Tibetan monastery, the first man from the outside world to be initiated into Buddhists' mysteries hidden even from many native lamas themselves." Selecting a few choice photos, the *Daily Mail* hailed Theos as the "young explorer" whose exclusive account they had secured was "the greatest adventure story of the year."

In the midst of his campaign, however, Theos received a telegram from Viola back in the States: after a relapse of cancer, her mother had died. Originally intending to accompany his books and artifacts home by ship, he instead had Viola wire him more money and indulged in the greatest extravagance of the day: flying by commercial plane back to England. Once there, with Viola's encouragement, he quickly reconnected with Younghusband, Lindbergh (who had recently written to him seeking help with yoga), and anyone else he thought could provide him with sufficient support for a successful application to Oxford. With Tharchin attending to the details of his crates, Theos took advantage of his presence in England to make himself a celebrity and attend as many social functions as possible, staying at the prestigious Ritz Hotel in London and even giving his first public talk, dressed in full Tibetan aristocratic clothes, and teasing London reporters when quizzed on his ethnicity: "I am not an American, I am a Tibetan!"

From the splash that Theos made in the British tabloids ("Secret Rites I Saw in Darkest Tibet, I Was a Lama"), claiming even to have been blessed by the spirit of the Nechung Oracle, even members of the Royal Asiatic Society became curious, if skeptical, about him and sought more information, wondering if he was just "another Illion."[5] Although this sort of exposure was actually damaging his attempt to attend Oxford before it had even begun, Theos still hoped to inspire everyone he met with his adventures. One man was so inspired that he left for India himself a mere month and a half later, determined to write Bernard's story—or at least a version of it. About Theos Bernard, his first putative biographer wrote:

> The man I am writing about is not famous. It may be that he never will be. It may be that when his life at last comes to an end he will leave no more trace of his sojourn on earth than a stone thrown into a river leaves

on the surface of the water. . . . But it may be that the way of life that he has chosen for himself and the peculiar strength and sweetness of his character may have an ever-growing influence over his fellow men so that, long after his death perhaps, it may be realized that there lived in this age a very remarkable creature.⁶

With those words, Somerset Maugham began his account of "Larry Darrell" in *The Razor's Edge*. Their meeting appears to have inspired Maugham to revisit one of his early unperformed plays, "The Road Uphill," and to travel to India to the ashram of Shri Ramana Maharshi, where he began to write a semifictional rendition of Bernard's life. Maugham's original play told the story of Joe Sheridan, who returns from World War I with post-traumatic stress. While his friends go on with their lives and his fiancée pressures him to get a job and marry her, Sheridan is unable to return to his old life. In the play, Maugham's lead character finally announces that he will go to Paris to study art. Incorporating these aspects of his earlier work into the narrative, Maugham made his new protagonist, still a victim of World War I, a man born into a life of privilege who forsakes it all to study in India and pursue a more authentic way of living. The myth of Theos Bernard had begun.⁷

Aboard the *Queen Mary*, bound for New York, Theos was one of the celebrities of the voyage, entertaining all around him with stories of his adventures and even being hosted as the toast of his very own "Tibetan Dinner." He hired an agent in New York, W. Coulson Leigh Inc., and subscribed to a newspaper clipping service, so that when the ship docked at the Cunard Line pier, Theos was greeted by newspaper reporters waiting for him to recount his story for an eager public.

"American Honored Guest of Tibetan Government," "Buddhist Worship in Tibet Pictured," "Arizona Scholar Finds Lore of Ancient Culture in Tibet." "First White Man to Live in Mysterious, Sacred Lhassa Found No More Danger Than in New York After Dark," and "American Details Tibetan Mysteries," ran the articles in *The New York Times* and *New York World-Telegram* in rapid succession, and more stories began to appear in syndicated newspapers across the country. Even the local Nyack paper, the *Journal-News*, which had been the bane of P.A.'s existence for many years, gave "Theo Bernard" positive coverage, proclaiming his activities to include "the greatest photographic record of Tibet ever made,"⁸ and as Theos and Viola's Christmas cards—now Tibetan New Year's cards—were sent out to their friends, the press accolades continued.[9] As he had hoped, Theos began receiving letters of inquiry from around the world, asking for details of his adventures and entry into Tibet and requests for recommendations and opinions on books. All this was wonderful for Theos, but foremost in his mind was his reunion with Viola after thirteen months. Both were excited and apprehensive, and, as almost eerily foreseen by both, their reunion was not what either had expected.

For Viola, the long months away from her husband had been a long-distance love affair in which Theos wrote constantly with expressions of love and an ever-changing sequence of grandiose plans for the future. Overworked and sleep-deprived, she constantly found herself having to reaffirm the spirit behind Theos's hopes and wishes, but at the same time provide a desperately needed "reality check" by trying to force him to see the difference between ideas that were "perfectly feasible" and those that were simply "pipe-dreams"—or perhaps, the effects of an oxygen-starved brain!

Theos, however, believed that he and Viola were about to embark on a new phase of their relationship. With more than adequate resources now at his disposal, he felt well suited to set up his own ashram, school, research center, or whatever he chose to call it. His uncle P.A., he felt, had committed professional suicide in the blow-up with DeVries; it was now clear that P.A. would never turn over the CCC to him as he had once hoped, but with the backing of Viola's money, he did not need it and was more than ready to break out on his own. Together, he fantasized, he and Viola could run a center that would put to shame his uncle's more amateurish operation, a place where rather than offering up his uncle's version of "bread and circuses," Theos would have Tibetan lamas, a massive library, serious students, and all the facilities he needed to make his dreams a reality.

Although these plans were grandiose by anyone's standards—"ye gods!" Viola declared, the first time she was confronted by "the multiplicity and scope" of his proposal—Theos had the secret for success. Not money, influence, fame, or personal connections—although all these would play a role and, he felt, were already in his possession, or at least well on their way. Rather, spiritual power, yogic attainment would make it all a reality. From his own ruminations as well as his father's research in India and ongoing studies on his behalf, Theos was convinced that the key to any success lay in fully awakening the "creative force of life." Of course, he felt, the way to do this was through yoga, and specifically, tantric sexual yoga. Having been practicing the necessary physical exercises to control himself during sex, Theos was eager to show Viola what he had learned and just as eager for them to put these techniques into practice. Viola, however, was horrified.[10]

As the realities of their radically incommensurate ideas for their future together began to sink in, the months that followed Theos and Viola's reunion became more and more unpleasant. Viola was consigned to remaining in New Jersey while she finished her internship, while Theos attempted to plead his case to his increasingly distant wife, making concessions when and where he could. But neither could find the happiness they had been looking forward to, only "unhappiness and a sense of insecurity" as their "actions . . . beliefs . . . standards . . . friendship . . . work" and other aspects of their lives all seemed to indicate "a widening divergence." Viola began devoting more and more time to her internship, while Theos tried to keep his public relations machine moving, joining professional societies, writing articles and doing interviews for newspapers and popular magazines, and continuing to play himself up as having been recognized as the reincarnation of the eighth-century saint Padmasambhava—though that was the Tibetans' idea,[11] he told everyone, reassuring them that he was "a serious scholar."

In response to his initial application to The Explorers Club, he heard that the rules of the club did not permit the use of their address by nonmembers. But after vetting Theos with his provided references, the club secretary offered him the option of applying for membership. Theos located and befriended Harrison Forman as a fellow Tibetan explorer, and Forman recommended Theos for membership, seconded by Lowell Thomas—the man who had made Lawrence of Arabia famous worldwide. By mid-March, Theos was a member of The Explorers Club; he even regaled his fellow members with stories of Tibet during their annual dinner and presented his own talk at the club later in the spring.

Playing many cards simultaneously, Theos wrote a letter to President Roosevelt, requesting the opportunity to meet with him and present the Tibetan letters he was couriering. He even offered to screen some of the movies he had taken in Tibet. The response from FDR's chief of protocol, George T. Summerlin, suggested that Theos simply forward the letters to him via the protocol office and be done with it. Determined to meet with the president personally, however, Theos contacted FDR's cousin, Frederic A. Delano, who worked for the Department of the Interior, who then contacted Eleanor Roosevelt on Theos's behalf. After more back-and-forth communications, Summerlin agreed to arrange a meeting, scheduling it for March 31, when the president would be at his retreat in Warm Springs, Georgia.

Theos hoped that this meeting would yield just the sort of publicity he desired, but larger forces in the world intervened. On March 12, 1938, German troops crossed the border into Austria, unilaterally annexing the country in violation of Article 80 of the Treaty of Versailles. The next day, Hitler announced "Der Anschluss" as the first act of the "reuninification" of the Germanic peoples of Europe. Although the United States had not signed the treaty,[12] the implications of the German chancellor's actions were abundantly clear: war was imminent. Immediately, all the president's social obligations were canceled, and with them Theos's hopes for an audience. The letters from Reting Rinpoche and the Sakya Hierarch would be put in a box and never delivered.

Meanwhile, pushed to the brink of a nervous breakdown by the stress of her work, the recent death of her mother, and the ongoing emotional trauma of her marriage, Viola left New Jersey—and Theos—the moment her internship ended that March, leaving him alone to sort out his life while she attempted to make sense of her own. At the same time, it became clear to Theos that he was probably not going to get into Oxford, so he needed to work fast. Completely unemployed, with his mining interests having failed, Theos decided to follow his father's initial advice expressed in India. Drawing on his and Viola's library of secondary literature, he quickly wrote and submitted a dissertation for a Ph.D. in philosophy at Columbia University.

Continuing to capitalize on his fame, when he received a letter from Lord Tsarong, Theos made the most of it. Lord Tsarong informed Theos that he had still not heard from Tharchin regarding the outstanding debt that Theos owed him from the previous summer, but he and his wife still thought fondly of him. Asking Theos to send him "some California apple seeds," Lord Tsarong also mentioned that no one had yet "found the reincarnation of the late Dalai Lama and the Paṇ-chen Lama, but hope they will be found in the near future."

Holding a private screening of some of his raw Tibet movies for the press in Manhattan, Theos used the opportunity to announce to a newspaper reporter that "No Dalai Lama May Be Found" and claimed that "the long reign of Living Buddhas may have ended forever." Moving the discussion quickly to himself, he convinced the reporter to describe him as "the young Columbia University graduate who in a few brief years has been recognized as one of the greatest Western authorities on what actually happens within the walls of a Tibetan lamasery." He was, the article further reported, staying in contact with his friends in Lhasa while "preparing a thesis for his doctor's degree at Columbia on this subject, which he describes as the basic philosophic concepts from which Buddha, and later Christ, drew their spiritual education."[13]

Entitled simply "Tantrik Yoga," Theos's "dissertation" sounded grand but was little more than a rehashed version of his earlier Columbia master's thesis, with additional information drawn from recent secondary literature and personal insights about religion, philosophy, and science from his India–Tibet trip thrown in. Sending copies to Evans-Wentz in Oxford and his father's friend Hans von Koerber in Los Angeles, Theos requested letters of support to be sent to Columbia. Evans-Wentz, writing to Theos's thesis committee, told them that he thought the dissertation constituted "a genuine contribution to the advancement of philosophical and anthropological learning." However, everyone else gave mixed responses, pointing out weaknesses, misspelled Sanskrit words, and the like. Von Koerber responded most negatively of all, pointing out that "the material presented in the dissertation is merely the compilation of what can be found in the Sanskritic and related Tantric Yoga literature referred to in the bibliography." He stated further that Theos's work showed "a highly subjective viewpoint in so far as he obviously accepted verbally the teachings given to him by Gurus or Lamas and simply incorporated them in his dissertation without first carefully weighing them." It was hardly the kind of support Theos needed.

Based on the reviews they received and their own analysis, at Theos's dissertation defense on Friday, May 20, the dissertation committee concluded that his dissertation "as it stands attempts more than it adequately achieves" and suggested three alternatives for reworking it into an acceptable document. Unrevised, they felt, the work was insufficient as an original contribution to the field, and did not merit granting him a Ph.D. Instead of attempting a rewrite, he decided to walk away from academia entirely.

Meanwhile, first at a resort in Virginia and then in South Carolina, Viola attempted to come to grips with her situation. Writing to friends and speaking with confidants, she eventually came to one inescapable conclusion: it was time for a divorce. Heartbroken, she informed Theos that she "no longer has wifely feelings" for him, would not consider the issue any further, and would not write to or see him again until after the divorce was filed, at which time they could divide their belongings. With that declaration, Viola boarded a plane for Reno, Nevada, where after a six-week residency, she would obtain the decree ending their marriage.

Although Theos continued to write to her, Viola remained true to her word and refused to respond to his letters and telegrams—until she heard that he had had a relapse of his teenage illness, "with his right leg paralyzed." Having vowed only not to write, Viola placed a phone call to their New Jersey home, but the voice on the other end was not that of a weak and ill man—indeed, he felt fine, he told her—but rather that of someone cold and emotionally distant. Determined to see her decision through, she saw that the decree paperwork was filed, and while she waited for the final judgment, received an urgent communiqué from her friend and lawyer in New York, informing her that Theos had begun to pack up large portions of their household, especially their library, and was moving to New York. But more startling to Viola was his specific destination. Theos was moving in with her best friend, Blanche DeVries, "to be near those whose love for me keeps an interest in my welfare in their heart," he told her.

At first, Viola was in denial, thinking that she was simply letting her mind "run away" with ideas, and convinced herself that she was only thinking the worst. But her fears were not ungrounded: having been just as enamored of Theos as Viola was when they both first saw him that spring day in 1934, and having been tossed aside by his uncle for another woman, DeVries had become Theos's new lover.[14]

Returning to New Jersey, Viola relocated to Grasslands Hospital to start her first psychiatric residency. Meanwhile, with no Ph.D., no job, no mining income, and soon no rich wife to support him, Theos was going to be in serious financial trouble, and although he could rely on DeVries to support him for the near term, he would have to find something else soon. Determined to make a career for himself, he contacted a public relations firm to begin negotiating for a speaking tour, but he had no track record, and no such previous experience. Having had his Tibet diaries retyped professionally that spring, Theos began to rewrite them as a manuscript to send to his agent in hope of a book contract, even going so far as to hire an out-of-work novelist as his editor. Dedicating his book to Viola, he submitted *Penthouse of the Gods* to his agent and got a book contract from a New York publisher.

Sitting in New York, Theos proceeded to edit his movies into a single narrative and prepared to go on the lecture circuit by practicing his speaking abilities, taking voice lessons,[15] and even having himself recorded at a studio in order to be able to listen to himself speak. Previewing his edited film at the Lotos Club in Manhattan, he received an overwhelming response: "Every one of them say that I have a fortune wrapped up in the story. . . . The president of both Fox and Paramount were there—Bob Ripley, one from N.B.C., etc. etc. in fact virtually everyone in the audience held some prominent position; so one in all, it is perhaps one of the best advertising things that I could have done."

Meanwhile, Viola had not forgotten Theos, for despite all the difficulties of recent months, he was being very friendly and amicable—she was still paying the bills for her "crazy 'X-'"—and she still had strong feelings for him. At the end of the summer, as her mother's estate was being settled, one final item remained: the provision of an inheritance of $100,000 for both Theos and Viola in lieu of the wedding present she had been unable to give them years earlier. Having expressed her "desire to help . . . not to hurt" Theos months before, Viola felt that she should honor her mother's original intent, and despite being divorced from Theos and under no obligation to him, she divided the inheritance in half and set up a trust fund in his name, from which he could draw up to $2,500 a year.

Despite the accolades he was receiving, Theos was still an unproven speaker, not yet star quality as far as his public relations firm was concerned. Consequently, the agency booked him in a series of local, relatively low-profile talks where he could hone his presentation of "the thrilling, gripping, true story of the land that time forgot—Tibet," offering audiences "the inside story of *Lost Horizon*."[16] His engagements were not very impressive, although by calling in a few favors back in Arizona, he managed to arrange an alumnus lecture at the University of Arizona close to the end of the tour. From October 1938 to April 1939, Theos traveled from small town to small town, speaking before Rotary Clubs and Women's Leagues, with the occasional college lecture hall or larger venue punctuating his journey. Crossing the United States four times in six months, he made sure to get as much local press as possible, even if only in the social register. It was a grueling schedule of ninety lectures, with appearances four and five nights in a row in towns hundreds of miles apart, being housed in local hotels and occasionally in organizers' homes.

Refining and perfecting his talk as the tour went on, Theos arrived in Tucson in March 1939 and pulled out all the stops for his appearance at his *alma mater*. When the curtains parted before a packed house, the audience saw Theos Bernard, religious scholar, explorer, and mystic, seated in a chair on a dais in the middle of the stage, next to a movie projector and surrounded by ritual artifacts and various Tibetan robes. "Come with me," he invited them, "in a flight in the Clipper Ship of the imagination from San Francisco across the vast Pacific . . . into the heart of Asia, the Land of the Lama—Tibet!" and proceeded to unfold his now well-polished narrative, filled with exaggerations and fantastic embellishments. His audience consumed the story without hesitation. The credulity of the American public at the time, it seemed, was going to work in Theos's favor. Only a week after he began his lecture tour, widespread panic and even suicides had occurred in parts of the country when, unaware that they were hearing a radio drama, listeners of the CBS radio network heard reports of a Martian invasion of New Jersey and the imminent takeover of Earth.[17] In such an atmosphere of gullibility and with enough care, Theos knew he could succeed.

A crucial part of Theos's plan was to remain constantly in the press. He tried to do newspaper and radio interviews in nearly every town he visited—both to promote his talks and to promote his forthcoming book. When initially interviewed, he presented himself as a matter-of-fact sort of scholar. "What is your own reaction to this explorative trip, Mr. Bernard?" one interviewer asked. He responded,

> I return a sincere friend of the Tibetans, devoted to them and to their religious teachings in a scholarly and critical sense. I subscribe to the philosophical teachings of Tibetan Buddhism not because of any esoteric or miraculous happenings, but on the basis of reasoned conviction. My experiences have given me an understanding and appreciation of Tibet and the religion inseparable from it.

As time passed, Theos would amend and enhance his story to include statements drawn verbatim from his book manuscript, such as his claim to be a Tibetan lama.

Returning to New York in time for the 1939 World's Fair, Theos prepared to attend the festivities. Writing to the fair organizing committee from Lhasa in August 1937, Theos had told them of his ongoing "researches in the Philosophical aspect of Tibetan Buddhism," claiming he had disguised himself as a Buddhist for that purpose. His proposal to the committee, as part of the larger "Hall of Religion," was for the construction of a representation of a Tibetan monastic temple "decorated with their intricate carvings and painted in the royal colors of Buddhism [that] will offer a thrill to anyone" and rival the set of *Lost Horizon*, which, he pointed out, "did not measure up to reality." The materials would not be difficult to procure; the key, he suggested, would be to import Tibetan Buddhist monks for the event. It was a clever, if not very subtle ploy to get Tibetan monks, presumably Geshe Wangyal, Gedun Chöpel, and a few others, to America. Unfortunately, Theos was told that his proposal was "entirely beyond the scope" of the planned events. In actuality, it was completely *outside* the scope of the organizers' vision for the convocation, which had been intended as a Judeo-Christian ecumenical gathering.[18] Still hoping to participate in some way, through his new friend, Harrison Forman, Theos managed to attend the fair under the auspices of the Ford Exposition, as one of the "celebrities" at the festivities at the "Road of Tomorrow."[19]

His first tour finished, Theos received endorsements sufficient to convince the agency to book him on their high-profile lecture package, and while the details were being arranged, he returned to California to spend time with his father, Glen. With the proceeds from the well-reviewed *Penthouse of the Gods*, he rented a house for three months in Beverly Hills and with Glen's help, began constructing a mythological prequel to his Tibet adventures set in India, hoping to capitalize on the reading public's enthusiasm for his story.[20]

No longer a student and explorer, he became, in his new writings, a religious visionary and pioneer. His life in Arizona was no longer a boyhood adventure; instead it became the tale of a secret yogi-in-training. Claiming to have been visited by an old Indian yogi during his convalescence,[21] Theos presented his experiences from the age of eighteen onward solely as a quest for the meaning of life. Instead of the struggles of a failed lawyer, his years in Tucson became sanctified as a conscious spiritual mission, with his hazing framed as a spiritual trial by fire and his illness and recovery as "sacred rites." From that point on, by implication at least, Theos maintained that he was thus qualified to receive yogic teachings. Claiming to have mastered all the preliminary practices and rituals of purification before ever leaving the lands of his adolescence, Theos was a man on a quest for "mental and spiritual realization"; indeed, he claimed, he had been on this path since before he was born.

His years at Columbia were no longer those of a scholar in training but mere background familiarization with his "own philosophical heritage,"

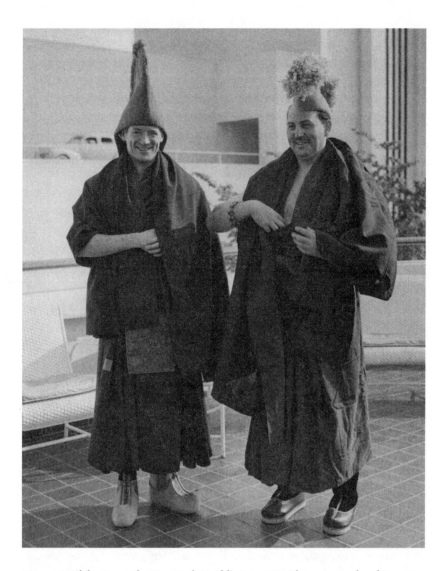

Figure 9.1 Celebrities at the New York World's Fair, 1939: Theos Bernard and Harrison Forman (BANC)

to allow him "to interpret the East in light of the West." Because, as he claimed, "I was still traveling in the Shadow of Truth rather than in its light," to attain the final levels of realization he sought, the only course of action was to go to India and be initiated at the feet of a true guru. With no one to disprove his story, Theos presented himself as the secret American student of an Indian swami and a boy prodigy of yoga whom his teacher and fellow students eagerly awaited in India.

Noticeably absent from this new rendition of his life was any mention of Viola, his father, his uncle, or the country club. Far from a delayed honeymoon or potential dissertation research, his trip to India was now a discovery of "a frame of mind and an attitude toward life," a new way of living that would "become a part of my very being." Mixing the facts of his father's life together with his own, he and Glen crafted a story in which, as a lone pilgrim to India in search of secret, sacred knowledge, Theos had journeyed around the world to meet his family teacher. In Calcutta, he waited for nearly two weeks to be contacted, only to learn that "his guru" had died "only a few days" before his arrival in India.[22]

But India, he claimed, was only the beginning of his spiritual quest, for Tibet was the true home of secret knowledge:

> The ancient teachers, preserved in the sixty-four volumes of the Tantra, books jealously guarded by the Lamas through the ages, seemed to hold an unaccountable lure for me, and I began to dream of going to Tibet and bringing back a set of these precious books. I asked my host why it was that some of those who had been initiated had not gone to Tibet and brought back the teachings to India. He explained that even the Indian was forbidden to enter the Forbidden Land; indeed, it was harder for a Bengali than for any other foreigner to get into Tibet. Moreover, nothing would be gained by going to Tibet unless one was first initiated as a Tantrik, as only a Tantrik was likely to get into contact with the true teachers.

And so, guided by his "tantrik friend"—a cross between Roy Chaudhury, who had aided Glen, and Glen himself, who later assisted Theos in a similar manner—Theos claimed he then traveled "long months . . . across the length and breadth of the strange land" to find a new guru. Eventually returning to Calcutta, he declared he no longer felt "a stranger," for "something of India had already entered my soul, and become an integral part of me."

Locating a "Swamaji," with aid and testimonials from his adoptive "family," Theos convinced this new guru to initiate him.

> I started early up the river, and on arrival stopped for some time on its banks awaiting the hour when I might put in an appearance before the

Swamaji. The gentle stir of the slow current on a warm evening, and the passing gusts of a cool breeze, filled me with unaccountable awe; my emotions ran high. All the yearnings I had ever experienced seemed on this evening to be dammed up in me, waiting for release in my first initiation, which was to be the gleaning of my first inner understanding. The purpose of this initiation was to awaken the creative flow within, to free the mind of prejudices, to make the soul receptive to all things in quest of Eternal Happiness.

It seemed so strange that I had come so far from the lonely deserts of Arizona to this devout land, from an environment so young to a culture so old. What had planted the seeds within me of this desire to come here? What had called me to this Land of Mystery? Why was I being accepted? It was clear, or so it seemed to me now, that all my effort to gain some understanding of the Laws of Life had not been in vain. . . . I knew I was on the verge of being liberated, on the path to verify by experience what I had learned in theory. Already I was realizing how the emotions expand while the intellect contracts; for I had almost become unaware of the passage of time. The initiation was to begin at midnight. It was to be the start of a new life for me, of spiritual rebirth. The shackles of the personal consciousness would be forever removed. I would directly perceive the universal manifestation of the Divine Law.

Of the subsequent "initiation" experience, Theos presented a highly polished and detailed account—at least, as detailed as his "vow of secrecy" would allow. Traveling by boat upriver, he "recounted":

As the master of the Chakra (sacred circle), the Swamaji was supreme, and his wish had to be obeyed in every instance during the ceremony of initiation. He was seated on a slightly raised seat before the deity of the Chakra. The rest of us were seated in Asana (sacred posture) in a semicircle about him; I was on his left, the second from the end. The Chakra was scented with the many flowers gathered for this rite, as well as sprinkled with scented water. Everything there was for the purpose of enabling the Sadhaka (worshipper) to awaken his inner consciousness. First there was a period of silence, during which I was to make an offering of my ignorance in order that I might become receptive to what the Swamaji was going to pass on to me. This is the natural law in the world of teacher and disciple. For, surely, there can be no need for a Guru (spiritual teacher) unless one is ignorant. One may be well educated in many subjects, yet be in complete ignorance in the field of Sadhana (spiritual practices). The pupil has not the least notion, or even the suspicion of a notion, as to what the Guru will teach him. Spiritual knowledge is not to be tested by the same standards as worldly knowledge. After I had meditated for a short while, the purpose of the ceremony was explained to me. Having sprinkled me with consecrated ritual water, the Swamaji then gave us a Mantra to repeat, following which he recited chants to cast a spell over me, in order to awaken the universal consciousness within. Then he made known the manifestation of the universal consciousness in its infinite number of forms. He took one aspect at a time, and before each, Mantras were recited, in order to induce a wholly different feeling, soon dispelled by understanding brought about by a simple truth that he would utter and dwell upon for a short while.

Thus the hours flew by, as I was being born into a new world of knowledge. Finally, the Swamaji's head and my own were covered over with a cloth, as the Swamaji whispered seven times into my left ear and seven times into my right the Mantra that was to be kept inviolate in the recesses of my mind, never to cross my lips in utterance. As the cloth was removed and I felt the dawn of this rebirth, the heart slowly awakened to a silent joy. The darkness of doubt was forever dispelled. I was free.

Returning to the home of his "Tantrik friend," he was received "with the welcoming arms of a father who meets his son after he has graduated from college." Perfect in mythic form, it was a story that no one at the time could confirm or deny.[23] Theos continued to recast his father's activities in India as his own. Glen's three-month retreat at Bhurkunda in the spring of 1936 became Theos's own stay at an undisclosed "jungle retreat" of a Maharishi. It was there, at the feet of an authentic Indian guru, Theos claimed, that he learned secret practices that led to "the realization of my early dreams," complete with its own final initiation.

Working the manuscript into its final form, Theos laced the chapters with illustrations drawn from Tharchin's block-print Tibetan book, photographed in Kalimpong, now billed as a precious "original handwritten Tibetan manuscript on the practice of Yoga which was given to the author by his teacher."[24] Appropriately dedicated "To My Father," Theos's new book, *Heaven Lies Within Us,* purported to relate one man's quest for the "Eternal Truth" buried in the heart of every man and woman. The title could just as easily have been a clever pun, referring to the fantasy of a sacred quest concocted between father and son and perpetrated on a gullible public. The book even garnered reviews—if mixed—before it was published.[25]

With another book under his belt and the success of his first lecture tour, Theos was in a much stronger position to negotiate with his agency, which printed four-color flyers and added Theos's lecture to their docket. Selling complete packages of lectures to venues around the country, W. Coulson Leigh secured its success by forcing a wide range of speakers on the hosts. For the 1939–40 season, venues accepting the tour package would have to present the great and not-so-great of the day. Attendees could look forward to seeing and hearing in person such notables as the First Lady, Eleanor Roosevelt; Charles Lindbergh; Carl Sandberg; Eve Curie, and other lesser-known names of politics, literature, and the silver screen.[26] Padding the list were the "illustrated" adventurers, including Theos Bernard.

Although other Tibetan scholars were busily writing and publishing books—Marco Pallis and Geshe Wangyal with *Peaks and Lamas*; Frederick Spencer Chapman with *Lhasa: The Holy City*; and Arnold Heim and August Gansser with *Throne of the Gods*—these were not the rivals Theos was concerned about. Rather, "the competition" were the Lee Keedick Stars and the National Lecture Bureau, agencies that made up for what they lacked in high-profile names with the promise of high-profile theatrics, often touring at the same time and in the same venues. In the still financially tough times of the late 1930s, success hinged on the ability to draw a crowd and Theos had stiff competition:

Carl Raswan with "His Life and Experiences amid the Black Tents of Arabia," offering the story of a European who was "accepted as a Bedouin"; "he hunted with them, he starved with them, he raided with them, he faced death with them in bloody battles against their enemies," supposedly even fighting with Turkish forces against Lawrence of Arabia;

Bwana Charles Cottar and "Cottar's African Attractions," presenting himself as "an old-time Western American plainsman, rancher, marshal, and sheriff . . . [who] moved to Africa . . . when our Southwest, the last American frontier vanished, and became too tame for him," and faced down "lion, as well as rhino";

Harlan Tarbell, of "Tarbell's Eyeless Vision"—a "Master of Impossibilities" and "World Famous Mystery Scientist," who had studied "magic and mystery the world over as practiced by the Witch Doctors of the Jungles, the Gulli-Gulli Wonder Workers of Egypt, the Magicians of the Orient and Occident, the Priests of the Pagan Temples, together with the Mysteries of Truth brought forth by the great Magi—the Wise Men of the Inner Brotherhoods";

Ruth Harkness, in "Pioneering for Pandas"—a "Chinese and Tibetan Adventure," telling how "a lone woman, without backing or previous experience in exploration, journeyed against all advice into the high mountains along the unknown Tibetan border and brought back the first live Giant Panda" and, in "the ancient Kingdom of Wassze . . . made her headquarters in a deserted Tibetan lamasery";

Jacques Charmoz's "Adventure in the High Places of South America" offering the story of "a brilliant young French explorer" who traversed "the High Andes, the volcanoes of Chile, and the ice fields of Patagonia" and who was a part-time artist, "handsome, talented, and altogether delightful," a "born raconteur," and "attached to the Chilean Army" as the trainer of "a special ski corps."

And the list went on. On these lecture circuits, Theos Bernard—now "the White Lama"—was in good company. Promotional flyers proclaimed him to be "The First White Man Ever to Live in the Lamaseries and Cities of Tibet," "Initiated into the Age-old Religious Rites of Tibetan Buddhism," to have "Passed Through Sections of Tibet Where No Other White Man Has Set Foot," and, of course, "Accepted By the Tibetans As One of Them." It was shameless and it worked.

This time on tour, Theos was playing the large venues—from the Pasadena Civic Center and Shrine Auditorium in Los Angeles to the National Geographic Society in Washington, DC, with tickets running from 75¢ to $1.50 (a substantial increase over the ticket prices for his 1938–39 tour, typically 25¢ to 50¢). Promoting himself beyond mere advertisement in the local press, he often did newspaper interviews and radio talk shows while on the road, giving at least three radio interviews in Los Angeles alone. Indeed, as Aimee McPherson was broadcasting Christian sermons throughout the day on her Los Angeles radio station KFSG, at night Los Angeles residents could tune in to other radio stations and hear a wide range of other subjects being discussed, such as Theos Bernard talking about yoga and Tibetan Buddhism. It was an apt metaphor for the era: Christian in the

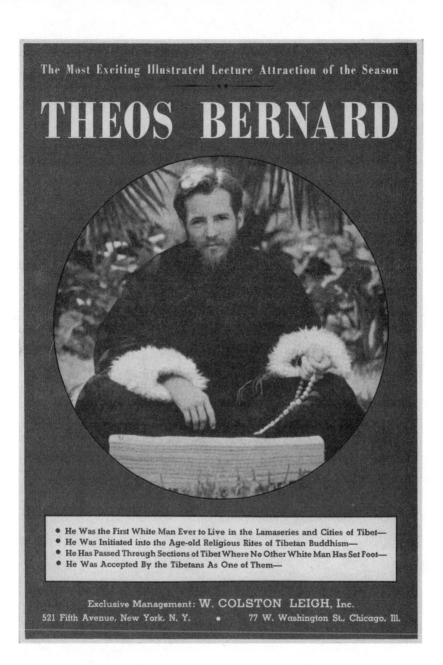

Figure 9.2 Bernard's tour flyer: the art of misrepresentation (HGPF)

bright light of day, with a nighttime counterculture that bore little resemblance to its diurnal counterpart.

Taking advantage of the momentum he was building, Theos used every scrap of paper or event as an opportunity for self-promotion. A letter from Lord Tsarong, written in English by his son, informed him of the outstanding balance *still* due on his expenditures two years earlier and of the arrival of the Schäfer expedition in Lhasa: "There came four Germans recently and now they have left," the letter stated, adding "one day I invited them for tea." Mere days after receiving the letter and only two weeks after German forces invaded Prague, Czechoslovakia, Theos contacted the *New York World-Telegraph* and broke the news: "Nazis and Fascists are Filtering Into Tibet As a Key in World Drive, Expert Reports," even garnering a photo of himself in the paper.[27]

Soon, however, all of it would backfire on him. That fall, *Penthouse of the Gods* was published in England under the title *Land of a Thousand Buddhas*.[28] Authoring a series of lengthy articles in the high-profile *ASIA* magazine, in his first article, he recast his visit to Ganden in late July as a last-minute summons by the Regent:

On the day before my departure from Lhasa, two lamas called on me. They revealed to me every thought I had had since my arrival in Lhasa and the nature of my reactions to the various ceremonies at the Tibetan monasteries. I had thought that this life was exclusively my own, but my lama visitors seemed to have some mystical power that gave them an insight into others.

They explained that all that remained for me to do was to go through with the final initiation ceremony, which would make it possible for me to make contact with my inner self at will, to the end of my days. They said that word had come from Ganden, the great monastery north of Lhasa, that the T'ri Rimpoche, the head lama of Ganden and next in rank to the Dalai Lama in Tibet, had returned and that preparations were being made to receive me there for this last ceremony.

It was not a question of whether I would go or not. It was a question of how quickly I could leave. There was no time to be lost. I had journeyed to Tibet hoping for this, the privilege of a lifetime, and here it had come to me on the day before my departure. It was a four days' journey east of Lhasa to the third largest monastery in Tibet. That very night runners were sent to the monastery to report that I was leaving in the morning.

Long before sunrise everything was helter-skelter in the effort to get the last-minute details taken care of.

Describing his arrival at Ganden and spending the night "in a sacred chamber in the main temple building," Theos purported to relate a whole other dimension of his experiences—proving his literary skills far more than his capacity for factual reporting.

There was unusual significance in this particular initiation. The fact is, I, the person about to be initiated into the Tibetan sacred mysteries, was no Tibetan, not even an Oriental, but an American, hailing from Arizona. And here, at the end of the ceremony, I should become a full-fledged Buddhist monk, a lama. This was for me the day of days: I was to appear before the T'ri Rimpoche, who was to install me with my vestments after this final ritual initiation.

The servants had brought my early morning buttered tea, which it is customary to take upon awakening. They appeared to be more excited than I. Never before had an American been accepted. It was, indeed, not as a stranger that I was being permitted to receive this divine benediction; I had been accepted as a reincarnation of a celebrated Tibetan saint. Fate had brought it about that I should be reborn in the Western World that I might learn of its forms and customs, and now the same fate had restored me to my homeland that I might have my inner consciousness reawakened. This was how they interpreted my action in leaving America and in coming to them. So it was not a mystery to them that I possessed a comprehension of their teachings. My subconscious self had directed my thoughts and guided my desires so that I was impelled to come to them, and each successive initiation was no more than a further reawakening of my true self . . .

The time had come for all to file into the temple room. I approached the great bolted door, which was guarded by a lama who waited until I had recited my *mantras* that I might purify myself before entering the holy sanctuary. For an instant I hesitated; as if there were another person within me, advising me, I paused on the threshold, my head bowed, while I uttered a silent prayer. The door slowly swung open.

As I stepped across the sanctified threshold, I found myself enveloped in a stream of sunlight flowing in from an opening above the first story roof. At once I prostrated myself in that cascade of sunbeams, and, while lying there in humble devotion, I dived for a fleeting instant into the innermost depths of human consciousness. An overwhelming emotion filled me. I rose to my feet, and stood aside. The great hall was vibrant with the prayers chanted by countless lamas seated cross-legged, heads bowed, upon rows of raised flat benches. . . .

It is taught here that there is only one force in life, but that it has an infinite number of manifestations; only through knowledge is it possible to direct this force. This vast chamber is always kept under guard and under lock and key so that the uninstructed may not have the opportunity to see these hideous forms; there is too much danger of their being interpreted literally. It is argued that the revelation they offer is esoteric, and that it is impossible to pass on knowledge until the individual is prepared to receive it.

We seated ourselves below the altar which pedestaled the image symbolizing the destructive aspects of energy. I heard the low rumbling drone of the high priest's chants, which he repeated for the purpose of preparing us. Then his assistants slowly joined in, intensifying the vibrant echoes of this dungeon of holiness. Soon I began to repeat the mantras which had been provided for me, until my entire being felt like the buzzing wings of a bumble-bee. I knew that I had to control and direct this energy which was being stirred up through the channels of the sympathetic nervous system. My months of training in the Yoga practices were useful here. The test was yet to come. Had I developed sufficient power of control to direct that energy so as to draw upon the hidden reservoirs in the subconscious? With each succeeding step the internal pressures of the body became more fierce, and I began to understand their power of destruction. It was only by sheer will power that I was able to hold on. The agony became terrifying, and had I given vent to the fears which were beginning to beset me I should have burst forth screaming and not stopped running until I either went mad or touched the borderline of madness. But I was determined to hold on.

I observed an assistant speaking to the officiating high priest. Then the vibrations were changed, and a new mantra was being chanted, and another was given me. Slowly I began repeating it after my mentor. Each line was the same, but a different syllable was stressed at the end of each phrase. My entire internal rhythm was changing, ever swelling. The walls almost seemed to sway with the ever increasing drone of beating drums, blaring horns and clashing cymbals. My imagination was beginning to run wild. I had learned by now how to sit apart and watch the inner self function. Yet I was in constant fear of being swept away by these mystical rites, which utilize every known emotional phenomenon.

In the midst of this spiritual storm, everything suddenly seemed dispelled as by some mysterious magic; the tinkling bells could be felt, when all receded, and we meditated in the dead silence of darkness. It will never be possible for me to express in words what actually took place. It was something beyond the realm of the mind and, therefore, beyond the expression of name and form.

The ceremony was over. Now it was for me to remain and reflect upon this volcano of subconscious power in the light of the teachings which had been previously given me, of which these fiendish plastic forms were symbols. Beginning with the first image which had caught my eye upon entering the chamber, I was deliberately to study each and to interpret its inner meaning. Not until then did I fully realize the wisdom of those who had created these hideous forms of devastation. Before me—so it had seemed at first—had stood a fiend of destruction; but now it had become a symbol of the greatest force of nature in the eternal battle to emerge from the subconscious into the conscious, giving intelligent guidance to each separate personality.

I had no way of telling how many hours had passed; for I was in a world in which the phenomenon of time did not exist. It was as if I had come back for a rebirth, memory of my past lives assisting me in my new orientation, with future experiences in prospect, since this was merely the beginning of that for which I was being prepared. It was, indeed, a test.

Now I was conducted to the altar below the dais, upon which sat the T'ri Rimpoche, shut away from the vision of all, yet in full command of every one within this vast temple chamber.

The officiating lama turned from the altar with a silver jar of holy water. This he poured into my hands, from which I sipped, placing the remainder on my head. Then the lama who had been conducting me through the ceremonies returned with a small image of Buddha, a Tibetan book and a sacred scarf, symbolic of the eternal truth, knowledge and the divine knot of life. This signified that I was to be accepted and permitted to receive the blessing of the T'ri Rimpoche, who, in some mysterious way, knew that I had gained the inner realization. . . .

"The Clipper Ship of the Imagination"

After a blessing from the T'ri Rimpoche, I left his presence, over-flowing with the energy which he had caused to be released from my subconscious.[29]

The only true statement in his entire account, perhaps, was that his "imagination was beginning to run wild." But Theos went too far in inflating his image—and especially at the expense of the British Mission. In a follow-up, highly political article, he articulated many of the idealistic "progressive" ideas he had heard advocated in Gyantse and Lhasa.[30]

Far worse than anything else that he did, Theos took the opportunity to ridicule the members of the British Mission in his book,[31] in the *Asia* article, and in British newspapers.[32] British Intelligence, who had maintained a file on him since his entry into Tibet, identified him as "an impostor like Gordon Enders and is presumably the same person who was permitted to visit Gyantse on a trade route pass in 1937." While they had "reason to think that he is genuinely interested in Tibetan Buddhism," it was clear that "he has apparently given the American public what he thought they would like—sensationalism, padded out with a good deal of obvious fact and Buddhist jargon."[33] The British authorities, displeased with his depiction of the Lhasa Mission, began sending communiqués to India demanding an explanation.

The obligation to respond to the home office was passed down the ranks to Gould in Gangtok. Tharchin was summoned to account for himself and his role in Theos's activities, and although grilled at length, was less than helpful, so, berating him, they barred him from ever visiting Tibet again. It fell to Rai Bahadur Norbu to respond. His letter to Gould in reply was a savage repudiation of Theos's account.[34]

In fact, Bernard's claims have no foundation and are exaggerated to make the stories interesting. If his publications both in America and elsewhere are being accepted without criticism, such can only be attributed to the wide-spread ignorance of the life conditions and religious customs prevailing in Tibet.

During his stay in Lhasa Bernard's behaviour was conventional and not unlike that of other visitors, except that he adopted the fine dress for visits to Tibetans, Tibetan theatrical dress of monks for monasteries. At no time was he seen associating with monks or carrying out religious Buddhist ceremonies.

He made several visits to the 'Potala' to take photographs of different shrines, but not as he states to take part in the daily ceremonies, but to routinely survey the items of interest with his camera when lighting conditions were suitable. Considering the enormous size of the 'Potala' and its numerous contents, this obviously would take many days in uncertain and dull rainy weather.

Bernard arranged to have himself quartered with Tsarong Dzasa in preference to accepting the offer of Mr. Richardson to stay with the Mission. This is significant, because in the light of what has transpired since his departure, he would naturally not be keen to have his actions and movements so closely watched or discussed by those in intelligent contact with the outside world.

His visits to the monasteries were arranged through the permission of the Tibetan Government and in the same manner adopted by any visitor, no matter whether he was a Tibetan, or a foreign official of a neighboring state. Bernard arrived in Tibet with plenty of money which he applied to great advantage in securing the services of monks.

The monasteries of course are institutions dependent to a large extent upon charity, and if a visitor makes a lavish gift of money to any one of them, it is quite obvious, he will be given all the polite and careful attention he desires for his purpose and exceptions would no doubt be made to show him every creek and corner of the monastery, if he so desired. In fact, this has been the experience of many visiting British officers long before Bernard's arrival in Lhasa.

Bernard has not seen or witnessed a ceremony or Buddhist worship which has not also been open to the British personnel.

Then, proceeding anywhere, Bernard always had a battery of cameras with him and was invariably accompanied by Tharchin, his interpreter and guide. His knowledge of the Tibetan language was very scanty indeed and he cannot even converse simple sentences freely.

His 'modus operandi' was to prepare the day with a handsome cash gift and advise the monastery officials when they may expect him. At the appointed time, he would arrive complete with Tharchin and the cameras and would be received with pleasure by the monks who would offer him the usual tea and sweetmeats, whereupon Tharchin would reel off as many film as possible from many angles. Normally the monks object to indiscriminate photography, but Bernard's clever generosity would, as he knew, over-ride such scruples temporarily and in many instances permission was readily given to photograph what he liked.

Another important part of his equipment was a complete monk officials robe and the yellow hat, all of which he had made for himself in Lhasa. Attired in this, he would, by arrangement with monk officials, mingle with the monks while at prayer, and Tharchin from various points, was busy creating one photographic proof of the 'caly White Lama'.

It may be of interest to point out that Bernard avoided as far as possible contact with the Cuttings, who left Lhasa just after his arrival.

Bernard was absent approximately a week from Lhasa visiting Sera and Ganden monasteries. Either on the journey out or returning would hardly allow him the time for the programme so ably arranged in his book the 'Penthouse of the Gods'.

It is quite apparent from the various articles appearing in the Press, periodicals and book publications that he is drawing upon a decidedly distorted imagination and sparing no effort in his superlative descriptions of the poorness of the people, the filth of Lhasa and the wickedness of the cult generally, to bring ridicule upon the religion he professes.

It was a carefully worded document designed to both discredit Theos and protect the British Mission with statements that were politically defensible, if not exactly accurate.[35] Norbu's letter was sent back up the chain of command and forwarded—indiscriminately, unofficially—to anyone who asked.[36] From that point on, Theos's name would be a joke in higher British circles and his official entry in British Intelligence files would be "Theos Bernard, an American impostor."

Meanwhile, back in the States, needing to move his new Tibetan library and temple artifacts out of storage at Viola's house, Theos rented a suite of apartments in the Hotel Pierre, just off Fifth Avenue on Manhattan's Upper East Side. It would be a place where he could set up his temple, lecture, and teach yoga, for interest in the subject was growing. In Europe, Aleister Crowley was getting into the act, publishing his *Eight Lectures on Yoga*, and it was even reported that the exiled former Emperor of Abyssinia, Haile Selassie, had announced he was moving to Ceylon (Śrī Laṅka) just to study yoga.[37] The mystique of yoga was in the air, and as celebrities and "respectable" individuals around the world began to embrace it, yoga began to enter the mainstream.

TEN
Yoga on Fifth Avenue

Yoga in Mayfair or Fifth Avenue, or any other place which is on the telephone, is a spiritual fake.

—CARL JUNG[1]

RETURNING TO NEW YORK FROM time to time during his first lecture tour, Theos began lecturing on the theory of "yoga" in the spring of 1939 at DeVries's "Living Arts Studio" on West Fifty-seventh Street while she and her students taught yoga exercises and related practices. Theos's talks were less a series of academic lectures than a mixture of John Woodroffe's ideas and a statement of Theos's own philosophy of life, recycling much of the content of the ruminations from his Tibet journals and his failed Ph.D. dissertation.

Everyone in the world is actually practicing one or another form of Yoga, but they lead lives of separateness, integrating nothing, and losing the value of their experiences. Yoga is designed to reach the creative flow, to conserve and then liberate it. . . .

In all forms of Yoga are found fanatics, who make their Way their end instead of the means. The Path is never the end, and there is as much danger of getting lost for the student of Yoga as for anyone else.

"Bhakti Yoga," Theos explained, is "the path of love and devotion," and Christianity, he added, "is a form of Bhakti yoga." Nonetheless, mindful of his audience, Theos always made a point of emphasizing the utility of the Living Arts Studio classes. Of the varieties of "yoga" spoken of in the Vedic texts, he told his audience,

The Tantras say that in this age of Kali Yuga, we are not vital enough to be aroused by any form of Yoga but Hatha Yoga. The Tantras teach that everything is energy, and Yoga is the means of releasing it. This experience cannot be described in words, but must be felt to be known.

After theoretical preparations such as these, DeVries and her students would give in-class demonstrations of breathing exercises and the various yogic forms—*āsanas*—from the most simple sitting postures to the more difficult poses.

Theos told his students that cultivating the religious life was the key to happiness, if not success: "An old saying explains that because the king of the land had everything, he needed to give no attention to himself, and could be good to his people. So with the Yogi, who may be called a spiritual king; having happiness, he can devote himself to helping others." Playing to his audience, he informed them that this was the common message of Hinduism, Buddhism, and Christianity:

The Bodhisattva (the perfected soul), having earned the right, may choose whether he will go on, or stay and help others. Since the Bodhisattva lives in universal consciousness, he doesn't wish to leave this plane until others have been helped. Christ is a soul who "arrived," came back to teach, and then went on. When the bodhisattva comes back to this plane of consciousness, he comes again within the scope of its laws. There are laws in the realm of bodhisattvas as well; as there are in every realm of consciousness. There is no great spiritual leader today; in the East, Gandhi comes closest; there is no one in the West; our consciousness does not seem to be directed that way.

Consequently, he encouraged people to change their way of life and to abandon their obsessions with themselves—with "name and form" (*nāma-rūpa*):

Money and sex are the motivating forces in the life we lead today. Our emotional relationships begin so pleasantly and easily, but soon we find trivialities become irritating. That is being concerned unduly with name and form. One may like classical music, and one a brass band. Understanding that this is a clue to the emotional nature within, we can avoid being lost in name and form. It explains why we gravitate to people of the same emotional nature, although their external characteristics seem not at all to be what we think we like. When emotional relationships are unsatisfactory, the weakness is in ourselves; lack of understanding.

Let us not follow name and form; let us learn to get at the essence of things. Truth is not to be found in what people say. Let us learn to search for that which is behind the words. Know people with your consciousness; not with your mind.

To illustrate what he meant, Theos cited examples intended both to inform and inspire:

Each ego is a complete universe in itself, and the gap between two egos can be bridged only by symbols, i.e., name and form. Now we are acquiring knowledge of the Yogic philosophy of consciousness, and the problem is to apply it in order to avoid the long, arduous path of hard knocks. Yoga in its truest essence is to see life intuitively. First purify the instrument; the intelligence is so delicate and precise that we are always in danger of getting lost in it. Let us develop our feelings, and then our knowledge will be of use. When great scientists grow older, and are preparing themselves for old age and death, they usually grow philosophical and idealistic. The Yogi knows that true knowledge is in the heart, not in the head. He knows that when a problem needs solution, the answer is in his consciousness, and by working at breathing and head stand, the consciousness will divulge the answer.

No matter how much he lectured, they would never truly understand the meaning of what he was saying until they had "arrived," and even then, "we can't put it into words, because it is beyond the mind. We want to help others get the same understanding; most people can learn only through feeling, and they require something concrete, therefore devices have to be used to arouse it."

Even though one could speak of "prayer" in the present day, he told them, it needed to be properly understood.

The inner revelation has been passed down through various religions which teach that through prayer all our desires will be granted us. Jesus said that if we pray and have faith our wishes will be granted. This must not be taken literally. Prayer, actually, is beyond name and form; it is the method whereby we can enter cosmic consciousness. Faith means feeling, and through feeling we can "arrive."

Thus, he explained, "Religion is therefore merely a device to enable people to have feeling," and since "today it is almost impossible to find the meaning behind the forms . . . let a new symbol come along, behind which we can find meaning and understanding, and there is our new religion."

As his lectures went on, Theos began to talk quite explicitly about new symbols for American religion: sexual yoga.

The Yogi starts out with the premise that we are no better than our sexual powers; it is the dynamic force that tells us how keen we are, and manifests itself as Kundalini. History shows us that the great men of the past had great sexual powers. Lack of knowledge of sexual powers results in failure to sublimate it, we get lost in it even more than in the economic structure. Yoga removes none of the beauty or idealism of sex; Yoga enhances it. The Yogi doesn't take sex blindly, he knows what it is, what its powers are and how to direct them. He has his physical channel and his sublimation. . . . The Yogi knows that in order for a wife to function as a full female, her natural sexual desires must be considered, and he satisfies them, although always under control. The Yogi has such control, that after emission, he can draw the semen back, thus not losing the ojuh. Women, because of their great intuitiveness could develop even greater control, but they lack the drive and the mental capacities of the man. The Yogi is not interested in the culmination of the sexual act; his system is first vitalized and consciousness spread throughout. . . . To gain control over the sexual powers, after culmination of the act, live in its ecstasy, and you are as close to heaven as you can be. Then go and meditate. . . . Sex is the closest thing in the physical world to spiritual realization.

Day after day, over the course of several weeks at the Living Arts Studio, Theos continued to mix Samkhya philosophy, Kundalinī yoga theory, Theosophical doctrines, Buddhist terminology, his father's research, and his own views, while students practiced āsanas and controlled breathing (prāṇāyāma) exercises. As his reputation increased, Theos began to accept (wealthy) private students at the exceptional rate of twenty-five dollars an hour.[2]

Before his first book had been published, Theos had begun to receive a substantial amount of fan mail from across both America and Europe, and it only increased once *Penthouse of the Gods* hit bookstore shelves. As ostentatious as the claims he made in his book and articles were, they often could not begin to compare with the mythic images of Tibet already in circulation. In his interviews, lectures, and books, Theos actively courted the "*Lost Horizon*" crowd of Tibetophiles and otherwise hopeful spiritual seekers. He drew on—and had to contend with—many people who had taken their inspiration from other sources: the readers of Baird T. Spaulding, Talbot Mundy,[3] Edwin J. Dingle, Theodore Illion, and others.

A self-proclaimed expert on Tibet, Baird T. Spaulding—who, more accurately speaking, was to Indo-Tibetan studies what Geoffrey T. Spaulding was to African ethnology[4]—had wowed the most gullible segment of "Eastern mysticism" neophytes with his series of books, *The Life and Teaching of the Masters of the Far East*—until it was discovered that he had spent most of his life as a gold prospector in Wyoming and a minor script writer for Cecil B. DeMille. Nonetheless, fans of Spaulding's *Teaching of the Masters* found inspiration from newspaper accounts of Theos's experiences in Tibet. One fan wrote to him, asking:

> I've read Baird T. Spaulding's books, "Life and Teachings of the Masters of the Far East." While you were in Tibet, were you privileged to see Jesus in person; to see food appear on the table, and to see people who were several hundred years of age?
>
> I like the teaching of these people as told by Mr. Spaulding, but would like to know more.

Careful not to alienate his consumer base, Theos had a standard form letter crafted for quick replies, thanking his fans for their interest in himself and informing them that "the answers to your questions can be found in my recent book, *Penthouse of the Gods*."

By the fall of 1939, with a lucrative business tutoring students—individually and in small classes—Theos was ready to break out on his own. Interviewed once again by his now friendly contact, Stewart Robinson at *Family Circle* magazine, Theos declared: "The general public is 99% wrong

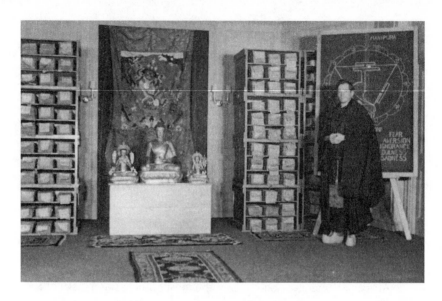

Figure 10.1 Bernard preparing to lecture at the Hotel Pierre (BANC)

about what Yoga is. It is not a religion, although it is most distinctly a way of life. No one need sacrifice an iota of his religion to engage in Yoga."[5]

Moving out of DeVries's studio, Theos expanded into the suite of apartments he had rented at the Hotel Pierre, on the Upper East Side, where he attempted to follow the model DeVries had used—a lecture followed by in-class demonstrations—offering daily yoga classes and Wednesday night seminars. Sending out flyers announcing "The American Institute of Yoga," Theos hired one of DeVries's old students, Claire Lea Stuart, to be a yoga instructor while he lectured, and his father manned the front desk.

In the present day and age, Theos informed his students, the only way to achieve happiness and spiritual realization was through the physical activity of yoga.

> We are constantly afraid of life. The mechanisms of a city drive us away from life. We can gain in this age thru action what Buddha did thru meditation, with what Christ did thru prayer . . . we must do it thru action. . . .
>
> In Tibet, vows of silence are common. A few hours of silence every day enables the mind to turn in on itself, and our spiritual development can begin. As it is, we hold ourselves back. When we lie to others, we lie

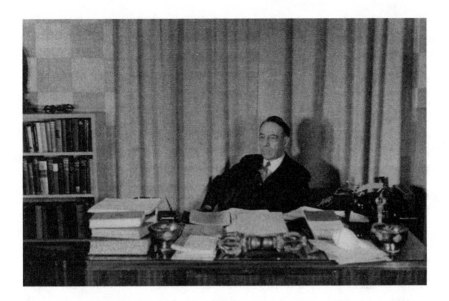

Figure 10.2 Glen Bernard at work in the office at the Hotel Pierre (BANC)

to ourselves; when we slander others, we are slandering ourselves. This is because we generally see in others the traits we ourselves have. Each of our friends sees us differently, for each sees himself in us. To help ourselves, we must speak the truth, praise our friends, and speak sensibly. If everyone observed this, they would all be in contact with the universal stream of consciousness and the world would be a peaceful and happy one. As we lift our own consciousness, we will have a corresponding effect on our friends. No one knew where Jesus went during his 18 years' absence; he was alone and in contact with universal consciousness, and he surely was the most unselfish man the world has ever known.

To be like the Buddha or Jesus, he told them, was completely feasible; all they had to do was learn yoga.

With Claire Stuart to give hands-on instruction and demonstrations of yogic postures, Theos was free to concentrate on his lectures. And with Glen's arrival, Theos once again had a ready research assistant. Drawing on his father's own writings[6] and the books in his library, Theos set a schedule of lecture topics—the Tibetan "Wheel of Life"[7] and Eightfold Path, Kuṇḍalinī yoga, recounting his adventures and experiences in Tibet—highlighting principles and philosophical observations that (he claimed) were validated by Western science. With Glen as editor and constant critic, Theos worked and reworked his notes for each lecture.

Although not the most pleasant of working companions, Glen was quite effective and helpful in acquiring resources. In addition to the various journals, posters, and assorted books and lecture materials[8] he could find, Glen brought in his own notes from his days with Sukumar Chatterji. More important, however, he had brought from California a copy of the privately circulated typescript of the Jung-Hauer lectures on Kundalinī yoga,[9] which he had apparently convinced Evans-Wentz to part with. Discarding Jung's psychological commentary, Theos and Glen proceeded to distill the transcript of Hauer's lectures into notes for Theos's own lectures on Kundalinī yoga to deliver at the Hotel Pierre.

Dismissing Woodroffe's translation of the ṣaṭ-cakra-nirūpaṇa that Theos had relied on for his master's thesis, Hauer had done his own translation of the text for use in his lectures. With both Woodroffe's and Hauer's perspectives at their disposal, Theos and Glen laid out a series of lectures, even reproducing a poster-sized version of Woodroffe's illustration of the bodily locations of the six cakras, complete with postlecture yoga exercises and breathing meditations.

Not all of Theos's students responded positively, however. Whether as a result of his lectures, the practice of yogic exercises, or simply her own disposition, the experiences at the Hotel Pierre proved to be too much for his private student Nina Donovan, who suffered a complete mental breakdown as a result. The woman's husband, Wilfred Donovan—a vice president at Abercrombie and Fitch—was not happy. Immediately having his wife institutionalized for her own protection, he next filed a lawsuit against Theos, "the Buddhist monk and yogi, and one of his women followers," Claire Stuart, the residents of a "sumptuous salon at the Hotel Pierre." The suit sought $25,000 in recompense for "damages sustained by me as a result of the fraudulent and negligent conduct of the defendants in injuring and impairing the mind of my wife . . . by teaching her Yoga philosophies and practices and by defrauding both of us out of large sums of money and personal property."

While Theos admitted to having received money from Mrs. Donovan in exchange for teachings, he maintained his innocence regarding her mental breakdown. Donovan claimed otherwise. "Bernard falsely represented himself to be a white lama (Buddhist priest) and an expert in teaching the theory and practice of Yoga philosophy" and, Donovan maintained, "said that he possessed spiritual powers which would be beneficial to my wife's mind and body." Nina Donovan, her husband claimed, had actually been "in a psychopathic condition which made her susceptible to suggestions like Bernard's and the yogi pair knew it."

Because the suit sought such a large amount in damages, it automatically went to the New York Superior Court, which caught the attention of William Randolph Hearst's newsmongers. More than a year later, lawyers for both sides had amassed over two hundred pages of depositions. When the details were finally made public, the story made headlines in Hearst's *American Weekly*, a newspaper supplement with nationwide distribution: "Wealthy Mrs. Donovan (Now in the Asylum) and Her Yogi Teacher."[10]

Harkening back to the "yellow press" days that built many a newspaper in New York City, the tabloid press picked up on the story and dug up every sordid detail connected with the name Bernard that they could, reacquainting the reading public with Barbara Vanderbilt's mental breakdown under the influence of P.A. years earlier.

Recanting large portions of his earlier statements—though reiterating that yoga *had* cured himself of an enlarged heart—Theos was not above disavowing and ridiculing his uncle in an attempt to distance himself from P.A.'s scandals of the past. Questioned by Donovan's lawyer, Theos was asked about the nature of yoga and his qualifications as a guru, or teacher of it; his relations with Mrs. Donovan; and his connection, if any, with Oom and the Nyack cult. Hoping to avoid guilt by association, Theos testified that

> he was unrelated to Oom by either blood or business. In other words, the fact that both have the same last name and are exponents of Yoga is nothing more than a coincidence.
>
> It is just coincidence, too, that Theos first met the woman who became his wife at the Clarkstown Country Club, Oom's place on the Hudson River; that after their marriage both lived there a good deal of the time; that they fraternized with Whittlesey and other Oom-bahs; that Mrs. Stuart had been a Nyack novitiate long before she began to instruct Theos' pupils in how to sit cross-legged; and finally that, after being introduced to Mrs. Donovan by a mutual friend, the White Lama recommended that she seek instruction at a New York studio then operated by Mrs. Stuart and Blanche DeVries.

In fact, he claimed, the only reason he associated with the Clarkstown Country Club was his then-wife's fondness for the place. He was casually acquainted with Blanche DeVries and others, but he let the world know that his opinion of P.A. was pretty low.

> Question (by O'Neill): What were the lectures that Pierre Bernard delivered?
>
> Answer: So far as I could tell they seemed to be nothing much but personal prejudices.
>
> Q: Against what?
>
> A: The world in general. The whole lectures were so long and involved that it was impossible to say afterwards what they were about for you usually were sleeping.
>
> Q: You slept through a number of his lectures, did you?
>
> A.: Every one I could, along with everyone else.

As for the issue of money paid, Theos claimed that Nina Donovan was not a very good student—hence the ongoing charges for classes and private instruction—and he had done his best with someone only marginally interested in what he had to say.

> When the twelve hours which the first $250 entitled her to had run out, the pupil handed over another similar sum, this time not for personal instruction but as the entrance fee to a class, or seminar, attended by a handful of people. . . . Five hundred dollars in an ordinary material market can buy quite a lot. Judging from Theos' remarks, its value in terms of spiritual things is not so great. A reading of the record suggests that Mrs. Donovan not only paid but, when it came to exchanging information, gave as much as she got. At least, her mentor hints that in the private meetings he had a hard job keeping her to the matter in hand, for at the drop of a hat she would start telling the story of her life.
>
> Even when they did get down to business, the return on the original investment seems to have been at a lower rate than, say, on government bonds. What Mrs. Donovan apparently got the most of was cold water: Theos himself implies that he was always having to throw this sobering liquid on her enthusiasms.
>
> "She would ask questions," he declared, "about the mysteries of religion . . . and I would then take it upon myself as best as possible to explain to what extent those things do not exist and do not obtain."

The same negative note kept cropping up again and again. The pupil wanted to known about levitation (floating in the air), apparently with a view to levitating herself somewhere, but once more the answer was: "those things do not obtain." She asked about "auras," and the master replied: "I don't know anything about it."

As for his other claims, Theos maintained that they needed to be put into the context of publicity. Nonetheless, the truth did come out.

When he first rocketed to prominence a few years ago, newspapers described him as a doctor of philosophy from Columbia University who had gone to the Orient and become the only white man ever to have resided for any length of time in Lhasa, the forbidden city of Tibet, the only one ever to have been initiated into the deepest mysteries of Tibetan Buddhism and actually to have become a lama. Why and how had this happened? Because, replied Theos in an article printed at the time, "they believed me to be the reincarnation of the God who founded that religion."

Under questioning in the present suit, however, he modified this colorful picture in a few particulars. It developed that his wealthy wife, Oom's disciple, had supported him while he was at Columbia and that he had not taken his doctor's degree but only studied for it.

And he disclaimed the appellation, "White Lama," as a figment of publicity, stating that he had not really become a lama at all but had merely gone through a preliminary initiation, on a level considerably below that of the final vows.

Bringing in his statements in *Heaven Lies Within Us*, Donovan's lawyer grilled Theos about the nature of his abilities. As a result, Theos was forced to testify

That he could not float in the air;
Or reduce his specific gravity ("still fluctuates with potatoes and gravy,"
    he admitted);
Or shed his skin;
Or bound about at will "like an inflated rubber ball!"
Or practise clairvoyance;

Or hold his breath for three hours;

Or even support himself on one finger—all of which attainments had been reported in his manuscript, later published in book form, as possible to those who had mastered Yoga.

He maintained, however, that he could do all the yogic postures himself, and on many occasions had demonstrated basic purification practices, such as using a *dhauti*.[11]

Despite his apparent financial success, 1940 through 1941 was a difficult time for Theos. The lawsuit was eventually settled out of court, but it did detract from his ability to draw students and continue his lectures. His personal life continued to be chaotic as well, and in the fall of 1940 he received another harsh blow: his mother had died in Tucson. Visiting Arizona briefly, Theos met with his half-brothers, stepfather, and uncle to sort out the details of Aura's will.

Upon his return to New York, Theos shifted his attention to one of his other students, the wealthy aspiring opera singer Madame Ganna Walska, who had been attending his lectures. Born Hanna Puacz in 1887 in Poland,[12] she had grown up under the care of her uncle in St. Petersburg and was by many accounts a beautiful young woman—reputedly selected by the Tzar of Russia as the most beautiful woman at one of his balls. At the age of nineteen young Hanna had eloped with a Russian count, Arcadie d'Eingorn, and moved to Switzerland. When the marriage fell apart years later, she returned to St. Petersburg, where she fell in love again, with a man she described only as "the second richest man in Russia." In the hope of being noticed by him—he was a patron of the arts, especially opera—she began singing lessons with the goal of becoming an opera diva. Still married to Count Arcadie when she performed in Paris, she adopted the stage name of Madame Ganna Walska[13] out of discretion, and used it for the rest of her life, often introducing herself as "Madame Walska," though she was known simply as "Madame" to her close acquaintances.

With World War I appearing imminent, Ganna followed the advice of friends to visit America, and with her knowledge of French, soon found employment as a cabaret singer at a French theater in New York. When she began to experience throat problems, she was referred to a specialist, Dr. Joseph Frankel. Ten days later, they were married, and Ganna began a rigorous course of training as a singer. Called "Baby" by her new husband, she had her every wish indulged. After a year and a half, she was ready for her debut alongside such notables as Enrico Caruso and the cellist Lucile Orrell. But after a disastrous operatic performance in Havana, Cuba ten months late, she returned to New York. Instead of redoubling her efforts at a music career, she pursue an interest in mysticism, from seances, Christian Science, and Rosicrucianism to yoga and meditation.[14]

Soon however, Dr. Frankel was diagnosed with a terminal "stomach ailment." Following his death, Ganna suffered from depression until the war's end convinced her it was safe to return to Paris. Crossing the Atlantic on the *Aquitania*, Ganna found herself the object of affection of not one but two millionaires—Alexander Cochran, "the richest bachelor in the world," and Harold McCormick, chairman of the board and son of the founder of the International Harvester Company. Wooed in silence by McCormick and repeatedly by Cochran, after several requests for her hand in marriage, Ganna relented and in the fall of 1920 married Cochran in Paris. The marriage was not to last long, as Ganna found Cochran to be a crass and insensitive man who preferred playing polo and hunting foxes in England over spending time with his wife.

Meanwhile, McCormick—still in love with Ganna—arranged for her to debut with the Chicago Opera Company in December 1920. The day before, Ganna fled Chicago without any warning, claiming that her husband's jealousy over her friendship with McCormick led her to return to New York and later, to Paris. Less than a year later, her lawyer appeared in New York with papers for divorce from Cochran. Cochran, whom the newspapers described with some glee as "formerly known as the world's richest bachelor," became the object of public scorn when Ganna's lawyer informed the newspapers, "if Mr. Cochran thinks he can dispose of his wife the way he disposes of toys and playthings when tired of them, he is much mistaken." When the divorce finally came—with Ganna retaining an undisclosed portion of Cochran's wealth—Ganna and Henry McCormick were free to wed, and did so in August 1922, making McCormick Ganna's fourth husband in ten years.

For several years, McCormick supported Ganna's desire to be an opera singer, even purchasing the Théâtre des Champs Elysées for her, but at every turn she met obstacles. At her Paris debut in *Rigoletto*, hissing was heard in the audience—sabotage by "some Russians," she claimed, who were trying to blackmail her—and her performances in Berlin were marred by "an illness" that affected her voice. In America, she fared no better. A shady Russian publicity agent charged her exorbitant fees, an arrangement that only ended in a lawsuit. Her scheduled performances with the Chicago Summer Opera were mysteriously canceled—the result of bribery by McCormick's ex-wife, she maintained—and the engagements she did have were punctuated by increasing episodes of stage fright that left her speechless or so ill she had to cancel or walk out on three separate performances, something the Chicago opera circle (and press) would not forget.

After nine years of marriage—most of which Ganna spent in France—in 1931 McCormick filed papers for divorce "on the grounds of desertion." Returning to her pursuits of vocal training and mysticism, Ganna spent the following years traveling back and forth between Europe and America. In the summer of 1937, she met the man who would become her fifth husband, Harry Grindell-Matthews, a physicist credited with the invention of sound motion pictures. They lived in France, but when German forces began their final approach to Paris, Ganna fled to America "on the last commercial passenger ship," leaving her husband behind. She claimed that she wanted to return to the opera world of New York but her voice lessons were proving difficult, and a friend suggested that she pursue training in yoga to improve her physical constitution. Thus she began attending Theos's classes at the Hotel Pierre.

According to her own words, Ganna Walska was initially not very impressed by Theos, finding him to be an "uninspiring teacher." Nonetheless, she continued to attend daily yoga classes "as a form of exercise and weight control," as well as his Wednesday evening lecture classes. She even engaged Theos for a series of private sessions, though she found them frustrating because of his refusal "to answer her questions, either about oriental philosophy or about himself." For these reasons, she was surprised one day in the spring of 1941 to receive a visit from him. During what appeared to be no more than a social call, to her amazement, Theos declared that he had fallen in love with her—the very first time she attended his lecture. Furthermore, Ganna claimed, Theos wanted to marry her the very next day "because it was the full moon." Informed that she was already married, Ganna later recounted, Theos became furious, demanding that she ask for a divorce. Only later, when she deflected his attempt at a good-night kiss, did she realize the depths of emotion he felt for her as she watched him break down and cry. "No wonder that my womanly, always motherly heart went out to this poor boy," she later recounted. "I was sorry I did not suspect his agony and pushed him away so cruelly." Claiming to not know what was troubling him—though certain that he was miserable—Ganna vowed, "I must help him because I am the stronger one" . . . and so their relationship began.

Ganna was soon in love with Theos as well, and in the process of completing her memoirs, gushed romantically over "the boy." "In the meantime, an extraordinary thing happened to me," she wrote, "that last winter, a young man—who taught me much about Forgotten Teachings—an old soul dwelling in a young Arizona boy, who already had time in flower of his youth to gather much knowledge in India and Tibet." Ganna thought that Theos was a dream come true, and a sign that she was finally on her spiritual path.

In this culminating year of finding myself on the right trail, I also most naturally was more ready and better prepared for the next step to learn, to meet the next teacher. For it is said that whenever a student is ready, the Master will appear! And that Master was the American boy. . . . He unfolded to my soul so much the Real Knowledge of Divine Law that I have stored up in my inner being enough food to digest and assimilate for the rest of this earthly life, that richness I was blessed to receive from this fortunate possessor of great undying Truth. Thanks to him, the concept of the Spiritual Law that governs us—simple in its greatness—now lies so clearly in my mental and godly being that already I can pass on those gems of purest water to those who, unlike myself, have not yet been priviledged to realize some parcel of Truth.

Learning of Ganna's aspirations to sing, Theos informed her that there were whole other potential dimensions to her voice that she was unaware of. "In the East," he told her, "there are still those who have voices developed according to the Great Law and who can by their sounds not only heal any physical illness but can even transfer spiritual knowledge to the truth-seeking soul deserving of such illumination." Reminding her of "certain vocal studies still practiced in India," Theos promised to help her train in them, and offered to introduce her to "a friend" in California—his father, Glen—a "Western possessor of this rare knowledge" who knew that, hidden somewhere in the mountains of Southern California, there was an expert, "a very strange old woman who is unwilling to communicate with the outside world." But his "friend" might be able to persuade her to see Ganna. This was only the beginning, Theos told her, both for themselves and for America. Although born in Poland and raised in Russia, from her studies of

Roscicrucianism, Ganna knew that America was a special place, "the haven for all souls inspired for freedom," she declared.

America—where the only restriction is our own limited expansion of consciousness.

America—the protecting Citadel of the High Ideal against materialistic concepts of happiness. . . .

America—where real houses are not meant to be sky-scrapers but eternal habitations of peace within ourselves!

America—where the work lies not in its fruit but in the resulting expansion of the consciousness. . . .

The founders of this country were . . . men of mystery and were directed by a Divine Force that, to the ignorant, almost took on the proportions of miracles. . . .

For what is America? And where is it? It is not a reality. It is only a place where reality can manifest itself and when that privilege is granted to each human heart, no matter what his race, color or creed—that is America. . . .

That is why America is the land where Men will build a civilization from which will come the greatest Spiritual Renaissance the world has ever known!!!

"Perhaps not all Americans realize that this country of the Future has been guided step by step by some Force," she continued, and "to the people with intuition it is quite evident that America was meant to be *the* Future World." This was all true, Theos informed her, but more importantly, it was but a prequel to greater things in store, in which she could play a part:

This so-called *new* world, America, has become *the* World, the safe deposit for all the best from the Old World, the new dwelling place of old civilization, the birthplace of a future spiritual empire, the root of Awakened Consciousness! . . . Only those who have lived away from the States for a while can appreciate the high awakening of the soul in this country!

Just as it was "historical fact . . . that a mystery man always appeared at the darkest moment in the construction of this nation to guide its builders," so too had Theos returned from India and Tibet for a similar purpose. But benefiting mankind was not something he could do alone; he need a companion, a "helpmate." Believing him, Ganna agreed to help Theos and work together on their great new mission. When they traveled to Southern California for her health and to consult yet another voice teacher, Theos was struck by the scenery of the coastal town of Santa Barbara, telling Ganna how much it "reminded him of Tibet," although not so much when a 5.5 magnitude earthquake struck the city shortly after their arrival.[15]

There they lived in separate accommodations while Ganna practiced her singing and Theos scouted the area for properties on which to set up an institute and make their plans a reality. Soon, he contacted Ganna when he had found two locations that met his requirements—one for a research center and another for his own residence. Ganna, expecting to see modest, ready-made establishments, instead was shocked that Theos has selected two massive properties: Cuesta Linda, a forty-acre estate nestled up against the foothills of the Santa Barbara mountains, which Theos declared would be the perfect home for his research institute; and, some twenty miles north in the St. Yñez Mountains, El Capitan, the former estate of George Owen Knapp (the founder of Union Carbide), a forested mountaintop resort with hot springs, tennis courts, a swimming pool, a lodge, and a cliff-edge castle . . . all of which, Theos told Ganna, would be the ideal place for his meditative retreat.

Taken aback at first, Ganna Walska eventually acceded to Theos's requests and purchased the two properties in June and September 1941. Theos renamed the downtown estate Tibetland and his new mountain home Penthouse of the Gods. Although not married, as far as he was concerned, Theos was once again rich. Back in 1937 in Lhasa, he had expressed interest in finding "people who have a sincere interest in this field of thought and willing to open mindedly work out the problems with me." Consequently, the first thing he needed, Theos told Ganna, was a research colleague, and he had one readily available and waiting in India, a man named Geshe Gedun Chöpel. With him by their side, Theos was convinced that he and his father could finally bring their work to fruition.

ELEVEN

Tibetland and the Penthouse of the Gods

Today they are in the process of translating these books into Chinese; so it will not be long before China can forget all about where they came from, and I hope that some day it will be the same for those in America. The chap who is undertaking the job of making the translation is about fifty, so if I am able to master this language in the next twenty years, there is still hopes of being able to carry out the ambition for the benefit of those who follow.

—THEOS BERNARD[1]

HERE WAS CALIFORNIA, Ganna Walska thought, "the seed of the new world which is the future America" and "the nourishment of the coming epoch."[2]

If the creative artists, the profound philosophers, the writers and the scientists and above all the deep Truth Seekers are choosing California as the place where their inspiration runs high, would it not be reasonable to think that it must be due to some condition, perhaps atmospheric, of that vast land, of that burning desert near the Pacific Ocean, of those valleys and that exhilarating air in those high mountains?

Is it not plausible to believe that something is attracting the mystical world—and all true artists are mystics, are avatars—to that part of the United States? Is it not credible to reason that this part of the United States is destined to become a spiritual capital of the future American Empire—the Vatican of all Spiritual Truth seekers? . . .

Great things are timeless, for during that period, so short but fertilized by many centuries, in this California wonderland—where God's creations flourish overnight—Truth of the Divine Law, old as are the worlds, had crossed the Himalayas, for the ways of God are impenetrable! crossed the Pacific, annihilated space and time and come to life again by depositing Living Knowledge in predestined Santa Barbara's "Tibetland" where the mystery of our being is to be unfolded to all Truth seekers.

The Spaceless, Timeless, Invisible Government has deposited through the medium of its Adept the Infinite Truth with its symbols—as in Shangri-La—and thus consecrated profane dwellings into a sacred Grail with its fantastic gardens where blooms the Divine Lotus, planted by unknown hands, and where the Powers-to-be built on the neighboring mountain heights the Penthouse of the Gods!

Through Theos's charm, Ganna Walska had bought (and been sold on) Tibetland and the Penthouse of the Gods. With the purchase of the Cuesta Linda estate—Tibetland—Theos was ready to put his plans into motion.

Over the years since his return, Theos had attempted to maintain contact with his various friends in India and Tibet. He received letters from time to time, from Lord Tsarong, Tethong Shapé, and Tharchin, asking for advice on the wool trade or conveying the latest news; he even got himself a subscription to Tharchin's *Mirror* newspaper. Theos sent out a simple "Christmas card" at the end of 1939 to most everyone he had met in India and Tibet, even the Ganden Tri-pa. For the previous nine months, Theos had been in contact with his friend in Darjeeling, S. K. Jinorasa. Asking Theos for a donation in support of his Young Men's Buddhist Association (YMBA), Jinorasa told him that the association was "growing popular day by day" and that he hoped "in the near future it will be doing immense good service to the humanity." Of greater interest to Theos, however, was that in addition to running "educational works," Jinorasa was hard at work translating Tibetan classics of literature into English.

I have two friends who are great scholars in Tibetan. One is Geshe Chhophel La and another is Geshe Tensing Gyaltsen. Both of them are well versed in Mahayana philosophy and Tantra. With their help I have translated the Bodhisatva-Cariya-Avatara by Shanti Deva in English and I shall try to publish it. This book is the sum and substance of Mahayana philosophy. And if one studies it he will know what Mahayana is.[3]

Contacting Jinorasa again mere days after the purchase of the downtown property, Theos informed him that he had succeeded in establishing

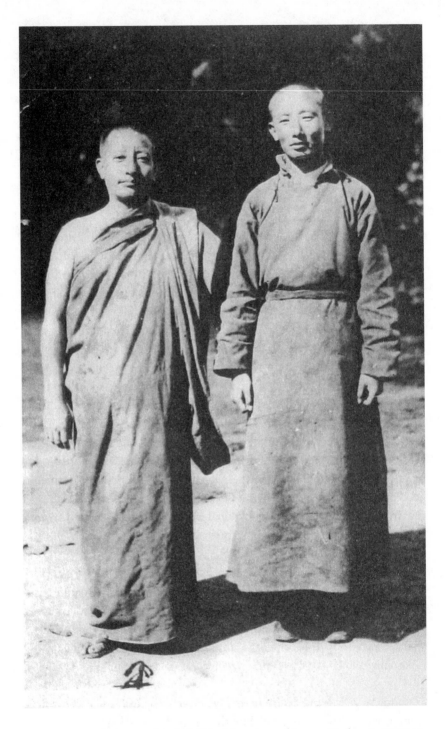

Figure 11.1 S. K. Jinorasa and Gedun Chöpel (courtesy of Amnye Machen Institute Visual Archives. Collection Tashi Tsering)

an institute in America and wanted Gedun Chöpel to come and join him at once. Jinorasa sprang into action and sent Theos a telegram with exact instructions to be followed on his end. He passed the information on to Ganna Walska, who had her lawyers begin to file all the necessary paperwork, from the visa application to affidavits of financial support. With money from Theos and Ganna, Jinorasa booked Gedun Chöpel passage on a steamship set to depart from Calcutta on August 3 for San Francisco,[4] while Gedun Chöpel's editor at the Mahābodhi Society proudly announced the geshe's departure for America to his reading public.[5]

But as Ganna's lawyer, Phelan Beale, attempted to get the paperwork through the U.S. State Department, he encountered no end of difficulties. Large parts of the world were at war—including British India—and though not directly involved, the United States was feeling the effects. Thousands from around the world sought to flee the growing conflict and were inundating American embassies and consulates worldwide. To make matters worse, the late nineteenth and early twentieth centuries in America had seen a marked increase in xenophobia. The vision of a Protestant Christian America seemed to be crumbling, and conservative forces in the U.S. government sought to stem the tide of immigration—specifically, Asian immigration—passing laws that enforced strict quotas and requirements for entry into the United States. By the 1940s, these laws had created a bureaucratic nightmare for the U.S. Department of Justice as hundreds of thousands of required documents were being filed by war refugees. As a result, two days before Gedun Chöpel's scheduled departure from Calcutta, Beale sent a telegram to Ganna Walska informing her that more affidavits and supporting paperwork were needed and Gedun Chöpel would not be able to leave as scheduled.

Convinced that Ganna's lawyers would still be able to finesse Gedun Chöpel's visa, Theos began the next phase of the project: the construction of a Tibetan temple on the grounds of Tibetland. Announcing the founding of an "Academy of Tibetan Literature," he gave an inaugural lecture in the grove where the new institute would be built. "The purpose of this talk," he told the assembled guests, "is to aquaint you with our plans as well as to give you a better understanding of that mysterious country, Tibet." Most important of all, Theos informed them, he was accepting students to learn Tibetan, and together they were going to translate the Tibetan Buddhist canon into English. He told them it would transform America.

It is our present plan to create here an Academy of Tibetan Literature in order that we can make these philosophical teachings accessible to interested students. Right now plans are being made to bring a Lama from Lhasa in order to begin the translation of the Tibetan Kangyur and Tengyur which is their encyclopedia of knowledge pertaining to every aspect of life. Presently this Lama is waiting in Darjeeling, India, a small town on the border, for our State Department to grant him permission to come on to the U.S. As is to be expected, the present international situation is causing many complications. However we are going right ahead with our plans to make it possible for sincere seeking students to come and further their studies as well as learn something about the Art of Yoga or the Art of Living Life.

It is natural to wonder why anyone would wish to undertake the task of translating 333 volumes of Tibetan Manuscripts. Obviously they must have something which we deem of vital importance to our lives. In the first place, this will be one of the greatest literary undertakings of this century, for it remains our last literary treasure of an ancient civilization. Secondly it records the knowledge of a culture that had its glory many centuries before the advent of Christianity. Here is knowledge that has stood the test of time. Its truths are as true today as they were when they were first written. With all the discoveries of modern science, at no time has it ever been necessary to revise any of their fundamental principles. . . . These principles are to be found in these Tibetan Manuscripts which we propose to translate and make it possible for students to obtain a more thorough understanding.

This was far from a mere whim—there was a very specific reason Tibetan literature was of value, and indeed, of crucial importance to America. The lamas he had met in Tibet

were men who had devoted their entire life to study and meditation on all that is of vital importance to the welfare and ultimate needs of man. Their minds have fathomed the fundamental laws behind every aspect of existence. Their knowledge extends from the movement of heavenly bodies to the simple relations between individuals. The mysteries of nature have become simple principles to them. Certainly the opinions of such minds should stir us to serious thought and reflection. . . .

It is conceded that the West has developed to perfection the applied arts and sciences. But what has been the price? We have invented, but what have we discovered? We have applied, but what have we attained? We have amassed, but what have we achieved? They say that we have learned to work, but we have forgotten how to worship, we have learned how to earn a living, but we have forgotten how to live. . . . Our triumphs in the mechanical arts have been at the price of failure to obtain spiritual insight. There has been no time to meditate on the life lived. The effect has been that our children are instructed but not educated, our people are assimilative but incapable of thought, we can rationalize but we cannot perceive. Convention guides our daily pattern of life, we go to church to appear religious, we attend theatres to appear cultured; we read best sellers to appear well read. Our homes are empty; our literature indulgences the most superficial aspects of human nature; our paintings only patterns in paint and not life in a frame. These are the reasons why the Tibetan says that western intelligence is misapplied, that our civilization is a huge machine out of gear with life.

What Theos offered his audience instead was the opportunity to discover for themselves a new way of living, a new philosophy of life that he claimed was only to be found in Tibet: tantric yoga. Not just yoga but the "very rationale behind Yoga" was what he proposed to teach "to those serious students who come here to further their knowledge in the realities of life."

As the weeks passed, there seemed to be little progress on Gedun Chö-pel's visa. Concerned about the delay, Ganna Walska, by then back in New York, pressured Beale, writing and sending him telegrams asking for information. They "must definitely know how many chances" there were for obtaining the visa, she told him, since it was unfair to Gedun Chöpel to keep him "all those months without benefit of his work."[6] Beale continued on the legal front while Ganna Walska contacted friends in the federal government. By November, prospects were not looking good. The U.S. State Department informed Beale that they could have no influence in the matter and that all decisions to grant or refuse visas lay with the consulates overseas, in this case, the American consulate in Calcutta.[7]

When the news finally came that Gedun Chöpel's visa had been declined, Theos chose not to tell Gedun Chöpel himself, but asked Jinorasa to break the news to him in person. Nonetheless, writing to Gedun Chöpel,

Theos reassured the monk that he was still hopeful that they would be able to sort out the difficulties with his visa. In the worst case, he might have to wait until the end of the war which, Theos told him, should only last a few months more; by the end of 1942 it would be over, and he could come to America. In the meantime, Theos offered to support him in India while he translated some texts.[8] Acknowledging the same request from Jinorasa, Gedun Chöpel agreed to Theos's offer, saying that he would remain in India for seven months contingent on Theos's support, and in July 1942 they could reassess the situation.[9] Theos sent money to Gedun Chöpel through Jinorasa, who offered to help in his research efforts, telling him that he could employ many lamas on his behalf in Darjeeling, and should he return to India, he would be more than welcome at the YMBA.

When Jinorasa broke the news to the young geshe, Gedun Chöpel was disheartened, and with the Japanese attack on Pearl Harbor and the entry of the United States into the new war, it was clear that the conflict would last far longer than a few months. Jinorasa informed Theos,

> I went to see [Gedun Chöpel] some days ago and showed him your letter and also requested him to stay here until the war ends. He was very sorry for not been [sic] able to go to America soon to help you in your works there. He told me he was very anxious to return home (Kansu in China) if he would fail to go to America very soon. I told him you were anxious to see him and to get his help in your work and that you were trying to come to India and that if you would get an opportunity you would come soon. He then agreed to stay here for one year more and requested you pay him monthly fooding, etc, charges of Rs 50/- . . . He says in the meantime if you want him to do any translation work or any other work in Tibetan literature here he would very gladly do it for you.

Trying to encourage Theos, as well, to not lose heart and remain hopeful and firm in his endeavors, Jinorasa told him:

> Mr. Bernard—we are ever ready to help you in your noble work if you are sincere to do it. Both of us have no desire for worldly fame and wealth. We have seen and enjoyed them and we find it [an] utterly useless thing to run after these worldly things. It is a sheer nonsense to waste this valuable human life after such mirage. Today you see quite clearly what the worldly fame and wealth mean. But if we can do some useful works

for the human beings we are ever ready to do it. Ignorance is bad and today the world suffers from ignorance. Wisdom is strength but the strength should be supported by selfless motives and then only the Wisdom can be used for happiness of the human beings.

In conclusion I must write to you again something about Geshe Chhophel La. I must tell you that he is the greatest Tibetan scholar I have ever met with in my life and he is one of the few rare best scholars in Tibet so you must not miss him by all means to help you in your Great Work if you really want to do real research works in Mahayana Buddhism. If you miss him I doubt very much whether you will again get another man like him. So do not miss him by all means. I shall do my best to keep him here till the war ends.

But someone else was doing his best to get the geshe to work with him: George Roerich. Jinorasa informed Theos, "Professor Roerich from Nagar, Kulu (Punjab, India) had also written several letters to Geshe La to go to Kulu to do some translation works from Tibet, but he did not like to go there as he prefers to await for your coming here or some instructions from you to do some works here for you."

While Theos thought it would be nice if circumstances in the world changed to allow Gedun Chöpel to come to America, he was not hopeful, so he began making backup plans. While they spent the winter in New York, Theos suggested to Ganna that they travel to India and Tibet together. There were some individuals dwelling hidden in India and Tibet, Theos told her, who could "transfer spiritual knowledge to the truth-seeking soul deserving of such illumination." Although he could not guarantee success—such masters were difficult to find—still such a trip would be worth trying to do. When he received a lukewarm response from Ganna, who instead suggested that he resume lecturing there in New York, Theos moved back to California. Accustomed to being the center of a man's attention, Ganna was more than a little upset when she discovered that Theos had packed *all* of his belongings and returned to Tibetland, leaving nothing of his in their New York apartment. She explained that she was far too preoccupied with writing her memoirs to travel to Tibet, and even if "Easter can see me in Tibet," she would be "most happy not only because I can be *there* but also because it would mean either that I advanced my work enough for the present or that I could advance it differently." But with food and gasoline rationing going into effect in parts of the country, such "leisure" trips were simply not feasible. By the summer of 1942, the war encompassed the entire globe, and it seemed little could be done to either bring Gedun Chöpel to America or get Theos to India. Gedun Chöpel, still hoping to return to his home on the Tibetan–Chinese border, was convinced to stay in India by Jinorasa. With Sānkṛtyāyana gone, he accepted George Roerich's offer to come live with him at his research institute in the Kulu valley and translate Tibetan texts.

Although he had reaffirmed to Ganna throughout the previous spring that despite being hard at work on his research, "the moment this is finished, I want to be where my heart is—with you," Theos remained apprehensive and concerned for the future with "Madame." As her lawyers were negotiating for Gedun Chöpel's visa the previous fall, Ganna had received word from Paris that her fifth husband, Grindell-Matthews, had died. Although she had rewritten her will, leaving the two properties in California to Theos in the event of her death, he repeatedly begged her to marry him.

Without Gedun Chöpel, Theos felt that he had no choice but to put the translation project on hold. Instead, he decided to return to New York and—with Ganna Walska's (financial) assistance—rematriculate at Columbia University to make a second attempt at obtaining his Ph.D. As they prepared to live together in close quarters in Manhattan, Ganna finally relented and after signing a prenuptial agreement, on July 27, 1942, in Las Vegas, Theos became her sixth husband.

Leaving the Penthouse of the Gods under the care of his "learned friend" and research assistant, "Mr. LaVarnie" (Theos's father, Glen), whom Ganna was asked to support, and the Tibetland estate under the care of maintenance staff, the two returned to New York, where Ganna spent her time putting the final touches on her memoirs. Life with Theos was a wonderful new experience, which she could not help but write about in the closing chapter: "It was only last winter—oh, how rich that winter was to me!—that I learned and understood, again thanks to my youthful teacher, for the first time the actual value of our physical body, the dwelling place of our spiritual being!"

Not only was Ganna personally happy to be with Theos, she was happy to be seen in public with him as well. She maintained a box at the Metropolitan Opera and added Theos to her entourage, though she still was unable to shake her operatic *faux pas* of the past.[10] Nonetheless, she was once again making the society pages: gossip columnist Hedda Hopper commented that Ganna Walska was seen in New York "showing the sights to the high llama [sic] who occupies one of her cottages on her Santa Barbara estate."[11]

With few other options, Theos re-enrolled at Columbia University and reconnected with his advisor, Herbert Schneider. At the time of his failed dissertation defense four years earlier, the committee had offered three ways to revise it, based on the three major themes they saw in his original 1938 submission, "any one of which might be developed into an acceptable dissertation":

(1) An investigation of the systems of Yoga teaching and discipline as they are found in Tibet (or India).

(2) A critical, "scientific" appraisal of the Yoga disciplines in terms of modern physiological and psychiatrical knowledge, examining the values and claims of these exercises.

(3) A detailed, "clinical" report of what the author has seen and heard, distinguishing the various Yogis and sects visited and what was gathered from each and interpreting the findings as far as possible in view of what other information is available on the subject.

Theos now told Schneider that he was ready to pursue the third option and willing to follow his suggestions.

For Theos, being back in New York was an opportunity to pick up where he had left off many years before in other ways too. When his younger brother Dugald passed through New York City, preparing to ship off to Europe to fight in the war, Theos took the opportunity to see him again and met his wife, Gretchen, for the first time. After Dugald had left, to try to cheer her up, Theos took her to dinner at the Waldorf Astoria and then out dancing afterward. Many years later, she recalled, Theos struck her as "the most debonair, handsome and meticulously dressed man" she had ever met.

Resuming his New York lectures, Theos began once again taking private students and teaching yoga classes. Rewriting his *Tantrik Yoga* manuscript as suggested, as a "clinical report," he refashioned it as a practical commentary on the core text, *The Small Lamp [Illuminating] Haṭha Yoga*, translated some years earlier.[12] Drawing on Swami Kuvalayānanda's illustrated *Yoga-Mimamsa* journal and posters that his father had purchased for him in Bombay, Theos replicated the various *āsanas* with a professional studio photographer for inclusion in his new dissertation. By the end of December, he had a completely revised manuscript, which he delivered to Schneider: *Tantrik Yoga: A Clinical Report*. Retaining the narrative of his father's retreat published in *Heaven Lies Within Us* and the spin on his activities represented by *Penthouse of the Gods*, Theos explained in the new preface:

> This study is the report of a Westerner who has practiced Yoga under a teacher in India.
>
> The primary purpose of the investigation was to test by personal experience the claims of Hatha Yoga. As part of the research . . . I surrendered to Eastern Traditional Training, yet tried to remain critical in order to appraise the results in the light of experience rather than theory. To this end I became the sincere disciple of an outstanding teacher and settled down at his retreat. For several months, under his supervision and guidance, I adhered to the rigid discipline imposed upon one who wishes to practice Yoga. . . . Any attempt to prove the merits of the "Art of Yoga" would be futile. If a thousand volumes were quoted in its favor, and all the rules of logic and sophistry were employed, the doubts and skepticism of modern man would still remain; therefore this study is not going to try. Instead, I will present a critical report of my personal experiences in learning and practicing several strange and mysterious techniques of Hatha Yoga.[13]

Confident that his new dissertation would meet the requirements spelled out earlier, Theos focused on teaching and lecturing, although the environment in New York for yoga teachers was starting to get competitive—the city was turning into the battleground for a turf war between counterculture religious groups. The Theosophical Society, which had seen its share of glory slowly fade after its repudiation by Krishnamurti and with the growing number of teachers arriving from the East, lashed out at rivals—P.A. and Theos included—apparently alluding to their respective troubles with Barbara Vanderbilt and Mrs. Donovan:

> In America, the religious groups which have been most successful in gaining adherents in recent years are those which relegate reason to an unimportant position in the scheme of moral life. . . . What of the hundreds of oriental seers, yogis and "spiritual teachers" who have invaded the shores of America during recent years, gaining for themselves immense personal followings? Almost without exception, their pro-

spectuses read, "Gain health, wealth, happiness by this new, easy, secret method! Develop your will, your secret powers, by learning from me!" The emotional exaltation produced in the devotees of these pseudo-spiritual teachers often ends in insanity and it cannot fail to warp the intellectual powers almost beyond repair. The native sages and prophets are not less numerous, nor less wily in their methods of exploiting the religious nature of their fellow men. Correspondence courses in spiritual development do a thriving business. The ignorant, the naïve and the miserable pay an annual toll of millions of dollars to purchase the "secrets of the ages." There is literally nothing that these merchants of psychic glory will not promise for a modest fee.[14]

Although clearly implicated by such criticism, Theos had a core of devoted students and could still draw a small crowd, so he remained unconcerned.

But on the academic front, there was an obstacle to Theos's graduation beyond his dissertation. Since he had decided on the third option offered to him, the one "regarded as most directly a contribution to the anthropology of 'religion,'" before his committee had even read his revised manuscript, they pointed out that the philosophy department at Columbia was not allowed to accept dissertations in "Religion."

Promising to see what he could do, Schneider wrote to the provost of Columbia University, suggesting that since a subcommittee had just recently been created to oversee graduate work in religion, the University Statutes governing "the Division of Philosophy, Psychology and Anthropology" should be amended to include the designation of "Religion." By the end of March, it appeared that the change to the philosophy department's bylaws would be accepted. Meanwhile, at the end of February, Theos finally heard back from his dissertation committee. Although it was a good step in the right direction, Schneider informed Theos, the manuscript he submitted in January still needed work, in terms of both documentation and the proper spelling of Sanskrit words. Determined to graduate that semester, Theos hired a private Sanskrit tutor and with only weeks to get a revised manuscript back to his committee, reduced his sleeping to no more than four hours a night, compensating with intense yoga sessions and daily massages, all the while rewriting and documenting the various statements in his thesis.

But Ganna was becoming convinced that his excessive yoga practices were having an adverse effect on his mental state. Having forced him to

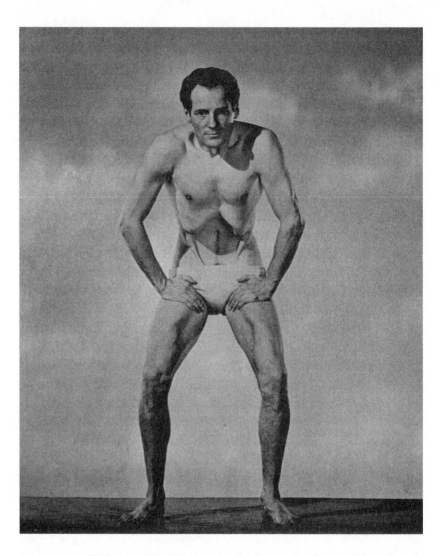

Figure 11.2 Bernard demonstrating the *uḍḍiyāna bandha* as part of his dissertation. Bernard, *Haṭha Yoga: The Report of a Personal Experience*

get a medical examination the previous fall, she wrote to him, pleading with him to stop his exercises, especially the headstand since given the increase in intracranial pressure, the doctors she consulted were amazed that he was not "completely insane." Ignoring her, Theos continued both his practice routine and his work on the dissertation.

Adding extra citations to the *Haṭha Yoga Pradīpikā*, *Gheraṇḍa Saṃhitā*, *Śiva Saṃhitā*, and the various works of John Woodroffe/"Arthur Avalon," Theos submitted his revised manuscript to his committee and on June 1, 1943 was awarded the first Ph.D. in Religion from Columbia University. He remained "in residence" at Columbia through the fall, and Ganna covered the cost of publishing his dissertation—now called *Haṭha Yoga: The Report of a Personal Experience*—with professional typesetting, a dust jacket, and thirty-six photographic plates, in gratitude for which he appropriately dedicated the book "To Ganna Walska."

Still, life was not entirely satisfactory for either Theos or Ganna. In public, Theos was the handsome young escort of Madame Walska at social functions, at the opera, or simply in art galleries, bidding on Tibetan and Buddhist artwork against their rival collector in New York, Jacques Marchais. In private, however, Theos was tired of the many social obligations that Ganna imposed on him. He told her that he could not stand Broadway musicals and the like, since "the vibrations are too gross" for someone of his sensitive constitution, so she found herself attending performances such as *Oklahoma!* alone.

Giving Ganna little notice, Theos suddenly left New York shortly after his dissertation was published, to visit his uncle in Phoenix and his friends and brothers in Tucson and Tombstone before heading to California to see his father. Ganna sent letters and telegrams almost daily, trying to locate him and objecting to his "mania about having General Delivery addresses." After returning to New York, Theos decided to take a room the Lotos Club, the famous literary and artistic club founded by Mark Twain. It was convenient on many levels, not only as a quiet space away from Ganna but also so that from time to time he could secretly visit Viola, who was still living in the city, and seek consolation from her for his difficulties with Ganna. It also afforded him additional privacy, for Theos had met yet another woman.

A few years older than Theos, Helen Park was the ex-wife of Arthur Brock Park, a high-profile partner in the American Life Insurance Company. Following an acute illness in Shanghai in the late 1930s, Helen began to have vivid dreams, which she believed were in some sense prophetic[15]— "for the benefit of mankind." She began dutifully recording all her dreams, occasionally adding interpretive commentary.[16] By the mid-1940s, Helen had been divorced from her husband (who had since remarried) for several years and was living and working in New York as an interior decorator. One mid-August evening, she had another dream, which she took to be of great significance. In it, she was commissioned to decorate a room, "to be done in Tibetan Style, very simple and austere."[17] Inspired, she sought out information on Tibet, and as a result came to meet Theos a few weeks later.

With the war clearly in its last days, Theos decided that the time was ripe for a return trip to India and Tibet, and even if Ganna Walska was unwilling to support him in this, Helen was. Two days after meeting Theos, Helen had another one of her "prophetic dreams," which she told him about the very next morning:

> I stood in the doorway and looked into a small room where a dozen Indian gentlemen (East Indian) were sitting around a table. Some had black beards and some were bald-headed and one sitting on the far side of the longtable had on a black homberg [sic] hat. As I stood there, this man got up and came towards me and we went off together.[18]

Interpreting the dream was not difficult for Theos. The man in the homburg hat could only be Geshe Wangyal, and it was clear that they were destined to return to India together to study with him. Theos sat down again at his typewriter that same day and wrote two letters.

Writing to Gedun Chöpel, Theos told his would-be collaborator,

> My Dear Geshe Chhophel:
> For many months I have planned to write, but world conditions have made it impossible for me to say anything definite, even now, there is no specific program that I can outline, save to say that I am still contemplating our work together. . . .
>
> Where are you living? Are you translating any material at this time? What are your plans for the future? I do hope you will continue to keep in touch with me, so that eventually, we can arrange to carry out our program. Have you been to Lhasa recently? Have you heard anything from Tsarong Shape? Have you contacted any other outstanding scholars who can help us? . . .
> As soon as world conditions will permit travel,[19] I will probably return to India in order to gather additional material for the library. At that time I want to contact you at the earliest possible date, so that, we can make preparations for the purchase of Tibetan manuscripts and arrange for our work of preparing them to be published in English. Once I am there, it will probably be easier to make plans for you to come to this country; however I *cannot commit* myself to any definite program at this

time. If the fates are with us, it will work out. The most we can do is to plan and try.

In the second letter, to Lord Tsarong in Lhasa, Theos told his former host that his Academy of Tibetan Literature was well on its way—although put on hold during the war—and once it was up and running again he hoped "you will be able to visit me here, for I am sure you would be inspired by what is being done, and certainly you would appreciate the beauty of this corner of the world. . . . I hope this message will tell you that my spirit still dwells at your fireside, even though I am far away."[20]

If he had to explain to Lord Tsarong that his spirit was with him, even if his physical body was "far away," he did not have to tell this to Ganna Walska, who could see it quite easily for herself. While Helen began practicing yoga, Theos decided to return to California, where he established legal residency. Once back in Santa Barbara, he rejoined Glen, who had been living at the Penthouse estate under the alias of Mr. LaVarnie, and they went back to work revising their research notes and parts of Theos's 1938 dissertation in the hope of publishing more books. By then they had several book-length works. Theos had four large manuscripts:

"Tibetan Saga": the third volume in Theos's story of his India–Tibet trip, picking up from his adventures at Ganden Monastery (where *Penthouse of the Gods* ended), covering his empowerment at Dra-yer-pa, travel from Lhasa to Sakya, and return to India and giving more detail to his "destiny" and "life-mission [that] was appointed, maybe aeons before my birth."[21]

"The Philosophical Foundations of India": an overview of the different Indian schools, extracted from Theos's 1938 dissertation.

"The True Nature of Things": a mixture of Saṃkhya cosmology, the Buddhist understanding of dependent origination, and subtle body *cakra* theory compiled from Theos's lecture notes.

"Yoga": a loose series of articles also drawn from his lecture notes.

Glen had two:

"The Rationale of Sex": a manual of advice on sex drawn from Ayurvedic and Kamic literature discussing aphrodisiacs, astrology, and moral laws and the conservation of "ojuh."

"The Art of Yoga" (a.k.a. "A Selective Treatise on the Theory and Practice of Yoga"): the manuscript Theos had drawn on for his lectures years earlier, as well as for his dissertation.

Theos's "Tibetan Saga" having been turned down for publication several years earlier, Theos and Glen decided to focus on editing the philosophy book.

By this time, *Hatha Yoga* was starting to get praise in the academic press for "striking through the mass of religious and supernatural barnacles which have attached themselves through the centuries to the essential practice of yoga." Ironically, the book was being seen as dispelling the popular image of yoga as "a method to gain occult powers in order to attain union with the universal spirit"—although that was precisely what Theos was attempting. Consequently, many saw it as a reaffirmation of the demystified secular perspective, in which yoga produced "better health and the normal mental conditions that accompany such a state of well-being," with the end result being "an improved human mechanism for life in this world rather than a mysterious union with Brahma."[22] With *Hatha Yoga* receiving favorable reviews—even if from friends[23]—Theos contacted the London publisher of *Land of a Thousand Buddhas* and delivered his draft manuscript of *The Philosophical Foundations of India* to their New York offices.

With two women now, Theos's personal life was twice as complicated, if not more so. Having been taken by Theos as his new "consort" in tantric sexual practices, Helen expressed a certain amount of guilt and apprehension about the affair with Theos, who would secretly visit her in New York when Ganna was out of town. Her guilt often manifested in her dreams as anxiety that "Madame" would "find us," though Helen felt comfortable that at "the worst she would kick the B.F. out of her house." The secrecy, however, was taking its toll on Helen emotionally, and she began to reveal herself to be far less gullible and manipulable than many of the other women Theos had dealt with before.

Joining him for dinner one evening, Helen tried to get Theos to make some concrete plans for their relationship together, such as when he would break with Ganna Walska—and her money. Instead, she was disappointed by his evasive attitude. Remarking the next day on their conversation and "things that were left unsaid and which I read between the lines," Helen felt he had made it quite clear that

He was going to stick to his present situation and he certainly was never going to go to work for a piece of tail because in order to have that one had to support a woman and pretty soon that wore out and what did one have of lasting value? . . . I'm sure [Theos] has no idea that he conveyed those sentiments between the lines . . . he's fighting being carried away by his own sexuality. . . . Somehow I'm beginning to understand the male reaction but I don't understand what it is that he fears or sees.

Still, Helen couldn't help feeling that Theos would be interested in pursuing a more substantial relationship with her if she "could support him . . . even humbly which is his concession."

Tired of having to pander to Ganna's wishes and of their fights, Theos returned to California, explaining that since he had injured his knee while skiing, the weather there would help him heal quicker. Having been abandoned by Theos as well, Helen became depressed and decided that she "was unhappy about always having to be mother to men." Moving out of her apartment, she went to the West Coast to spend time with her family in Washington. With a change of scenery, Helen began to question the air of authority that Theos liked to project. He had ignored her since their last visit together in New York, and because she had received "no word since he left a month ago," she was beginning to have doubts about their relationship.

Maybe he knows what he is doing . . . and maybe he is just being selfish and spoiled. I don't know what is going on in his mind. I only know what is going on in mine and I don't like it. Somehow there is much too much libido tied up in this situation and I am not free. It looks like I shall always be socked in the jaw when it comes to getting affection and love and I might just as well never count on it or expect it from anyone . . . not even an ardent lover, in spots.

Just the same, Helen did have sympathy for him: "it's pretty tough on a guy who was born and raised to be a God . . . but literally." Although he was, he told her, "born at four A.M. which is the time Gods are born," whatever significance that may have held for Theos, for Helen it remained a weakness.

I also noted in last night's mood, a depreciation of D. and a great realization of his "weaknesses," his weakness of character . . . but I also realize that he can do nothing without having suffered the split in the Western Soul. But is he strong enough to overcome it? I wonder. He's pretty blind and opaque to this side of himself and on the other side he is a God.

Her conflicted emotions and thoughts aside, she was "getting to the point where I realize that I can't leave my thinking to others . . . there isn't anyone that bright that I have met."

Meanwhile Ganna, also unhappy about being abruptly abandoned, lashed out at Theos, telling him that she had never loved him. Attempting to assuage her feelings from afar, he initially was not very successful. In response, Ganna told him further,

> When I wrote to you that I never loved you I meant that I was never in love with you, as people would say: "she is crazy about him." I could not love anything ugly & from the beginning I could not have respect for your lying to me even when it was not necessary. But I thought you will get better in another atmosphere. And naturally I loved your beautiful soul that is part of the Universal Soul & can be only beautiful. But carefree atmosphere made you uglier & spoiled you completely, nothing counted but your fancy, your wishes, your self-indulgence & life with you was a *hell*!!! You wanted only servant or someone to talk with or mother who would listen to you. You used me as a servant secretary, between secretary, shop girl—everything, nurse, somebody to go to movies with because you do not like to go alone. . . . Small wonder that you do not like to be with yourself! Who would ? If I would have lived with an idiot or the great invalid or a child, I would have felt the same. Never myself, I could not express my views, my opinions without you being furious or mad so for all those years I kept all these thoughts and feelings to myself, unable to express my ideas to commune with an intellectual companion. I had to swallow all unjust criticism, all suspicion, all condemnation & never open my mouth, much less my heart, my soul in order not to contradict a madman, a great invalid, or a mentally sick person. This winter it was so bad that finally one drop was too much as past never will be again. No matter what happen in future I *never* will be your servant any more.

She continued for another sixteen pages, telling Theos what she thought of his selfishness and his inability to help or teach others, much less answer a simple question. It was his "demonical ego" that led to his jealousy and arrogance toward everybody, herself included, she declared. In short, she told him, "you walked on me, on my soul, on my heart as one walks on the invisible worm," and unless he spoke the truth to her from that point on, he would not see her again.

Writing her back, Theos attempted to plead his case in terms of his spiritual nature and greater purpose in life as a reincarnated Buddhist saint—though still with human failings—but Ganna was not buying it and unleashed another tirade on him.

In order to save yourself much misery in the future . . . you must try to see yourself in a real light & not as circumstances or flattery as my 5 years of spoiling make seem to you that you are but what *really* in actuality you are . . . if he was a saint & you are his reincarnation then why are you not a good man, but beastly animal? . . . You fool yourself that you are exceptional & nothing is ordinary about you, that all was predestination even your birth, your parents were chosen *highly spiritual* purposely to conceive the great soul. Judging by the result, it does not look *at all* plausible . . . because if you are a great old soul—it must be hidden so well that even you yourself cannot perceive it (after your own discouraging admittance) . . . if we want to be logical we have to admit that you are like thousands & thousands [of] other ordinary American boys who happen to read perhaps [too] early books which just as today's boys become detectives or bandits after seeing movies, you wanted to play—unfortunately not Budha [*sic*] right away because it was not so comfortable—but Milarepa because it excused your lack of heart. It encouraged your selfishness, your cruelty, having excuse that later, later when you would be old man (you told me this yourself) you will à la Milarepa become saintly.

Perhaps you omit one calculation in order that your plan would be fulfilled? Suppose you die at 40? What then?

Not about to let Theos play the spiritual master, she told him, "Milarepa didn't plan in advance, he was just bad until he saw better, but you know . . . *know* that you are bad—therefore you cannot—with *your knowledge*—escape the consequences—unless the Law you preach is not a *Law* & I believe it is!!"

Again she continued, for another eighteen pages, telling him that even though he preached Buddhist ideas, he lived his life in precisely the opposite way, and this was "the reason why people do not want to hear you."

It was a source of misery for her because despite her efforts on his behalf "it did not save you," and if she was miserable and crying, it was because she was "thinking how unhappy you are & will be still more without real friends, and a companion." While she still considered herself "his friend," Ganna was done trying to save Theos from himself, and absolved herself of his "spiritual suicide." Feeling that the situation was completely out of his control, Theos wrote and even telephoned Ganna to plead his case. After many words were exchanged, he felt that he had succeeded to a sufficient degree, but it would come at a price.

At almost the same time, Helen decided to come down to Santa Barbara for a visit, to get some clarity on their relationship. Spending time together once again, Theos and Helen enjoyed their time in the mountains and at the beach. Once she returned to Washington and she had time to reflect, however, she saw their relationship as problematic again. Her move from New York back home to Washington was an attempt to gain perspective on her life and her relationship with her father, and in general "to get my mental house in order." Theos was making things difficult since it seemed he was only "interested in sex." Following his tumultuous exchange with Ganna, Theos wrote to Helen, telling her that he had had a rapprochement of sorts with "the Madame" and the future was uncertain. Now it was time for Helen to get angry. As usual, her anger expressed itself in her dreams. The morning after receiving his letter, Helen was forced to deal with her conflicted emotions.

This is all the result of receiving a letter from D. saying that he was all fixed up again and happy with his missy . . . or words thereabouts. He still hoped he could get inspiration from the Fountain[24] but his work came first. So once again I am thrown back into my "insides" and now I shall have to work it out and work hard . . . circumstances have finally forced me to this and all the day-dreams have gone for nothing but I was happy and I know now that love does rest within myself. Just now I have the hurt rejected feeling again . . . but it's not out of control and I know that I have brought it on myself because I have something to learn.

Adding to her stress, however, was the fear that she had accidentally gotten pregnant by Theos, even though he was "a yogi . . . I thought who had control over his seed." Attributing her concern to larger irrational fears on her part, she decided to visit Theos in Los Angeles again. Arriving at the end of June, however, she was disheartened to find him gone—or at least inaccessible—which sent her into a fit of depression before becoming angry again. As a result, she was determined "to be able to go about my business without a spiritual guide because this guy is weak . . . and will not leave his mama . . . without being sure of another same to attach himself to."

Meanwhile Theos, having traveled north to UC Berkeley, had met with linguists there in an attempt to garner support for a new series of books that he and his father hoped to launch. Having decided to make the English translation of the Tibetan canon a reality, Theos pitched his ideas to faculty members and received a favorable response. Glen, meanwhile, had been making inquiries about facilities for typesetting Tibetan-script texts, contacting Horace Poleman at the Library of Congress as well as the Harvard-Yenching Library, and had located a publisher in Southern California, the J. F. Rowny Press, while Theos spent time with Ganna in Santa Barbara.

Once Ganna returned to New York, Theos and Glen assembled a few friends and close students and held the first meeting of the board of directors of the Tibetan Text Society of Santa Barbara.[25] Having gone through Sarat Chandra Das's and Herbert Hannah's Tibetan grammars—the same ones he had studied in Kalimpong, Gyantse, and Lhasa—together with Kroeber's Sino-Tibetan linguistics survey and others, Theos attempted to summarize the essential points of Tibetan grammar. The result of these efforts, a small pamphlet, *A Simplified Grammar of the Literary Tibetan Language*, would be the first publication of the Tibetan Text Society. Feeling that the peace he had negotiated with Ganna would not last long, Theos began taking steps to secure as many of his belongings as possible. Taking an illustration from one of his books,[26] he designed a bookplate stamp for himself and began stamping every book in his possession with it.

Within the month, Theos and Ganna began fighting again, mostly over money. Following the war, the costs of America's involvement in Europe and the Pacific had necessitated a revision of the tax codes, and Ganna was beginning to feel the financial pressure. Having managed throughout the war by taking out loans, she now found herself in a difficult financial situation. Theos, however, continued to maintain his lifestyle, traveling to San Francisco and making secret visits to Helen—and routinely passing the bills on to the managers of the California properties for them, and Ganna, to pay. As Ganna repeatedly reminded Theos that he would have to be responsible for his own bills, his disregarding her wishes and reneging on his promise to join her in New York was almost the most insulting thing he could do.

He had, in fact, just done something more insulting and humiliating to her: accidentally sending a letter intended for Helen—talking about his difficulties with "the Madame"—to Ganna herself. Intending the letter for Helen, Theos had written, "Cleomé is having Gateway send me those Sanskrit works of which I have spoken to complete my set. The Madame told me to have them ordered a couple of years ago; and then when Gateway found them, she refused to let me have them."

Writing of her own studies, Theos had given Helen an extensive reading list and said he was impressed by her ability to work through a substantial portion of it, though he encouraged her to put her questions on hold until they were in India.

When you are in India and there is free time so the mind can reflect clearly on these problems, it will be soon enough to go into detail. Until we can be together, do not be concerned about results, merely strive to charge the mind with all the available data; the insights and understanding will come later—such is the progress of growth from which there is no short-cut. . . . I will be with you again soon—always yours, Theos.

Ganna responded to Theos by returning the letter to him with her own comments. It was not the intimate nature of his words to Helen that hurt Ganna so much as his dismissal of Christmas. Referring to a book given to him by Helen, Theos had remarked,

Call that my birthday and Christmas gift—you know how much I dislike the material acknowledgment of those events. The birthday one cannot help, but I am certainly opposed to insulting my intelligence by recognizing the ignorant superstition of Christmas; especially in view of the fact, that I am devoting all the energies of my life to enriching the inner world of understanding.

Ganna wrote back to Theos:

You will get this on your birthday but I will not offend you by silly wishes knowing that all those years—contrary to all evidence you disliked any fuss about it. I still remember how every Xmas, Thanksgiving, etc. you almost cried when I tried to get out of it & last year I jumped on [the] excuse not to make Xmas dinner & free when Cody invited us to their house but you wanted *so much* to have that *at home* that I had no heart to deprive you of this pleasure. I did not know I was *insulting your intelligence*!!! I wanted to send you a little birthday present—naturally I cannot know your inner vibration by such superstition. On the other hand, as I cannot afford an expensive present, I do not want you to have good opportunity to write to your friends complaining on my meanness, stinginess as I do not suppose you told them that last year for your birthday & Xmas presents I sold my bracelets & earrings!

She continued,

It is a painful mistake that you made by putting my letter to "Helen's" or someone else envelope & mine to "Helen" or someone else. The only advantage of your secretive nature was the fact that you never spoke bad about me to others (also I thought you are the *only* one who *should* not have spoken badly on account of your behavior). I see that my good Karma wanted me to know that even in this I was mistaken.

Calming down slightly, Ganna reflected for a while and then continued:

Most painful of your mistake is the idea that *my* letter would be read by others who probably would laugh never believing that you could write *sincerely* "my dear one" or any beautiful thing you could have written to me. Normally they must think you are hypocrite [*sic*] with me and for purpose because & quite naturally they could not think you can have affection for someone about whom you speak & think of so badly, because, dear one, they *do not know* you as *you are*, as I *know* you!

Realizing the seriousness of his mistake, Theos and Glen discussed its implications for the future. With Ganna now painfully aware of his continued duplicitousness, they concluded that it would only be a matter of time before the financial (if not marital) ax fell.

Leasing a house in town, Theos and Glen began grabbing everything they could carry from the Tibetland estate and moving it all to the house for temporary storage while they decided what to do. They called another meeting of the Tibetan Text Society, worked up a formal mission statement, and filed articles of incorporation with the California Secretary of State. Contacting his California friends from over the years, Theos and Glen asked a number of them to be on the board of directors of their new society.

Telling Helen that he had decided to leave Ganna Walska, Theos offered her the choice of staying where she was or joining him on his return to India and Tibet. Helen was torn. It appeared that her life continually offered her a choice: "one either took that path of material security and boredom or the path of the spirit and love and non-security where one had to live dangerously." After thinking long and hard, in the end, Helen decided to join Theos. Telling her to wait for word from him, Theos went back to other matters at hand.

After receiving feedback on his *Philosophical Foundations* draft manuscript, which questioned the absence of any mention of Buddhism in a book on Indian philosophies, Theos informed his publisher that his next book would be a "complete analysis of this doctrine [Buddhism] and Karma." As a result, he received an official contract, and while making last-minute revisions to the manuscript, he dedicated the book to his father, now in the guise of "my teacher." With one book out of the way, Theos went back to work on finalizing his *Simplified Grammar of the Literary Tibetan Language* before sending it off to be published as well.

Hearing from Ganna that she was planning to come to Santa Barbara to visit for the first time since their last fight, Theos wrote and sent telegrams, telling her of his recent trips north and assuring her that if she would send him the specific details of her arrival, he would be waiting for her "regardless what hour." Unbeknownst to Ganna, however, having registered the names Tibetland and Santa Yñez Mountain Lodge (the new name for the Penthouse of the Gods), Theos and Glen were preparing for the biggest challenge of their lives: legally seizing control of the California properties from Ganna and being rid of her once and for all. After receiving the her itinerary, Theos sent a telegram to New York, telling her, "WE ARE ALL JOYOUS TO LEARN THAT YOU ARE ARRIVING ON THE 21ST. I WILL BE WAITING FOR YOU AT BURBANK."

When she arriving at the Burbank Airport in California, however, Ganna found not Theos but rather his lawyer, who "callously and publicly" served her a court summons. Shocked, embarrassed, and abandoned at the airport, Ganna was forced to take a taxi to the Tibetland estate, where her shock would only increase. In addition to reading in the papers she'd received that Theos was suing her not only for separate maintenance—alimony—but

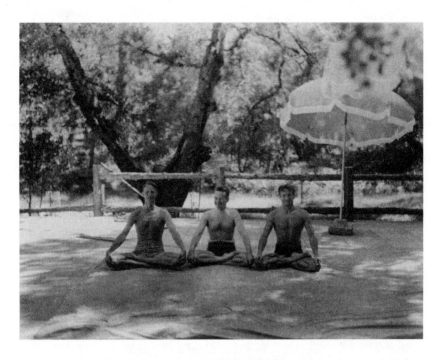

Figure 11.3 Bernard (right) giving "intensive and highly advanced spiritual meditations and exercises" poolside in Santa Barbara (BANC)

also for possession of the two estates, Tibetland and Penthouse of the Gods, she was dismayed to find that the houses at Tibetland had been stripped nearly bare and were little more than empty buildings. Making her way to the Penthouse, she discovered "Mr. LaVarnie"—Glen—living with Theos in the mountain lodge with "several years worth of provisions" stockpiled in the buildings. Telling Theos that she had no intention of providing him with separate maintenance, she vowed to do everything within her power to keep any more of her money from reaching him.

Ganna contacted her lawyers and prepared her deposition for the Santa Barbara County Court. Within days, reporters had heard the news, and it began to spread across the country: "Suit Discloses Fifth Ganna Walska Marriage," the *Los Angeles Times* headline read. Recounting that Theos in his suit "declares he is physically unable to support himself and recites that his wife is a person of wealth," the newspaper went on to list the succession of Ganna Walska's lucrative past marriages.[27] When depositions were heard a week later, Ganna's lawyers prepared to file a cross-complaint naming Glen as well, charging that he and Theos were using the estates purely for "materialistic enjoyment and pleasure" and not the occasional summer weekends of "intensive and highly advanced spiritual meditations and exercises" that Theos claimed. When the contents of the depositions were made public, newspapers around the country would have a field day.

Theos claimed that after years of living with Ganna Walska, he had been "spoiled by the life she provided him," and that in addition to having a rheumatic heart—he was certified 4-F by his physician, exempting him from service in the war, the newspapers pointed out—"he was no longer able to support himself." At the same time, he informed the court that Ganna had treated him "in a cruel and inhumane manner"—citing her letters to him from a year earlier—and that she "no longer loved him," wished him harm, and had threatened to defeat his lawsuit for the purpose of "embarrassing, hindering, and delaying the satisfaction or payment of any Order or Orders" that might come about as a result. Consequently, Theos asked not only for separate maintenance and legal fees but also that the court act swiftly to permanently restrain Ganna "from selling, transferring, conveying, encumbering, and disposing of, the properties, both real and personal . . . which the defendant now owns within the jurisdiction of this Court"—essentially fixing in perpetuity Ganna Walska's will, which still stipulated Theos's inheritance of both Santa Barbara properties.

With such claims, Theos became the new headline in newspapers across the country: "He Can't Work But He Stands on His Head For 3 Hours."[28] But it was Ganna Walska's countertestimony that sent the reporters—and undoubtedly more than a few readers—into fits of laughter. Ganna herself had a long litany of deceptions and charges to place at Theos's feet. Speaking with regard to "Theos Bernard," her lawyers made it clear that in addition to being the son of Glen Bernard, "sometimes known as La Varnie," Theos was "the nephew of Dr. Pierre Bernard, sometimes known as Ooom the Omnipotent." As for Theos's own claims, Ganna herself recounted them, one by one:

(1) That he, said Theos Bernard, was conceived and born into this world of parents specifically chosen as his worldly parents; and,

(2) That he, said Theos Bernard, was so conceived and born a white child into this world endowed with the power to become and be the spiritual savior of mankind.

(3) That he, said Theos Bernard, was in fact and truth the spiritual and physical reincarnation of Guru Rimpoche, also known as Padma Sambhava, an ancient Buddhistic Saint of Tibet; and,

(4) That he, said Theos Bernard, had occult powers giving him control over the mind and body of men and women and over the physical universe as well; and,

(5) That he, said Theos Bernard, was a great Yogi of rare and highly developed spirituality, a duly consecrated White Lama and the possessor of the esoteric knowledge and learning of the aforementioned Guru Rimpoche, the great Tibetan tantrik; and,

(6) That he, said Theos Bernard, was one with the Universal Consciousness of Life and as such the knower of ultimate truth; and,

(7) That he, said Theos Bernard, if assisted by this defendant [Ganna Walska], could and would use his powers and knowledge aforementioned to advance and perfect the spirituality of his own soul, of the soul of this defendant and of mankind in general.[29]

It was quite a résumé, and one that, when called to testify, Glen affirmed in its entirety!

Not to escape scrutiny himself, Glen was also targeted by Ganna and her lawyers. Asserting that Theos was engaged in "a planned concert of action"—aided and abetted by his father—she further claimed that Theos

consistently and deliberately, selfishly and with materialistic avarice . . . sought to gist and enrich himself by living off this defendant and coerce her by his display of a nasty and mean temper and by threats of force and violence and the exercise of the harmful powers of Kundalini, into providing him, the said Theos Bernard and his father, usually referred to by the said Theos Bernard as "Mr. La Varnie", with funds and luxuries far beyond their respective needs and requirements.

Maintaining that she had believed Theos based on his sincerity and her continued belief in "the Doctrines of Karma (Destiny) and Re-incarnation," she stated that only when she began to question his needs did Theos show a different side of his personality. As time progressed, she told the court, he had become insufferably rude, mean and insulting toward [her and] . . . in rage and fury at [her] insistence that the plaintiff [Theos] work and labor to advance his spirituality, that of this defendant and of mankind in general and in further rage and fury at this defendant's unwillingness to grant every monetary request and to satisfy every materialistic whim and wish of the plaintiff, has in demonaical frenzy and anger choked and well nigh strangled unto death this defendant.

Claiming that he repeatedly boasted of his yogic powers, Ganna revealed to the court that

Theos Bernard has threatened her with dire and awful consequences by his use and energies of the Power of Kundalini and with which said Power of Kundalini . . . [Theos] claims and has stated . . . that he, the plaintiff, said Theos Bernard, shook the City of Santa Barbara, California, and the aforementioned Tibetland estate of this defendant by the earthquake experienced in this City of Santa Barbara and at said Tibetland in June of the year 1941.

Trying every angle, Ganna accused Theos of every form of duplicity she could identify, even calling into question the legality of his first divorce, claiming that Viola had falsely established residency in Nevada solely for the sake of obtaining it. If she could prove this to be true—and consequently that Theos was still legally married to Viola—she could have their entire marriage annulled. Finally, stating for the record that Theos and Glen had ransacked the Tibetland estate, removed "art works, artifacts," and the entire library, and placed the articles "beyond the power" of Ganna to reclaim them, she asked the court to issue a restraining order against Theos and his father and sought to have them evicted from her properties immediately. This may have been a lot for the court to take in, but the court newspaper reporters swallowed it all with glee, and their stories rapidly made their way across the country.

Chicago readers learned about the "lurid tale of alleged deception by Bernard,"[30] Los Angeles headlines proclaimed "Ganna Walska Fights Mate's Support Suit," and in his hometown of Tucson, the papers read "'Buddhist Monk' Sued By Singer."[31] Agreeing to accept a "temporary alimony" of $1,500, Theos waited for the outcome of the court case, but when the time for the official hearing arrived, Ganna's lawyers were ready. They

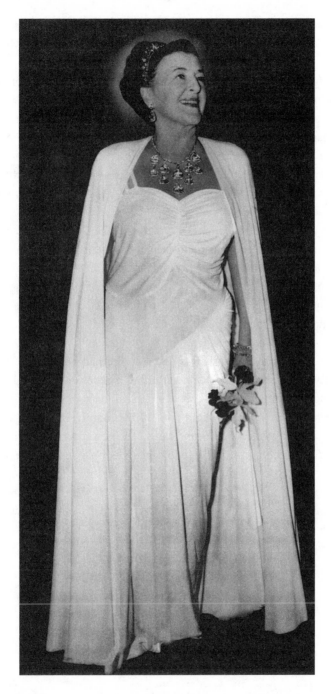

Figure 11.4 "Ganna Walska—free and wearing 'diamonds as big as pigeon eggs.'" (Patrick A. Burns/*The New York Times*/Redux)

questioned Theos about his "inability to support himself," and when he re-affirmed his poverty, Ganna's lawyers revealed to the court that Theos had failed to mention his $40,000 trust fund from Viola, as well as his Arizona mining rights and $5,000 in war bonds. Theos was found guilty of perjury, and his lawsuit was thrown out. Hurriedly refiling legal papers, Theos's lawyers repetitioned the court for a simple divorce with no maintenance—as proposed by Ganna. Ruling in favor of Ganna Walska, given the impossibility of sorting out each other's possessions, the judge ruled simply that "all property whatsoever" in the name or possession of each party should remain as such, and gave Theos and Glen four days to vacate the mountain estate.

There was little that Glen and Theos could do. They had succeeded in securing all of Theos's books, manuscripts, and assorted art and ephemera long before by placing them in an undisclosed storage locker in Los Angeles, but they had little more to show for their efforts. Renting a small apartment for Glen, Theos contacted Helen, trying to put the best spin on things and telling her that his relationship with "the Madame" was finally over and now they could be together.

Ganna Walska, in contrast, was ecstatic. She had been faced with the possibility of massive financial obligations and losses, but through Theos's own bungled conniving, she had been released from any obligation to him, for the comparatively slight cost of one month's alimony and legal expenses. Ganna Walska had been "freed," the newspapers declared,[32] and she decided to celebrate that freedom in style, once again attending the season's opening performance at the Met, wearing "diamonds as big as pigeon's eggs, 10 at her throat and two dangling from her ears."[33] But while Ganna was celebrating her successful divorce, Theos and Helen were preparing for their first big adventure together: Theos's return to India and Tibet.

TWELVE

To Climb the Highest Mountains

The Himalayas . . . the great saints and sages of India, her seers and seekers after truth have been, from immemorial times associated with this mountain range and, even in these days of gathering unbelief and sordid endeavor, men are occasionally to be met, who, after brilliant achievements at Oxford, Cambridge or Harvard and successful careers thereafter, turn to the Himalayas, in their moments of introspection, with thoughts of relief and retirement, to seek on its snowy plateaus the peace and contentment, which no other refuge can supply.

—M. R. JAYAKAR[1]

BEFORE THE JOURNALISTIC DUST had even settled in California,[2] Theos and Helen were in New York. In early August 1946, Theos and Helen were rapidly attending to the various details associated with a trip to India, from purchasing camera equipment and getting vaccinations to insuring the new equipment. Getting new portrait photos of themselves taken professionally for their visa applications and Helen's new passport, they made a point of having enlargements made as "publicity shots" in anticipation of Theos's return, sending copies to Glen.

Earlier, Theos had contacted Dagobert Runes, an editor at the Philosophical Publishing House, telling him that he was embarking on a trip to India and pitching the idea for a book to be called *Twentieth Century India*, a survey of the current state of knowledge in various fields in the subcontinent. Given the approval to proceed, Theos had his father send him a detailed list of contacts in India who could serve as potential contributors to such a volume, while Runes provided Theos with a letter of introduction presenting him as "a member of our editorial staff . . . leaving for India on our behalf" with even letters addressed specifically to Gandhi and Nehru.

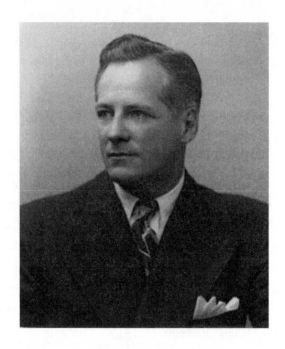

Figure 12.1 Bernard's visa photo, August 1946 (HGPF)

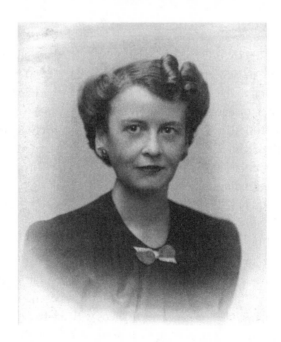

Figure 12.2 Helen Park's visa photo, August 1946 (HGPF)

Outfitting themselves with the latest travel clothing, Theos and Helen packed the bulk of their belongings into trunks and had them shipped on ahead. Seeing to last-minute details, Theos visited his bank and investment firm in New York, giving his father full power of attorney over his finances, and a lawyer, drafting a new will that left everything to Glen.[3] He even took time out to have dinner with DeVries and her sister, Franci, and to pay a quick visit to Viola.

With the war only recently over, however, many families were trying to reunite, and ships and planes were booked solid. Although they were wait-listed on five different ships, they were told it could be months before they could get passage. Having maintained friendly relations with her ex-husband's business partner, C. V. Starr, Helen arranged for both Theos and herself to claim affiliation with Starr's U.S. Life Insurance Company by taking a commission to redecorate Starr's personal home in Hong Kong the following March while Theos went to Lhasa. Having had one flight canceled on them already, through the company's influence, Theos and Helen managed to secure another and by the end of September were en route to Bombay.

Following up on Glen's list of contacts for the book, Theos and Helen spent the better part of a month in Bombay before proceeding to Delhi, where Theos received permission to see both Nehru and Gandhi. But both meetings were less than productive. Nehru told Theos that he was far too busy to write an article for a book, and Gandhi told him that he was an old man and had "written his last"; he wished only "to withdraw from the world, but must do what circumstances demand" in regard to the ongoing struggle for Indian independence. Nonetheless, Gandhi offered Theos the freedom to take whatever he liked from his previous writings for the anthology. Theos had to console himself that "it was enough that [he] was able to manage interviews, realizing that [he was] actually arriving at what is probably the most critical time in the history of the career of both these men." From there, Theos and Helen continued their journey across India. They toyed with the idea of an extended stay at Rishikesh so Helen could learn yoga, "especially if she is going to help run a school for Yoga in the U.S." Instead, thinking something better might come along, they decided to continue on to Sikkim, and so returned south and east toward Calcutta. When they arrived, however, the city was still reeling from the aftermath of the riots only three months earlier.

Over the course of three and a half centuries, since the arrival of the first merchant ship in 1608, India had slowly been incorporated into the British

Empire. But for the previous half century forces had been mustering in order to reverse that tide of history. Although initially confined to the intellectual class of Western-educated Brahmins, for more than twenty years the Indian independence movement had been gathering popular support. But the movement was far from unified. Factions had formed an uneasy alliance in the face of a common foe, but as success loomed closer and closer, that cooperation was beginning to break down. The biggest split fell along religious lines: Hindu versus Muslim. The de facto leader of the Muslim faction was Mohammed Ali Jinnah, inspired by Rahmat Ali, who, in 1933, had put forth the idea of an independent Muslim state to be carved out of British India, a state called Pakistan, meaning the "land of the pure."

Committed to bringing about this vision at all costs, Jinnah had proclaimed the previous August 16th, 1946, to be "Direct Action Day," a day on which the Muslim populace of India would make their presence felt. Consequently, while Theos and Helen were in New York getting more vaccinations to protect themselves from India's smallest inhabitants, the human populations of several major cities in India were actively trying to kill each other. Within twenty-four hours the streets of Calcutta were littered with corpses—both Hindu and Muslim. It was an ill foreshadowing of things to come.

Making their way through the city in late December, Theos and Helen stopped to have their horoscopes drawn: 1947, they were told, would be "a great year." Proceeding northward to the Himalayan hill station of Kalimpong, the two settled into a small suite of rooms at the Cawnpore House. Theos found many familiar faces in Kalimpong, and even some of his old possessions, which had lagged behind on his return from Tibet and been held for him by Frank Perry.[4] David Macdonald and his family were still running the Himalayan Hotel. Tharchin was still busily at work on multiple ventures and publishing his newspaper, and even had a large contingent of employees. Twan Yang, who had been Johan van Manen's manservant when Theos and Glen visited them ten years earlier in 1936, was now working for Tharchin in Kalimpong. With him were several others, including a strange Mongolian monk named Dawa Sangpo.[5]

Some members of the aristocratic families, having seen trouble ahead for Tibet since the first Chinese invasion of 1909, had begun to divest their wealth and move their holdings out of the country. Some went to Bhutan and Sikkim, others to India. The Tsarong family had made their home in

Kalimpong, and Theos finally had the opportunity to meet Lord Tsarong's son, Dundul Namgyal, who had been in school in Darjeeling the summer Theos stayed with his parents in Lhasa.

But one man was missing, the main object of Theos's return to Kalimpong: Gedun Chöpel. Unbeknownst to Theos, much had transpired in his ten-year absence from India. Over the course of several years in the Kulu Valley with George Roerich, Gedun Chöpel had dictated a translation of the massive historical work on the history of Tibet by Gö Lotsawa called *The Blue Annals*, which Roerich transcribed in his notebooks. But following this undertaking, Gedun Chöpel had little to show for his efforts. He had been living in Kalimpong, but ten months earlier—just as Theos and Helen were committing to a trip to India—had decided to return to Tibet.

During his time in Kalimpong, Gedun Chöpel had befriended some of the town's more ambitious Tibetan expatriate residents. One of the founding members of the Tibetan Revolutionary Party, Pangdatsang Rabga—one of the younger, disaffected sons of the wool merchants Theos had met in Kalimpong in 1937—convinced Gedun Chöpel to "travel through Bhutan and Tawang to Tibet . . . drawing maps of the country,"[6] much as Sarat Chandra Das had done seventy-five years earlier.

Arriving in Lhasa in early January 1946, a few weeks before Heinrich Harrer and Peter Aufschnaiter,[7] Gedun Chöpel did not make the maps he had been asked to create, but nonetheless, six months later he was arrested and imprisoned as a political subversive in the wave of hysteria gripping the Tibetan plateau, as many in the central government saw the threats to their autonomy—real and imagined—closing in fast all around them.

Writing to his father back in California, Theos told him how "the chap we were bring to America" had returned to Tibet and was now "in Prison in Lhasa and will probably remain there as far as I know." It was a terrible situation, in fact, for both Gedun Chöpel and Theos, as he was well aware.

Our former contact, the Geshe we met at Jinorasa's has been placed in the dungeon in Lhasa for life, being taken out and thrashed every so often. As far as I can gather it is because of some sort of political ideology that he seems to be promulgating as the result of his association with Rahula [Sānkṛtyāyana]. . . . It is interesting to reflect on the workings of fate in this case, for had the Geshe come to us in America as we had planned, he would not be where he is now—and I probably wouldn't be as I am.

But luckily for Theos, Geshe Wangyal was living in Kalimpong again. Geshe Wangyal remembered all too well what had happened to his homeland when the Soviets invaded in 1921. Indeed, even as he was sitting in England with Marco Pallis in 1937, Stalin was on a mission to purge the Soviet Union of any and all he considered undesirable. Geshe Wangyal's teacher, Agwan Dorjiev, had been arrested and interrogated as a leader of "the counter-revolutionary Pan-Mongolian insurrectionary terrorist organization, the ultimate aim of which was the overthrow of the Soviet people"; he would die in prison. At the same time, all across Russia his promising students, Sergey Oldenburg, Eugene Obermiller, Andrey Vostrikov, and others, having established identities as Buddhist lamas or scholars, were being rounded up and imprisoned. Accused of similar "political crimes," they would be tried, convicted, and shot all on the same day.[8]

Seeing the Communists gaining ground in China and eagerly eyeing Tibet, Geshe Wangyal had tried to warn those around him. But his concerns went unheeded, for the most part. "Don't worry," he was told, "we know how to deal with the Chinese." But these were *not* the same Chinese that the Tibetans were used to dealing with—these were Communists, he tried to explain, but few would listen. The fate of Tibet was being written on the wall and although Geshe Wangyal could see it, he soon realized he could only save himself. He left Lhasa and headed south to India again, where he settled, for the time being, in Kalimpong.

Telling his father that Geshe Wangyal was still there and had agreed to work with them, Theos and Helen began their study of Tibetan anew. Theos immediately expressed his desire to study the Tibetan texts on tantra and in particular, Tsong-kha-pa's mammoth esoteric treatise, *The Great Exposition of the Stages of Secret Mantra*. Geshe Wangyal, no doubt amused, told Theos that before he could study tantra, he would first have to study *sūtra*, and instructed him to first translate the topical outline to Tsong-kha-pa's exoteric masterpiece, *The Great Exposition of the Stages of the Path to Enlightenment*, which he did.

Not to be dissuaded from his goal, with Helen as fellow student and assistant, Theos acquiesced to his teacher's instructions and with his guidance, began to translate and compile vocabulary lists on the introductory texts. Over the months that followed, Theos prevailed upon the young geshe to help him move along toward the study of tantra. From their conversations, however, it was clear that Theos did not even understand the simplest foundations of the *sūtra*-based presentation of the Path to Enlightenment, such as the "Wheel of Life," so Geshe Wangyal began by explaining the three poisons of desire, hatred, and ignorance, and the workings of karma. Jokingly, Theos asked him what he would do if he found himself reborn as "a Christian in the next life thereby making it extremely difficult for his mind to awaken to its rightful state." Relating the geshe's response to his father, Theos recounted,

> He said, without hesitation, that he could never be born a Christian. Such a thing was absolutely impossible according to the laws that govern the birth of an individual. Only an undeveloped mind could ever be born in a Christian world with the single exception [of] a mind that had not only been enlightened but also had a disposition toward teaching and leading others toward the doctrine of the dharma, and this disposition he did not have in this lifetime.

Eager for philosophical discussions, Theos quizzed Geshe Wangyal about a wide variety of subjects, asking him to confirm what he and his father had discovered on their own. Setting Theos straight on the basic structure of the "Wheel of Life," Geshe Wangyal told him that the subtle body *cakra*s played no role, nor did "various astrological conditions," contrary to Glen's imagining. Indeed, Geshe Wangyal was often perplexed by some of Theos's notions about religion and religious practice and could not "figure out how one ever learned ideas like the ones [Theos] put forth" and as were found "in the West."

Helen also took advantage of the opportunity to study with Geshe Wangyal. In addition to learning the Tibetan script, she asked him for his opinions of her own ideas, such as her belief concerning the import of her dreams. Geshe Wangyal bluntly told her that "dreams were so much nonsense and made no sense unless one got to the point where one could control one's dreams as advanced Yogis could." Disheartened, Helen recorded her last dream that February and would not record another for twenty-six years.

Despite Geshe Wangyal's brusque Mongolian nature, Theos and Helen were both duly impressed by the man, feeling that they were "very unlikely to ever contact anyone who will ever have a better grasp of the subject." Nonetheless, Theos found studying with Geshe Wangyal to be frustrating at times, sometimes feeling that he "must eventually get [himself] another Geshe." This was not because Geshe Wangyal was overly serious about their studies; if anything, the exact opposite. Geshe Wangyal, Theos said, thought

> it is more fun enjoying life than worrying about all these intellectual problems—especially after one knows the fuller working of the entire scheme of problems as this one does from the philosophical angle—I can see his point and probably when I am as only as he and have covered the field and finished my writing I will meet the enthusiastic enquiries of a beginner with about the same sort of solicitude.

Beyond his studies, however, Theos still hoped for the sort of adventure that would make a splash in the American papers upon his return, since one magazine had already promised him "$700 to $1200 [for] an article illustrated with color photographs." So one of the first things he did upon his arrival in Kalimpong was to send a large number of telegrams to Lhasa and—as he had done ten years earlier—get Tharchin to print an extensive article on the front page of his newspaper, recounting his adventures with Theos in Tibet and spreading the word of Theos's return to Kalimpong and his desire to visit Lhasa in time for the New Year's (Mön-lam) festival.[9] Laying the foundation, as he had done before, Theos petitioned the British Residency in Gangtok for a travel permit to Tibet. But this time no amount of cajoling would convince the British authorities to allow Theos past their checkpoints for travel to Lhasa, while in Lhasa itself, Hugh Richardson advised the Tibetan government against granting his request.

In February, Theos was given "the final verdict on the trip to Lhasa," with the British authorities citing the current political situation as their excuse.[10] Hoping to bypass them and possibly go to western Tibet instead, Theos sent a request to Kathmandu asking the Nepalese authorities for a permit to enter Tibet. But, suspecting that Theos might try this, the British authorities had already contacted the Nepal government and advised them of their opinion of Theos; consequently, that request was rejected as well. Theos appeared to be stuck in Kalimpong.

Instead, Theos and Helen decided to make the best of the situation. Theos convinced Helen to postpone her trip to Hong Kong and remain in India to help him "dream over the various avenues of approach" that he and Glen could pursue to start their school back in America. Theos told his father he was "sure that she is the one I have been looking for in order to further these other ambitions." By the time of their return, he thought, one of DeVries's students, Clara Spring, would have finished her book on yoga and the four of them "should be able to start something there on the Coast." Having talked with Geshe Wangyal about his education, Theos felt that "something along the line of the training of the Lamas at Drepung monastery" would be the ideal model for a Tibetan studies school in either "Beverly Hills or Hollywood." In the meantime, he would "devote [his] energies to getting the material and organizing it." Indeed, he was quite hopeful, given the popularity in America of things Tibetan, because "it seems something along the Tibetan line will have the necessary religious or rather emotional appeal, while sticking to the philosophy will give it the needed strength to enable it to endure." To that end, Theos decided that it was most likely preferable to restrict attendance to yoga classes. Geshe Wangyal advise him that basic "stages of the path" teachings were suitable for all, but Theos was now of the opinion that "Yoga and the like should be used only for those special students who are serious and willing to settle down to the sort of routine and discipline that it requires."

From his time studying under Geshe Wangyal, Theos's command of the Tibetan language was improving, and by mid-March he was overjoyed at having "translated a small work . . . on the Sipa Khorlo"—an excerpt from Tsong-kha-pa's *Great Exposition*—"and this I have done all by myself," he proudly declared to his father. Giving Theos a portion of a "stages of the path" text that "Tharchin happened to have," Geshe Wangyal,

> after reading it over hurriedly to me left it and told me to do it myself otherwise it would be of no value. If he did it, I would never learn; so I buckled down and finally waded through it. For the most part I got everything all right; but it was a lot of sweat. . . . I went through it alone and it did not make too much sense; then Geshe gave me a rule which he pointed out that they all had to learn and without which no one could understand the writings of any of their literature—that is philosophical literature; so with this rule I went back over and everything fell into entirely different categories and began to make much more sense.

The problem, Geshe Wangyal explained to Theos, was that "in the last analysis all of their literature is talking about one and the same thing, and the confusion of the outsider is that because there are so many different books talking about what seems to be so many different subjects, they are never able to get the pattern straight." For the first time, Theos was beginning to feel humbled in his knowledge compared to his teacher's, and although he felt slightly annoyed at the geshe's low opinion of Indians and Westerners, Theos had to admit that the Tibetan Buddhists "have a fairly accurate estimate of human nature and have all mankind divided up into a few simple types of mind," with a clear estimate of "what kinds of knowledge . . . should be given to each type."

Around the same time, Theos received word from Tharchin that a "high lama" had come down from Lhasa and was going to be giving teachings on Tsong-kha-pa's *Great Exposition* at the nearby monastery of Tharpa Chöling. When Lord Tsarong had heard from his son that Theos was back in Kalimpong, he asked his good friend Dardo Rinpoche[11] to invite Theos to attend the proceedings so that he could receive both the oral and explanatory transmissions, a process that would run from noon to 6 p.m. every day for a month. It was quite an experience for Theos to attend and be accompanied by Geshe Wangyal, who sat next to him to help him with the chanting. Thoroughly enjoying the experience, Theos found the daily teachings an inspiration to persevere in his studies, memorizing vocabulary since "already I can hear endless things he is saying, but I do not have enough of the connective tissue to be able to follow the ideas in their continuity." During the occasion tea breaks, Theos was able to ask Geshe Wangyal to summarize what had been said since "they do not go so fast that we can't keep up in this way" and Geshe Wangyal had "the work virtually memorized."

Still, while the *Great Exposition* teachings would help Theos understand the fundamentals of Buddhism, he would never master the philosophy unless he understood the basics of logical reasoning. For months, Theos had asked Tharchin to do his best to find him a copy of the text Geshe Wangyal recommended, Pur-bu-jok's *Collected Topics*, an introductory textbook on epistemology, logic, and reasoning. When one of the geshes working for Tharchin managed to locate a copy for Theos, he ran to see Geshe Wangyal the next day to tell him the good news, only to learn that his teacher was leaving town. Geshe Wangyal told him that under ordinary circumstances they would be able to read through the entire text in a couple of months, but without help, Theos would find it impossible to comprehend.

Disheartened, Theos decided to try to read it on his own, hoping he could occasionally ask Tharchin's geshe for help even though the man spoke no English. Although he made his best effort, it was a rough experience for Theos. Starting to translate the work by trying to crib from Vidyabhusana's English translation of Dharmakīrti's *Drop of Reasoning*,[12] Theos soon realized that his Buddhist "Nyaya" text was "the hardest [thing] I have ever tackled and probably the hardest I will work on again" since "there is nothing in the dictionary to help."[13]

Determined to pursue his own interests in addition to Geshe Wangyal's recommendations, Theos asked Lord Tsarong's son George to help him locate more books for him, including more works on the twelve links of dependent origination, the bardo, and yoga. Theos told him that he was "interested in everything that pertains to the control and discipline of the breath and also the various physical exercises that are used for the control and discipline of the body." In the meantime, he continued to try to work his way through Pur-bu-jok's primer without Geshe Wangyal, and even took a stab at retranslating a section of the *Tibetan Book of the Dead*, which Evans-Wentz had already translated and published.

Shipping books back to America as he acquired them to be put in storage until his return, Theos was constantly receiving mail as well. In addition to the letters he continued to receive from his family and even DeVries, one day Theos received a package from the Rowny Press: his *Simplified Grammar* was finally out. After an intense few months of study with Geshe Wangyal, however, Theos was surprised by his own reaction upon seeing his grammar book: it "attempts to outline the structure of the language and this it does with considerable clarity, in fact, it is most deceiving, for it would lead one to feel that after reading that analysis, one could set right to work and read any text by merely looking up the words in the dictionary . . . and this is far from the truth." As an example, he told his father, after three months of steady work on Pur-bu-jok's primer, though he knew most of the words, he still lacked "the vaguest notion what it is all about except that they are arguing about whether or not apples exist or do not exist etc." It was clear that he would need to do more language training.

While the grammar was far from ideal, as far as his scholarly career was concerned, it was still a worthwhile publication, though none of his studies, he admitted, would contribute to the larger concern of making another public relations splash upon his return. Without a trip to Tibet, any fame he managed to garner would be minimal at best. Hoping at the very least to obtain some otherwise rare manuscripts, Theos began experimenting with photographing books and confirming the camera settings necessary to ensure their legibility.

Through informal channels, Theos learned that as he suspected, it had been the British authorities who had squashed his application for a visa. He realized that "so long as they have any influence, [he] might as well figure [his] chances are out," but with the announcement of Indian independence, Theos was confident that they would soon be out of his way. However, it was clear that the solution would not be ideal, as factions comprising the authorities who would replace them were already choosing sides. Guru Golwalkar, the leader of the Rashtriya Swayamsevak Sangh (RSS), a right-wing Hindu nationalist movement, declared defiantly before the announcement had even been made that they would oppose partition of the country into India and Pakistan, while on the other side, Jinnah and the Muslim League remained determined that Pakistan would become a reality. As Jinnah informed Lord Mountbatten, the last Viceroy of India, the idea of a unified India was little more than a fiction, since "the only thing the Moslem has in common with the Hindu is his slavery to the British."[14]

Even in Kalimpong, Theos and Helen felt they might not be immune from trouble as rumors spread throughout the hills.

> Here in town guns are being smuggled through to Lhasa, Kham, Bhutan, and Sikkim. The idea is that Bhutan is going to take over Kalimpong and on down to Siliguri, and Sikkim is going to take Darjeeling by the force of arms if need be before India gains its independence and the British move out. Anyway the bazaar is a bee-hive of talk and we see various moves by people which are indicative; so apparently it is just as well that I am not in Lhasa at this time.

On a personal level as well, things were proving less than satisfactory. Although it was an unusually dry summer, the summer months in Kalimpong meant monsoons, and by the middle of July, both Theos and Helen were suffering from diarrhea and dysentery and losing weight. Despite taking all the prescribed doses of ayurvedic medicines, neither saw any improvement, so they decided to simply vacate Kalimpong and resume their travels with the hope of eventually relocating to the paradisaical "vale of Kaśmir."

Informing his father of this, Theos wrote that there was "no way to calculate our plans, but if all goes well we should be in Europe until the end of 1948, returning to New York toward the very end." When Theos told Geshe Wangyal, who had returned to Kalimpong, that they were leaving for Kashmir and western Tibet, Geshe Wangyal advised against it, saying that such a trip would be too dangerous and that he should simply stay in Kalimpong. But this was not something Theos was willing to do, so he continued his preparations for travel to the northwest.

Theos wrote a letter to Nicholas Roerich in the Kulu Valley, expressing his disappointment at not having met him in 1937 and saying that he anticipated visiting Kulu soon and would like to meet him. Theos then approached Dawa Sangpo—later discovered to be a Japanese spy who had been[15] maintaining his disguise as a Mongolian monk working for Tharchin—and asked if he would accompany him as a guide to Ladakh and western Tibet. This was appealing to Kimura, who felt that such a trip could be beneficial for him, but Tharchin vetoed the idea, telling Kimura he had "other things in mind" for him, namely espionage for the British.

Instead, Tharchin sent one of his employees, Dorje Senge—a monk from Kalimpong who had never been to Calcutta, much less Kashmir—to serve as Theos's guide. Setting his plans in motion, Theos reserved a "first-class coupe" for himself and Helen on the Darjeeling Mail leaving for Calcutta at the end of the month (and third-class accommodations for Senge), and had his travel agent in Calcutta draft an itinerary for them, hoping to be in Kashmir by the 10th of August. Resting at a friend's house in Calcutta, Theos and Helen withdrew 5,000 rupees from their bank account before boarding their train for Delhi a week later. But with the announcement of the pending partition of Britain's "Jewel in the Crown" into two separate countries, India and Pakistan, the great migration of Hindus, Sikhs, and Muslims had begun. As a result, Helen's "Trip to Paradise" proved problematic within the first few days. Having reached Amritsar, the trains running north and west were stalled, overburdened with passengers; just the same, Helen and Theos headed toward Kashmir full of optimism.

It was August 9, 1947, and they had little suspicion that this would be "the last day of peace on the plains of the Punjab." For, hundreds of miles to the south, Sir Cyril Radcliffe sat in a government office in New Delhi. Having been charged by the Lord Chancellor, Viscount Jowitt, with drawing the boundary lines between the two new countries of India and Pakistan, Radcliffe was at a loss what to do. Having just arrived in India for the first time in his life, the ex-barrister had never had the chance to visit the Punjab and indeed, had only seen a detailed map of the region for the first time weeks earlier. Nonetheless, he was ordered to partition 175,000 square miles and 88 million people, with no knowledge of the landscape beyond what he could discern from a surveyor's map. His efforts would have vast and long-lasting repercussions for the world, the subcontinent, and Theos and Helen in particular.

Arriving in Pathankot at midnight, Theos, Helen, and Senge had to wait at the station until 4 a.m., when their connecting train arrived. Passing through Kangra and changing trains, they finally arrived, in the rain, at Jogindernagar. Negotiating truck transport, first to Mandi and then up the Kulu Valley, along sheer cliff-edge one-way roads that Theos likened to "the canyon going up to Taos," they arrived in Kulu at the Mayflower Hotel as recommended by the Roerichs, only to discover that it had been years since the hotel had served Western guests; now it was for Sikhs only. Following the manager's recommendation, they continued up the valley to the small village of Katrain, where an old dak bungalow was being run by a British couple as a guest house: Tyson's Riverview Hotel. After a long day riding in a truck and an unceremonious "here" as their driver exhausted the bulk of his English vocabulary, Theos, Helen, and Senge (along with their twenty-five pieces of luggage) were deposited at a small cluster of buildings at the river's edge by the side of the road.

Theos wrote to his father,

> Having taken a through train all was well until our destination at Amritsar and from the moment we arrived in Kulu I was never certain we would ever make it. You should have seen us with baggage stacked up like cord wood standing in the station surrounded by teeming hundreds—perhaps thousands—of refugees running from what was to be Pakistan to Hindhustan—and vice versa. The Sikhs, of course, all carrying those long sabers—three feet or more long. It was a rather dangerous place to be for no small amount of rioting has and is going on there and on numerous occasions they have been dragging people out of the trains and beheading them right there at the station. . . . They have police all over, but they would be of little avail in the event of real trouble. One never sees British police anymore and you know what the others are like.

Recovering from their journey, Theos and Helen settled into the relaxed life of the privileged classes in the last days of the British Raj. With three days to go before India received her independence, the valleys and plains were host to an endless stream of farewell parties, and the Kulu Valley was

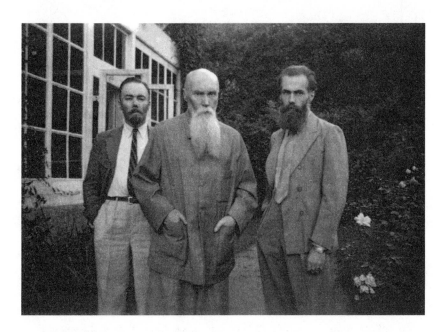

Figure 12.3 The Roerichs in Kulu (courtesy of the Nicholas Roerich Museum, New York)

no exception. Arriving just in time for a party, they heard that the local British "D.C." (district commissioner) was leaving, saying good-bye to his Indian post for the last time, and so attended the festivities. Sending "a chit"[16] to the Roerichs in Naggar and receiving a chit in return, the next day Theos and Helen hired a car for a short day trip, up and over to the other side of the valley to Naggar, where the Roerichs had established their research foundation. Where only two years earlier, Gedun Chöpel had sat beside George Roerich translating the *Blue Annals*,[17] Theos now sat discussing Himalayan research with Nicholas Roerich and his sons.

The patriarch of the family, Nicholas Roerich had established a reputation in Russia, America, and India. A painter, scholar, and mystic, he had run a research institute in New York out of the Master Building on Riverside Drive, just a few blocks from Columbia University. With his wife, Helena, Roerich had advocated an interpretation of Buddhist sources that bore a closer resemblance to Theosophy than to any orthodox form of Buddhism; just the same, it had attracted many adherents, from artists and writers to government officials and political candidates. Following financial troubles in the late 1930s, the family had packed up their belongings and moved to the Kulu Valley in northwest India. When Theos arrived at the mountaintop estate looking out over the Kulu Valley and Beas River below, Nicholas Roerich was nearing the end of his life.

Telling the Roerichs of his hope of locating rare manuscripts at his primary goal, Hemis Monastery in Ladakh, Theos quizzed them about possible leads to follow in the nearby Spiti Valley. They had a number of recommendations. Indeed, Nicholas Roerich had published an article some years earlier on this very subject. Recalling his travels through Khotan along the Silk Road, Roerich wrote:

> On the mountain trails to Khotan we saw several caves which once served as retreats for Buddhist anchorites. Their dark entrances opened on perpendicular cliffs so that there was no access to them. Earthquakes or landslides have obliterated all approach so that these secret hermitages are now suspended in air, sharing their mysteries with the eagles and vultures. To reach them from the heights above would be a very complicated undertaking. . . . The approaches have crumbled away and the lower levels have been filled up. When you walk through the upper caves you gather from the hollow sound that there must be other compartments beneath. . . . It is fascinating to tap the walls and floor and speculate about hidden retreats. There are probably whole libraries yet to be discovered.

Writing about similar research potential within the Lahoul and Spiti valleys, he claimed, "Here in the Kulu Valley are said to be hidden some very ancient manuscripts. . . . What lucky 'chance' may lead to their discovery? According to the accounts of Chinese travelers there were once fourteen monasteries in this valley. Where are they to-day?"[18]

This was precisely what Theos was looking for: a single rare manuscript, if not an entire cache of texts, thousands of years old. If he could return to America as the discoverer of a "second Tun-huang," his reputation would be secured.

Roerich recommended heading north and east, over the Rohtang Pass into Lahoul and Spiti. A valley in the farthest reaches of western Tibet—not so far from Tharchin's birthplace, Khunu, south of the Spiti Valley—this was where the great translator of the eleventh century, Rin-chen-sang-po, had established a series of monasteries. The most famous of them, Ta-bo, had been studied by Tucci and Francke some years earlier, so in Roerich's opinion, the hilltop monastery of Ki, the next largest in the valley, offered the best chance for success.

Returning to Katrain, Theos immediately sent a telegram to the Kangra District Commissioner in Dharamsala, prepaying for a response:

FOR THE PURPOSE OF RESEARCH STUDIES OF TIBETAN LITERATURE I WOULD LIKE TO VISIT THE KI MONASTERY AND THEN PROCEED ON TO LEH LADAKH WILL YOU KINDLY GRANT ME PERMISSION TO CROSS THE INNER LINE.

DR. THEOS BERNARD, TYSON HOTEL, KATRAIN.

Since receiving a permit would probably take a couple of weeks or more and it would be a difficult journey to Ki Monastery, it would be best for him to go there alone, he argued to Helen, and only take Senge as his guide and a few porters. By the time of his return, they should have received their Inner Line permits and could head to Ladakh together.

In the Kulu Valley, as the day of Indian independence approached, there was little evidence that anything had changed, nor any reason to think anything would. Tea parties continued, and even the local Muslim butcher, Golam Mohammed, had been relaxing, rehearsing for his performance in a short play from the *Ramāyana* scheduled for that night.

Discussing the trip to Spiti with Senge, Theos compiled a list of necessary supplies and arranged for Senge to go down to the town of Kulu the next day to begin purchasing them while he, Theos, began assembling his own equipment. Just another research day for Theos, the fifteenth of August was a momentous one in world history, for that evening all across the Indian subcontinent the Union Jack flag was lowered for the last time and the sun finally set on the British Empire.

Attending the play being put on in town, Theos and Helen sat at the back of the makeshift theater with their new friends, the Banons, the Tysons, and Vicky Noon. The festivities were a welcome relief from the past week's adventure and an opportunity to socialize and talk about their own research there in the valley and the role Buddhist philosophy played in their lives. Still, despite all the reverie, there was a palpable tension in the air. The festivities, Theos told his father,

lasted to well past midnight and after that I suppose the villagers had their other forms of amusement for such celebrations. And so Helen and

I saw the birth of a new India—we will probably not feel the impact of this change until we begin to move about a bit again on the plains when we will have to travel from Hindustan to Pakistan and vise versa and thereby encounter the new order of things. Actually, I would prefer being here than anyplace I can think of for tension is high throughout the land and I prefer to stay away.

Still, there were indications that not everyone viewed independence as a simple political transition. The next day, as the new Indian flag was raised, "speeches were made by local officials, who were violent in their expressions of patriotism and who made many references to their feeling that only Hindus should be allowed to live in India."[19] Senge had returned from Kulu with provisions and supplies—a camp stove, starter fuel, some extra tarps, knapsacks, and the like—but also with news from the south. The details of the Partition had been announced, and throughout the Punjab, Hindus and Muslims were preparing to relocate. But there were stories that the situation was already turning violent.

Unconcerned and ready to go north, Theos wrote one final addition to his letter to his father before leaving Katrain. "Dear Dad," he wrote,

Everything is now set for an early departure next Tuesday morning. We could make it a day earlier, but I prefer to delay and make certain, for once we are off there can be no changes and we are heading into the barrenness section of this part of the Himalayas so everything must be in order. For the next twenty-one days, at least, I will be sleeping under the open skies unless I can stay in the monastery during the days I am there. I have tried to locate a tent, but there is not one to be had—this was also the case in Calcutta—however I prefer the open skies except in the case of rain and for this we have enough tarps to get under cover for the few hours it may rain.

Closing his letter, Theos wrote, "This is my first message from Kulu—the next will be in about a month, shortly after my return. Until then much love, Theos."

Theos told Helen to expect them back around September 9, but if they were delayed, it would be because he found the library at Ki to be exceptional and hence would probably spend an extra week at the monastery.

With all the details taken care of, having hired seven ponies from a local Muslim contractor, on August 20, Theos and Senge, along with the man's son, Faiz Mohammed, another friend, and a Lahouli, saddled their ponies and headed up the valley toward the Rohtang Pass, carrying camera equipment and more than two thousand rupees in cash and traveler's checks.

For the next few days, Helen occupied her time practicing horseback riding in the valley, in preparation for her trip to Ladakh with Theos, and socializing with local families—some British visitors to the valley having intermarried with Kulu families over the years while others remained simply perennial guests. But by the 24th, stories were beginning to filter up the valley: shops and houses were being burned in Kulu. Though everyone still hoped that the violence engulfing the rest of India would pass them by, it was slowly coming to be seen as a naïve dream. Recording events in her notebook, Helen began to feel scared as the situation in the Kulu Valley got progressively worse.

25th—Burning in Manali . . .
Next afternoon we had a ride planned—Ponies hired—boy came back to say 2 rps per hour. Received—we wondered if they would come—Later we heard all the M's [Muslims] had been asked to leave
Midnight. the fire at quarter of 12—All of us up dressed. Paraded down road—little flash lights.
26th—Rumors of shops in Kulu—Cook disappeared
27th—Bus from Manali brought news of same—Pada said he couldn't answer for safety of M's [Muslims]. Tisheries' man agreed the watchers should keep guard. Major Holmes sent telegram asking protection.
28th—Vicky here most of day—no ponies as M's [Muslims] had been asked to leave—rains—
12^{55} Called out of bed by Pada telling us that Brahmacharis' houses were on fire—Golam Mohammed, butcher & carpenter, Mohammed Singh—shopkeeper—parading in the torches all night.

As frightening as it all was for Helen, her new friend Vicky had much to worry about as well. Austrian by birth, as a young girl she had fallen in love with an Indian man she had met in England, Firoz Khan Noon, a Muslim from one of the more wealthy and powerful families in what would be the new Pakistan.[20] As his wife, Vicky Noon had become a target of the anti-Muslim violence that was unfolding in the Kulu Valley, and she soon discovered that the perpetrators knew where she was. "They are coming to your house tonight," she was told.

> She had two shotguns and a revolver which belonged to her husband who was already in Lahore. She armed her two trusted Moslem servants with the shotguns. Although she'd never fired a gun in her life, she kept the revolver herself. As darkness fell, she could see bursts of flame flare up in the valley leading towards her home, the houses of her Moslem neighbors being set ablaze by Hindu mobs. Slowly that chain of fires crept towards her.

Twenty-seven years old, the only thought that kept occurring to her was something that Helen and Theos had told her about the Buddhist view of life: "Everything is transitory."[21] But Vicky was lucky that night. For months, a drought had plagued the Indian subcontinent as normally heavy monsoon rains failed to appear. But that night, the weather changed and almost as if with a vengeance, the monsoon rains began to descend on the Indian northwest. As usual, when the storm clouds hit the Himalayan mountains, over which they could not pass, they dumped their force on the valleys below. Vicky had been saved—for the night, at least—by the rains that doused the fires in valley and saturated those who had lit them. She sent word of her situation, and the next day the Roerichs came to her rescue, while throughout the valley the Indian officials were rounding up all Muslims in trucks and, it was said, sending them down to a detention center in Kulu.

> 29th—Vicky sent her paintings first thing & asked Tysons to come—Packing and off in Roerich's car with servants. Pogees of M's [Muslims] en route to Kulu. Bearer sure they were to be killed. Tessaldar and officiating Thanadar came to tea.[22] informed us not to interfere. our torches hindered proceedings last night—Tonight: Patli Kuhl. We should be safe if we heard or saw nothing.
> 30th—Stories of murders on way to Kulu—Hindus in Manali. Shree Kote & Dicksie Cote—Patli Kuhl—our house not program—Guards Laksmi Kunt & Harichan
> 31st Big Day—M's [Muslims] going up to attack Kulu—MacDonald had killed five H's [Hindus]—

> 1st Gautam Singh showed up with letter from Vicky who had arrived in
> Mandi not without incidents—He had wired Jalunda to his cousin the
> Commissioner—Gautam took pictures & dog

Making it halfway down the valley, Vicky took refuge with the Hindu Raja
of Mandi in his palace. But her route had been noted and passed on. Soon a
message was received by the Raja: send out the English woman or his family would suffer the consequences.

Gautam Saghal, a Hindu cement dealer who had been sent by her husband to ensure her safety, with the help of the Raja, would get Vicky to
safety. The Raja's Rolls Royce with its curtains drawn was sent at high
speed out of the palace at sunset, and the race was on. But Vicky was not
in the Rolls. Having taken a bath in potassium permanganate to darken her
skin, she was dressed in a sari, her face painted with brown shoe polish, a
bindi on her forehead and a gold ring in her nose. A few minutes after the
Rolls left the palace, Saghal's 1947 Dodge proceeded southward at a relatively unhurried pace. The ruse appeared to have worked. With her flight
from Mandi, Vicky's trial would be over. But Helen's was just beginning.

For five nights, fires had burned in the valley below as the homes and
shops of Muslims were set ablaze. Promised protection, bus drivers offered
to convey Muslims to safety, but what they found on their arrival in Kulu
was something far different.

> Muslims were asked to take to the hills and their houses were burned
> at night. After this was finished, Muslims were invited to go to Kulu
> where they would have protection and be conveyed to a safer place. Af-
> ter the Muslims had gathered in Kulu they were placed inside barbed
> wire enclosure.
>
> A crowd gathered armed with swords, guns and sickles then gath-
> ered around the barbed wire enclosure where the Muslims were con-
> fined. Buses loaded with ex-soldiers equipped with firearms then circled
> round the enclosure firing into the crowd until all the Muslims were
> exterminated.[23]

All across India, the stories were multiplying: riots and burnings in one
city, protests in others, trains filled with migrating Hindus and Muslims
being attacked en route and arriving at their destinations filled only with
the dead. The situation was spiraling out of control with individual attacks

by small groups—burnings, beheadings, and all forms of violence—taking place everywhere, despite the efforts of the woefully inadequate "Boundary Forces." Only Calcutta, of all places, seemed to be calming down. Horrified by the violence unfolding around him, at almost seventy-eight years old, Gandhi took the only action he felt capable of and on September 1 announced that he was entering a fast unto death unless the violence in the city came to an end. He would succeed three days later, saving thousands of lives by his actions, but the Kulu Valley had no such protector.

Although for more than a century, the valley had been home to British residents and their descendants as well as Hindus and Muslims alike, with the Partition and the migration of Muslims to Pakistan, some realized that there was more to be gained than religious and ethnic homogeneity—there was also money. All across India, Muslims were abandoning their properties and shops and now, in the chaos unfolding, some Hindus saw the opportunity to take by force what a few had been unwilling to abandon. Although the Banon family had been intermarried with local Kulu Hindu families for more than a century, they still maintained many British habits. As they were one of the more wealthy landholders in the region, their properties were eyed enviously. Declaring that the Kulu Valley should be purged of not just Muslims but all "cow-eaters"—the British, most notably—ambitious Hindus from the south made the Banon family and others the new targets for attack.

> 2nd Lieut. Henry Banon called—fairly scared
> 3rd rumors

Many in the valley were in denial, refusing to believe reports that those who had been their servants were coming to kill their former employers. The Banon family was not taking chances, though, and sent word north to relatives and friends in Lahoul that they needed help to defend their lives. As time went on, Helen was beginning to get worried about Theos—his return from Spiti was imminent, and no one could predict what he would find. Hoping to warn him, Helen hired a runner to meet Theos with a letter about conditions in the valley.

> 6th. Balak Ram. MacDonald never fired a shot. house looted—letters came—Build up for [Theos]—try to rescue. everyone scared—letter sent

Within days, the violence that had been washing up the Kulu Valley like a wave of fire and blood finally reached its upper limit. As the mob that had set out from Jagatsuk gathered on the east bank of the river at the Manali Bridge and prepared to cross, on the western side stood the Banon family, and their friends and relatives who had gathered in their defense. In between them stood only a narrow bridge from which, by then, hung the corpses of dead Muslims. Prepared to perpetrate a massacre, the men on the east bank were now faced with the prospect of a vicious, bloody battle and after an extended standoff, finally turned and headed south, back down the valley. With this showdown, the violence seemed to have peaked in the Kulu Valley. There was still difficulty for Helen, however, as Theos failed to return. Worse yet, the bodies of Theos's three Muslim porters and been found; they had washed downstream and were discovered with their throats cut. Hoping that he had escaped a similar fate, Helen could only believe that the porters had abandoned Theos and Senge at the Rohtang Pass to proceed to Spiti alone, and had met their fate on their way back down the valley.

As India descended into bloody chaos, the new government was at a loss for what to do. Finally, three weeks after receiving independence from the British Empire, the new Prime Minister, Jawaharlal Nehru, and Deputy Prime Minister, Vallabhbhai Patel, did the unthinkable: they asked Lord Mountbatten to resume leadership of the country. Stunned, Mountbatten agreed to act as the head of an Emergency Committee, but only if they promised him complete secrecy and complete and unquestioned assent to his decisions. And so, for the time being, Lord Mountbatten would assume the role of protector of India, second only to the man he considered more singularly powerful than himself, Mohandas Gandhi.

Even with a seasoned military command in charge of the country and requests sent south for assistance and evacuation, it would be almost two weeks before help would arrive in the Kulu Valley. Until then, everyone was on their own. Helen had already begun to hear rumors of Theos's troubles returning from Lahoul.

15th Hasan the butcher converted to Hinduism
16th—10th Gurkhas arrived with Capt. Wilson—Met all foreigners here on return from Manali—Besharis had seen Dr. Bernard. trouble at border—news brought by Roerichs—

17th Via Pada sent letter of inquiry to [Jagatsuk]. No news—except
through innuendos from Balak Ram.

18th Sent for Capt. Wilson. met Henry Banon on road—Bad news—

The monsoons that were drenching the valley with rain had piled the
mountains deep with snow, and reports were coming in that the Rohtang
Pass was unnavigable. Stories, unreliable perhaps, were coming through
that Theos and Senge had headed east, back up the Lahoul Valley toward
Chatru, where they were going to try to cross at the Hampta Pass, which
would bring them out in the Kulu Valley somewhat south of Manali. This
in itself was troubling, since while the Rohtang Pass was easily negotiable
from the Lahoul Valley, the Hampta Pass was much more difficult. Located
deep in the mountains, the path from Lahoul to the Hampta Pass was in-
direct and punctuated with many dead ends; only an experienced guide, it
was said, could successfully navigate that trail.

Even worse, it was possible that they had been attacked near Chatru, but
it was "a vague rumour and from sources who were terrified for their lives
and households for having breathed that much."

19th Thanadar sent police to Hampta for information. upper house
found looted.

21st sent telegram to Amer. Consul to help speed investigation as Capt.
Wilson wouldn't do anything with Civil Authorities request.

With each passing day, more information slowly sifted down the valley.
Theos and Senge had been spotted a week earlier by some shepherds at
Chatru. Running low on food, the man had given them dried cheese (*atta*),
but they were without horses and the man was unable to fulfill Theos's
request to find coolies to carry their things across the pass.

24th Heard of Shepherd coming through said he had given atta and dev-
astated coolies at 10 Rs. a head per day—

Taking what money she had, Helen purchased food and supplies and
hired coolies to head toward the Hampta Pass and Chatru, hoping to in-
tercept Theos and Senge. But every encounter, it seemed, only brought
additional conflicting information.

Other rumours state that he has returned towards Spiti. Still others have it that a group of Khampas (who seem to be traveling nomads) have helped him out but the direction they took seems to be questionable. The Dak runners have returned from Spiti saying they did not see Dr. Bernard and they passed through Chatru on September 15–16th.

Although the 10th Gurkhas had arrived in time to protect her, with trouble up and down the valley, they soon left but just as quickly returned. They had succeeded, or so they thought, in sending Helen's letter to the American consul in Delhi, following up on her telegram and giving the consul—now ambassador—as much information as she could.

Having acted on her first telegram, Eliot Weil at the American embassy in Delhi contacted Arthur Hopkinson, the British Political Officer in Sikkim—the same man who had rejected Theos's application to visit Lhasa—asking for information that would help them with the situation. Hopkinson, however, informed Weil that "Theo [sic] Bernard is an eccentric who had made himself persona non grata in the course of a previous visit—or visits—to Tibet. The question arises whether he is now in Tibet without the approval of Lhasa authorities."

Meanwhile, back in Katrain, Helen continued to hear encouraging news.

25th Heard from Naggar that B. [Bernard] alive & alone due tomorrow—Capt. W. [Wilson] off to Manali with 20 men in 3 trucks—Trucks returned in pouring rain at 6 or so.

But the next day, Theos did not arrive. Instead, there came only an unrelenting, torrential downpour.

26th Sound of river terrifying—Trees falling like matches. All bridges washed away. Roar of rocks from Hillsides—Crops destroyed—

The rains that had been falling steadily for weeks had reached flooding proportions, and soon all the bridges in the valley had washed away. Everyone was now stranded, while to the south, lines of communication were breaking down and messages were not getting through, including Helen's letter of request for help for herself and Theos. It would be another two weeks before the American ambassador would hear that the efforts he had requested had failed. Helen and her friends would have to fend for themselves.

> 27th Walked to Dobhi bridge
> 28th Anna's birthday—walked to Patli Kuhl—Tessaldar & party called—
> cooperative stores—Food prices exhorbitant. 12 rs. for box of matches
> 29th Heard that Capt. Wilson unable to leave Manali because of washed
> out bridge—from 2 returning Gurkhas—news of floods Lahore & Delhi.
> 30th Maylor came—picnic tea Patli Kuhl—shopkeepers left.

By this time, word had still not reached the American Mission in New Delhi, but even if it had, it would have made little difference. For some time, directives had been in place to secure the safety and well-being of American citizens in India. But those measures were intended only for the staff of the American missions and their families, detailing how to take refuge in the official compounds in New Delhi, Bombay, Madras, and Calcutta. There were no exceptional provisions made for any U.S. citizens out in the field.

It was now October and as another week passed, Helen remained adamant that she was not leaving without Theos. But soon word came that more violence was on the way: Muslims were coming to the valley to seek revenge. Helen would have to leave whether she liked it or not.

> 1st left early—talked & talked—not leaving
> 2nd Dippy building
> 3rd Rumors of 50 escaped M's [Muslims] threatening valley—
> 20 Gurkhas arrived from Manali
> 4th Major Hotz on way to Kulu to arrange leaving via Simla
> 5th left early morning—Capt. Wilson arrived 2 o'clock with 2 Gurkhas.
> Said he questioned everyone including Lama priest—no news—
> 6th hot cakes. Captain left—I decided to be on my way—
> 7th Major Hotz returned & I made arrangements to go to Simla with his
> party—
> 8th Heard shops looted in Kangra.
> Busy packing—writing letters to be mailed in Simla—

As she prepared to leave, finally news came through:

> 9th A note from Hilary to the effect that Naggar rumor has it that [Theos] has returned to Spiti & will try to get through to Leh—Suspected bridge building—200 pack ponies going down with wool etc.—so the road must be open—

Thinking to stay and wait for Theos, Helen was advised against it by her friends. With a Gurkha escort present, that would be the only way of guaranteeing safe passage out of the valley. Furthermore, the locals were saying that the local oracle had declared that the Goddess had more storms to send.

> Fri—10th—News that the Rei of Rupee (Raja of Kulu) has consulted the Devta who has said that she has worse things in store for the valley. So far she has only used a little stick but a big one will be coming by Desera [Festival time]—Floods & earthquakes—Got suitcases done up in gunny.

Given no other choice, Helen finally left Katrain with Major Hotz and his party, but as the bridges were washed out, it was going to be a long walk out of the valley.

Major Hotz had decided that since it would take weeks to walk along the only major road in and out of the valley—not to mention being conspicuous and dangerous—the party would head south along a trade route, believing it to offer the quickest path to Simla, and sent word ahead to officials there. But first they would need to cross the now swollen Beas River. Near Naggar, it was said, the local village had begun constructing a new bridge, but it would be not be completed for close to a month, so "in the meantime, Balak Ram felled a tree a few miles up the river," and the party was able to cross successfully, if precariously. On their way south, the route they had chosen would be a rough road, only portions of which jeeps and army trucks could negotiate under the best of conditions.

Just as they were setting out, Helen received a note from Helena Roerich, saying that she had heard that she was leaving and wished her luck, adding that she had heard a rumor that "your husband was trying to get through Ladakh and onto Kashmir from there," which would take a few weeks at best. At the same time, word of their plans had reached Simla, and the Ministry of External Affairs replied to the American embassy that "protection has already been afforded to Mrs. Bernard" and that she was not in "any imminent danger," though it would be up to the embassy to ascertain "from Mr. and Mrs. Bernard what their future plans are." With little help coming from the south, Major Hotz's party set out on their journey.

Oct. 13—Mon—Left Katrain with Major Hotz + Mrs. Hotz
Mr. John Hotz
Mr. + Mrs. Robertson
walked 12 miles to Kulu.
14th—Capt. Wilson took us to Aut, 18 miles in army trucks—
walked 2 miles—Largi [Larji]
15th walked to Baujar   12 miles
16th " "   Soja 9 miles
17th " "   Ani 16 miles—over Jalori Pass, 10,000 ft.
18th " "   Luri 15 miles—elev. 2,000 ft.
19th " "   Narkunda 13 miles—top of pass 9,144'
20th " "   Matiana 11 miles—road into Simla, 28 miles—bus.

Only when she reached Simla did Helen become truly aware of the magnitude of the events unfolding around her. The city was overwhelmed with refugees fleeing the violence all around them. Lord Mountbatten had taken control of the government, but when his aerial patrols reported that lines of people migrating from one country to the next stretched for hundreds of miles and individual caravans alone numbered close to a million people, even he found the situation daunting.

All but declaring martial law, Mountbatten ordered that all the railways be put under "dawn-to-dusk" aerial reconnaissance and that military escorts be provided for all trains, and that furthermore, should a train be attacked, any member of a military escort arriving unwounded was to be court-martialed and shot on site. But even that level of safety was contingent on getting on a train. Although she had arrived in Simla on October 20, it was three days before Helen could board a train bound for New Delhi, and then she was limited to one second-class ticket for herself, one third-class ticket for her servant, and "three mounds of luggage" on the next available train bound for Delhi on the 23rd.

Meanwhile, on the east coast of India, the Roerichs had reached Calcutta. Svetoslav paid a visit to the American vice consul, telling him that "an American citizen, Mr. Theophile Bernard, is lost in the Himalaya mountains between Spiti and Lahaul." Since Naggar was on the east side of the Kulu Valley, the Roerichs had been able to leave by car and although only able to transport themselves, were carrying letters and messages from various people in the valley. Svetoslav went on to report,

Fearing that Bernard might have met with an accident, a Captain Wilson of the 7th and 10th Gurkha Regiment, located in Kulu, on October 4th left in an attempt to trace him. After nine days, however, he returned having found no trace. A Captain Boyce of the same regiment informed Roerich that Captain Wilson, in his questioning of the people of the region, had determined inconclusively that Bernard's caravan was attacked in Spiti as a result of the communal disturbances which had then just broken out in that region. No one, however, could tell what had become of Bernard.

Nonetheless, Svetoslav asked "that the Embassy intercede with the Central Government in order that [Helen] may attempt to find Bernard and have him returned safely."

Arriving the next day in Delhi, Helen wrote another letter to the Embassy Counselor, Howard Donovan, acknowledging receipt of the ambassador's telegram five weeks earlier and asking him for an update on the situation, pleading that "even just a few words from you may save much fumbling around on my part + waste of time on the part of your office."

Obtaining a meeting with Eliot Weil, Helen passed on Helena Roerich's information that Theos was most likely headed toward Leh in Ladakh, asking him to convey this to Donovan, along with her request that they contact the Ladakh government, inasmuch as there was one, to see what could be done. Brought to see Donovan himself, Helen told the counselor that she was leaving a suitcase full of Theos's clothes with the manager of her hotel, and since he would most likely contact the embassy looking for her upon his arrival, asked that this information be entered into his official file. Donovan, intent on doing all that he could, even allowed Helen to send a telegram from the embassy to Theos in Leh, informing him that he should contact Donovan for further information, and provided her with a letter of introduction to the American Consulate General in Calcutta. As a precautionary measure, given "the remoteness of the region in which he was last seen, the uncertain state of communications, and the generally disturbed conditions prevailing in northern India," Donovan forwarded

Helen's account of events surrounding Theos's disappearance to the U.S. Secretary of State in Washington, as well as to the consulates and embassies in Lahore and Karachi.

That night, Helen met a travel writer, Nicol Smith, who was working in Calcutta for the Associated Press newspaper syndicate. Fascinated by Helen's story, Smith wrote it up in detail and wired it back to New York, where each of the tabloid newspapers in the city broke the story in rapid succession the next day: "American Feared Slain In India" (*New York Sun*), "U.S. Scholar Feared Killed in Indian Raid" (*New York Post*—Sports Edition), "Fear Indians Kill Bernard, Tibet Expert" (*New York Journal American*). The next day, dozens of papers around the country were running the story, and Glen learned of his son's possible fate from the *Los Angeles Times*.

Taking the train to Calcutta on October 30, Helen returned to the Great Eastern Hotel, where she and Theos had stayed only three months earlier. Still carrying Senge's personal belongings with her, Helen wrote to Tharchin in Kalimpong, asking for his help and advice. "Theos is not with me," she wrote.

> He is somewhere in Spiti or Ladakh and not able to get back or communicate with me. He and Senge left Kulu on August 20th to visit Kyi Monastery and planned to return to Kulu [valley] and then we would all go through Lahul to Leh. It seems that he got back to the Hampta Pass about the 12th of September or thereabouts and there ran into transport trouble as his muleteers were Mohammedans and all the Mohammedans in the Valley had been polished off by then and they [Hindus] were out after the stray ones. There were all sorts of rumors back in the Valley that he had been attacked and looted and his servants all killed, etc.—but that Sahib was unharmed. Whether that means Senge, too, I do not know. I haven't heard from him since. Other rumors say that he has returned to Spiti and is attempting to go to Leh—I guess he can't get out through Kashmir at this stage anyway. . . .
>
> I also have Senge's best clothes here and his silver charm box [the *dablam*], etc. and newest fur hat, etc. Can you suggest any place where I could leave them or send them so that they would eventually catch up with him if he is still alive and kicking? I somehow can't believe that anything could have happened to him. I'm sure that he will turn up in Kalimpong one of these days. I could leave them at the [Calcutta] apartment where we lived after we left Kalimpong as I think Senge could find that

and he knows the servants there. . . . Perhaps I could leave the dictionary there for safekeeping, too, until the situation and the postal service
improves. If I don't hear from you, this is what I shall do.

Sure that Theos was still alive, but thinking that even Kashmir could
have been problematic, she wasn't sure he wouldn't try to head east toward Lhasa—a journey she was told would take at least three months. "It
is entirely within the realm of possibility that Dr. Bernard will have found
company going to Lhasa from the monasteries in Spiti and joined them.
There is a regular trade route, centuries old, between the two countries
which formerly were one."

Helen then contacted Donovan, asking him to contact the State Department about informing the Tibetan government of the situation, since she
could guarantee that the Tibetans were eager to please the American government in the wake of their high-profile participation in the Asian Relations Conference as an independent country the previous spring.[24] She
even sent a telegram to Lord Tsarong in Lhasa, asking for his assistance in
looking for Theos.

TSARONG SHAPE
LHASA TIBET
THEOS BERNARD FORCED TO RETURN TO SPITI BY COMMUNAL TROU-
BLE ON PUNJAB BORDERS AFTER VISITING KYI MONASTERY STOP COM-
MUNICATION IMPOSSIBLE VIA INDIA STOP IF YOU SHOULD HEAR ANY
NEWS WOULD YOU PLEASE INFORM THE AMERICAN AMBASSADOR NEW
DELHI AS THEY ARE MOST CONCERNED ABOUT HIS SAFETY AND WEL-
FARE STOP BEST REGARDS TO YOU AND FAMILY
HELEN BERNARD

But just as they had blocked Theos's application to visit Tibet, the British
authorities—who still controlled Sikkim and the borders of Tibet, if no longer India itself—blocked Helen's telegram as well, and Lord Tsarong never
received the message. The embassy offered to send their own telegrams as
well, with written follow-up letters, but were advised by Hopkinson that
there was no need, since he doubted that the Tibetans would be inclined to
help Theos. Reiterating his previous statements about Theos having "made
himself very unpopular with the Tibetans when he traveled in Tibet some
years ago," Hopkinson added that they had rejected Theos's application

since they felt he might give all foreigners "a bad name" if he should go to Lhasa again. Not willing to defy the U.S. ambassador, however, Hopkinson reluctantly forwarded Donovan's cable to Lhasa, and a few weeks later received their reply:

REC'D YOUR TELEGRAM. WE HAVE NOT HEARD NEWS OF THEOS BERNARD'S ARRIVAL IN TIBET. WILL ASSIST HIM IF HE COMES.
TIBETAN FOREIGN BUREAU

Still pursuing her own avenues, Helen wrote to Theos's publisher, Dagobert Runes, a few days later, telling him that she was sure Theos was still alive. Receiving her letter, Runes contacted the New York Times, and once again, the news wires were buzzing: "Theos Bernard Reported Alive."

Theos Bernard, American author and Tibetan scholar who on Nov. 2 was reported as having been killed in the Punjab by tribal raiders, is alive according to word from his wife received here yesterday by Dr. Dagobert D. Runes. Dr. Runes, head of the Philosophical Library, Mr. Bernard's publisher, said that Mrs. Bernard had written to him from New Delhi, India, on Nov. 5 that her husband was safe. She said that the marauding tribesmen had attacked her husband's expedition and had slain most of the carriers but that he had escaped. His present whereabouts are unknown, she said.

But before this story had even been printed, the report of Theos's disappearance had become a media sensation, and Helen was being hounded by the press, all producing conflicting reports and misinformation—he had been attacked by Hindus in Kulu, he was killed by Buddhists in Lahoul, he was being held hostage by "tribal raiders," he had been buried in an avalanche, and so on. In no time, the media frenzy that had put her in "the limelight" with the story of her "fleeing 126 miles on foot" proved too much for Helen, for she was "having no peace or privacy" and so would "be glad to get out of India."

Contacting her old boss back in New York, C. V. Starr, she told him she was now ready to go to Hong Kong to work on remodeling his apartment there. And so, booking a flight with Pan American airlines, at midnight on the 10th of November, 1947, Helen boarded a plane on the outskirts of Calcutta and left India behind.

THIRTEEN
The Aftermath

When everyone is dead, the Great Game is finished.

—RUDYARD KIPLING[1]

WHILE MANY IN INDIA WERE convinced that Theos was dead, his father, Glen, was not. Even more than a year later, he declared to a local reporter that he was sure that Theos was still alive and would be returning any day with the greatest story of adventure anyone had yet heard. But as time went on, Glen's hopes slowly began to fade. Years later, as Theos's *Haṭha Yoga* continued to be reprinted, Glen would finally be forced to publicly state the bare facts of his son's disappearance.

In 1947, Theos Bernard was on a mission to the KI monastery in western Tibet in search of some special manuscripts. While on his way, rioting broke out among the Hindus and Moslems in that section of the hills; all Moslems including women and children in the little village from which Theos departed were killed.

The Hindus then proceeded into the mountains in pursuit of the Moslems who had accompanied Theos as guides and muleteers. These Moslems, it is reported, learning of the killings, escaped, leaving Theos and his Tibetan boy alone on the trail. It is further reported that both were shot and their bodies thrown into the river.

To date we have not been able to get any authentic information on the entire circumstances of his death, nor have we any line of the effects

Theos had with him. That region of Tibet is so very remote that it is unlikely we shall ever learn the full details.

A young woman named Eleanore Murray who had read Theos's *Heaven
Lies Within Us* contacted Glen asking how she could find Theos to study yoga
with him, but Glen simply informed her that his son had gone missing and
was most likely dead. Pursuing the issue of yoga with him, Eleanore convinced Glen to teach her the basics and some fundamentals of philosophy
in exchange for housecleaning services. Eventually, Eleanore simply moved
into Glen's home and became not only his student and research assistant
but also eventually his heir and common-law wife. Going by the "secret"
initiation name that Glen gave her, Kamala,[2] Eleanore, who claimed to be
psychic, spent the following years "attending to his needs and studying
yoga and Buddhism with him, in the role of a *chela*." For reasons he never
specified, in his later years Glen simply considered her insane.

Although Glen was understandably sad at Theos's disappearance, his
half-brothers had mixed feelings. His brother Ian never saw Theos after
their Arizona days. Despite being divorced from Theos, Viola had continued to support the Gordon brothers financially and in other ways as well.
Making recommendations and phone calls, she had succeeded in getting
Ian into the arts program at the progressive Black Mountain College in
North Carolina. But having lost an eye due to a slingshot accident as a child,
Ian had become depressed when he began to lose sight in his other eye and
committed suicide while his brothers were away fighting in Europe.

Although Dugald had seen Theos in New York while en route to the bat-
tlefront in Europe, after he returned from World War II, Dug felt somewhat
disappointed and let down by Theos. Indeed, as early as the years following
his return from Tibet in 1937, Dugald and the rest of the family came to feel
somewhat abandoned; Theos, he thought, seemed very self-serving, leading a flamboyant lifestyle and surviving in New York as a "flim flam man."

Of all Theos's brothers, it was his youngest, Marvene, who never stopped
idealizing his older brother. Drafted out of law school, Marvene had fought
in the American invasion of France at Normandy before entering the Judge
Advocate General's corps in the 1950s. From his youngest days, Marvene
could remember many impressions of Theos:

watching him play football . . . [he was a] splendid [athlete] . . . teaching
me to swim . . . having him teach me to dive off a 20 ft. tower . . . having

him out there in the water to pull me out. . . . I was just a little kid, I was six years old. . . . he came home from the university and he was the lifeguard at the Tombstone municipal swimming pool. And of course everybody thought the world of him. . . . He wrote his mother a letter every week and it arrived to her in Tombstone or Tucson . . . it just exemplifies his love and concern for his mother, which I feel was the same for his brothers, 'cause I have never known it to be otherwise.

As for Helen, she spent those first few months attempting to recover from her ordeal. Staying for most of the winter in Hong Kong, she received condolences and an outpouring of emotional support from her friends. Doing her best to cope with the situation, she spent her time alternately trying to keep occupied with work, hiring people in the Kulu Valley (through the Tysons) to try to locate more information about Theos, and simply consoling herself, remembering that Theos had predicted his own death and that when the time came, he had told her, she should simply "kick his body aside and move on." Making her way east, first to the Philippines and then to Hawai'i, she eventually arrived in Los Angeles, where she was able to see Glen again.

Having kept in contact with the American embassy in Delhi, Howard Donovan had forwarded to Helen what little communication they received from the various government agencies in Tibet, Ladakh, and Pakistan. She appreciated their efforts, but although she might not have believed it, Theos was *not* the most problematic American citizen at large in the Indian northwest at the time.[3] Nonetheless, investigations in the Kangra district continued. In Kulu, the chief of police paid a personal visit with a detail of men, questioning every inhabitant of the small village of Koksar located just over the Rohtang Pass, but no one had seen any sign of Theos and Senge. The police could only conclude that they had returned to Spiti when they found both the Rohtang and Hampta passes snowbound. Being informed of this, the district commissioner in Dharamsala sent a message to Spiti, "inquiring about Dr. Bernard," but by the time the message went out, the snows had rendered all the mountain passes insurmountable and communications were cut off for the winter. When Donovan finally wrote to Helen at length a year later, the news was not good.

After an extensive investigation by the police and military in Kulu "questioning everybody," even "drinking with the local inhabitants (all Lahoulis)," they were convinced that no such rumored attack had taken place in the region. Nonetheless, they were forced to conclude that Theos must have "met with some fatal accident or incident." And so, expressing her disgust at individuals in Kulu who claimed to have heard from Theos, Helen resigned herself to the fact that he must be dead. Heading to the Catskills in upstate New York, Helen tried to regain a sense of peace. But the experience of the previous two years had taken its toll, and by the time she returned to New York City, her hair had turned completely gray. She and her friend Lucien David opened their own business as registered architects, under the name David and Park, with Helen specializing in architecture and interior design. Still committed to finding out the truth, three years later, Helen embarked on a second trip around the world as part of a larger "business trip," visiting Karachi (Pakistan), Bombay, and Calcutta, seeking more information about Theos's fate.

Throughout this time, news of Theos's disappearance had been slowly spreading around the world. In Lhasa itself, reports were being read in foreign newspapers, and even Heinrich Harrer learned of Theos's disappearance. Running a radio program out of Lhasa, Lowell Thomas, who had seconded Theos's application to The Explorers Club, broadcast the news on one of his shows, claiming that he had been "killed in a drunken brawl while trying to sneak into Tibet illegally." After returning from Tibet with his son, Thomas wrote a high-profile article for *Collier's* magazine recounting their adventures, telling American audiences of the small but distinguished list of Americans who had ever succeeded in reaching Lhasa, among whom, he claimed, he and his son were only the sixth and seventh (they were in fact twelfth and thirteenth).[4] Thomas wrote about Theos:

> The third American to see the Potala, and the last man pre-war, was Theos Bernard, an Arizonan, who thought that in the mystic East he might find a solution to the physical and mental problems that beset him. . . .
>
> Upon his return he announced that he was a "white lama." Theos wrote about his journey in a book call *Penthouse of the Gods*, and dreamed of building a typical Tibetan monastery in the mountains of California. But on a second unauthorized attempt to enter Tibet, some months before our visit, he disappeared mysteriously. Although his body was not found, it is fairly certain that he was murdered.[5]

Bad enough that he had claimed Theos had died in a "drunken brawl," but when Viola read this description of Theos and his "mental problems," she was livid. Months later, when Thomas contacted Viola inquiring about Theos's fate and introduced himself as "a friend of Theos's," he received an understandably cold response.

Others contacted Viola as well when they heard the news. With the kindness and consideration that seemed to be her strongest traits, Viola responded to each of them, expressing her lack of optimism and thanking them all for their concern. For her own part, Viola felt that Theos had put himself in a "do or die" situation, and later remarked, "you can't go on being the first 'White Lama' forever without refurbishing your resources and doing some more, and my impression was that he was going back to catch up with things and get more data, perhaps, and build up his reputation." She was not hopeful of his return.

Both Viola and DeVries had heard about Theos's disappearance early on. Although they had not spoken in close to ten years—ever since Theos's affair with DeVries—after his apparent death, DeVries contacted Viola to express her sadness over his fate and declare her contempt for Lowell Thomas and his "stinking jealousy." DeVries told Viola that she had seen Theos in New York just before his departure for India. Since he was dead, she felt she would no longer be betraying his trust, and told Viola that during this visit Theos had "broken down" and confided in her that Viola was the only woman he had ever truly loved.

Back in California, word of Theos's disappearance had reached Ganna Walska, a woman Theos had apparently never loved, or so she felt. The gossipmongers in Los Angeles were speculating that Ganna herself, still furious about all he had done and tried, had hired men in India to have Theos killed. It was an outrageous accusation, but the sentiment was not far from the truth. Converting Tibetland into a horticultural museum—now called Lotusland—Ganna Walska gave orders to her staff that they were never to so much as utter Theos's name, much less discuss him with anyone. Her orders remained in effect until her death in 1984.

In Germany, Ernst Schäfer learned of Theos's disappearance. As there was still substantial animosity between the British and German Tibetologists, and the feeling that the British still held deep resentment toward him for his 1939 expedition to Lhasa—he had been snubbed by Hugh Richardson at the time—Schäfer theorized that standing orders had been left for him to be killed should he ever attempt to visit Tibet again. Because both he and Theos were bearded and often seen with cameras around their necks, Schäfer suspected that Theos had been mistaken for himself and been killed at the behest of the British.[6]

As time went on, some people speculated on more mystical reasons for Theos's disappearance. Taking his claims of being a yogi as an indication of a higher commitment, some people felt he had faked his death in order to "leave the world as he knew it in a way that no one would follow him" and live out his life undisturbed in the Himalayas. But the Himalayas were proving to be anything but a haven for those wishing to be undisturbed. Prevailing in the civil war against the Nationalist government of China, Chairman Mao and his Communist forces had defeated Chiang Kai-shek and his army and declared the Peoples' Republic of China. In one of his first speeches after the victory, Mao declared that the "liberation" of Tibet was next,[7] and four months later, on October 7, 1950, Chinese Communist troops crossed the Yangtse River into Tibetan territory and destroyed the small garrison at Chamdo. The Chinese invasion of Tibet had begun.

Even though a year earlier, members of the Tibetan Trade Commission had visited New York,[8] now Tibetan representatives were there to petition the United Nations for membership for Tibet. Although the British government had privately concluded "since Tibet has from 1913 not only enjoyed full control over her internal affairs but has also maintained direct relations on her account with other States, she must be regarded as a State to which Article 35(2) of the UN Charter applies," in public they remained uncommitted, waiting to see what Nehru and India would decide. Similarly, for some time, members of the American embassy in New Delhi had been debating the situation with the State Department and what action they should take, if only to monitor the situation from inside Tibet and broadcast reports to the rest of the world.

If we are to take any action, it must be speedy. It is possible that our people in the Far East might take the view that the dispatch of such a group might prejudice our relations with the Communist government of China. I myself am inclined to believe that the greater the difficulties encountered by the Chinese Communists in conquering all of China, the better for us. Furthermore, it would be well for the peoples particularly in Asia to receive broadcasts regarding Communist endeavors to conquer Tibet.

If people are sent in, they should, of course, understand that their mission is hazardous, that in the event of a sudden Communist uprising they might lose their lives, and that they might even be taken prisoner and subjected to tortures. Nevertheless, it seems to me that the enterprise is worth considering.[9]

Two months later, the project received authorization, and Krishna Menon from India's Ministry of External Affairs communicated the U.S. government's intention to send a CIA officer into Tibet. Since there was already one in Urumchi (Eastern Turkestan), a locale the Chinese Communists were closing in on fast, the decision was made to send him south to Tibet and Lhasa. Menon warned the embassy, however, that "a direct line from Urumchi is very difficult and thinly inhabited by nomads, addicted to banditry [and] there is little active Tibetan administration there."[10] Concerned about the fate of Tibet, Eleanor Roosevelt, the former First Lady, who had chaired the drafting of the UN's Universal Declaration of Human Rights, asked to be kept personally informed about the situation and the possibilities of providing "American aid to Tibet," including land and air routes, coordinating with India and Nepal, and even using Khampas as guerrilla fighters.[11]

While still waiting for some official word of Theos's fate, Helen saw an article in *Life* magazine with a picture of Tibetan border guards awaiting punishment by whipping for "killing an American." Helen saved the article, although the American was in fact Douglas McKiernan, the CIA officer authorized by the State Department (the first to be killed in the line of duty), who had been on his way south to Lhasa when he was shot and killed by the border guards before the authorization for his safe passage had been received.[12] It fell to the Tibetan Foreign Minister to apologize to the U.S. government for "the unfortunate incident which occurred at Nagtshang," express "deep regret beyond measure," and advise them that the Tibetan government had given "appropriate punishments to all those men who are responsible for this unlawful action."[13] But the damage had been done. Even though the American ambassador had received permission to offer asylum to the Fourteenth Dalai Lama and a hundred-person entourage, in the end only two visas would be extended from Calcutta: one for the Dalai Lama's older brother, Thubten Norbu, and one for a single servant. Two months later, the American ambassador in New Delhi was forced to concede in a private informal statement to the Secretary General of India's Ministry of Foreign Affairs that "the Government of the United States has never and is not now irrevocably committed either to support or oppose any particular political group in China" and could only hope that "the Peiping Regime will not engage in aggression against any of China's neighbors in the Far East."[14] From this point on, the U.S. government would be first and foremost concerned with Chinese aggression in Korea. Only after the Korean conflict had been settled would Tibet be a major issue for the U.S. government again.

Fearing for the future themselves, the Tibetan people expressed their belief that only divine guidance could protect their country. After repeated incidents of public outcry, on November 17, 1950, as Chinese forces were pushing farther and farther west into Tibet, the Tibetan cabinet agreed to break with precedent and at the age of sixteen, two years ahead of schedule, Tenzin Gyatso, the Fourteenth Dalai Lama, was invested with full powers as Tibet's spiritual and temporal leader. Fearing for his safety should the Chinese reach Lhasa, the young Dalai Lama, accompanied by the Tibetan cabinet and his German friend, Heinrich Harrer, headed south for India, leaving Tibet for the first time. Photographs of the new Tibetan leader made headlines, and the "Flight of the Dalai Lama" was splashed across *Life* magazine in full color for the whole world to see.[15]

Hearing of the arrival of His Holiness the Fourteenth Dalai Lama in Kalimpong, David Macdonald immediately left his residence at the Himalayan Hotel and began walking into town to try to see him. Halfway down the road, however, Macdonald was startled to see a party of Tibetan monks coming toward him. The central figure in the group called out to him in Tibetan and said, "David Macdonald, it has been a long time!" Realizing that it was the young Dalai Lama himself, Macdonald dropped to the ground, doing three full prostrations in the middle of the road. Taking Macdonald by the arm, His Holiness the Dalai Lama walked back up the hill with him to the Himalayan Hotel where, surround by Macdonald's family, they "reminisced" about the many times they had shared during his lifetime as the Thirteenth Dalai Lama. Although raised Buddhist, David Macdonald had converted to Christianity as a young man and had raised his family in the Christian tradition. Following this audience with His Holiness, however, some in the family found themselves seriously questioning their previous opinions of Buddhism, and David Macdonald himself subsequently repudiated Christianity altogether and returned to the Buddhist tradition of his youth. Heinrich Harrer remained at the Himalayan Hotel for several months, and inspired by Macdonald's account of his time in Tibet—*Twenty Years in Tibet*, which he found on the bookshelves of the hotel—began writing his own account of his experiences on the Himalayan plateau, which he decided to call "Seven Years in Tibet."

Given assurances by the Chinese of their peaceful intentions, the young Dalai Lama and his entourage eventually returned to Tibet. Meanwhile, back in his home country, having served his time, Gedun Chöpel had been released from prison, but the nearly three years he had spent there had taken their toll on his health. His return to the small house in Lhasa where he had lived was a sad homecoming. Prior to his arrest Gedun Chöpel had been hard at work on a history of Tibet as well as other works, but despite his old residence having been sealed by officials, his books and other papers were missing, and he came to find comfort only in alcohol and cigarettes. He had been supported by monks from his old monastic "regional house" while in prison, and upon his release many visitors came to see him, but, content to lecture to the walls of his home, many times he gave almost no acknowledgment of their presence. Often, in fact, there would be a crowd of monks gathered outside his home, listening to him talk—rant even, occasionally throwing things at the crowd—about whatever topic motivated him at the time. When the Chinese Red Army reached Lhasa two years later, Gedun Chöpel asked friends to carry him to the roof to witness their arrival. Hearing the blaring Chinese loudspeakers and seeing large banners and pictures of Mao lofted high, Gedun Chöpel knew the Tibet he loved was doomed and soon would be gone forever. He died that October. Far from fading into oblivion, however, from that point onward his notoriety would only increase as the books and poems he had authored were printed and published by his friends, creating a stir in certain quarters.

Back in America, over the years that followed his disappearance, Theos's reputation seemed to be growing as well. Glen continued to receive fan mail from around the world from people who had read Theos's books, as well as regular royalty checks in Theos's name. Carl Dorese, a ghost illustrator for *Ripley's Believe It or Not!*, had read Theos's *Penthouse of the Gods* and wrote that he was interested in doing an illustrated adaptation of the book, even sending illustrated letters as samples. Meanwhile, *Haṭha Yoga* had come out in paperback and the hardcover was about to go into its second printing. With full power of attorney over his son's affairs, Glen could continue to manage Theos's estate, including its income, but the legal issue of Theos's disappearance remained unresolved.

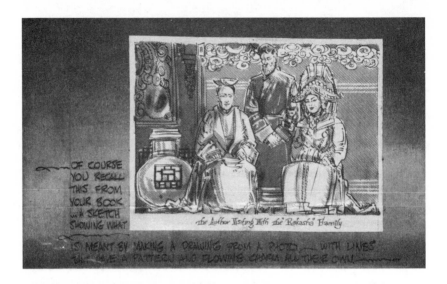

Figure 13.1 Illustrated letter (detail) by Carl Dorese (HGPF)

Although he and Helen had maintained a friendly relationship, Helen had expended a substantial amount of money on her trip with Theos, and a large amount of that was tied up in book purchases sitting in a storage facility in Los Angeles—in Theos's name only, that neither Helen nor Glen could access. Helen had spent a considerable amount of additional money as well trying to find any shred of evidence concerning Theos's fate that she could. Although there was little to show for her efforts, one small item was recovered: a receipt made out to Theos for a donation to Ki Monastery, indicating that he had in fact reached Spiti, at the very least; this corroborated, in her mind, that it was on his return trip from Spiti that he had met trouble.

Over the years Helen had heard more and more news coming out of India. Major Hotz, who had led her and the others out of the Kulu Valley, was still running the Cecil Hotel in New Delhi. Hotz had continued to coordinate efforts to find Theos on Helen's behalf, or at the very least, to obtain whatever information he could.

Others besides Helen were searching for Theos as well. Back at The Explorers Club in New York, his disappearance had become a topic of discussion, and though he was "regarded by fellow members as somewhat of a mystic," they were still concerned about his fate and "an informal inquest at the long oak table concluded that he had been caught in a mountain avalanche." If that was indeed what had happened to him, they concluded, "there's no use even searching for his body."

One of the members of the club, Prince Peter of Greece and Denmark, decided that he would go looking for Theos. Visiting Kulu the following summer, he reported his findings:

> I have since obtained quite reliable information as to how he died. It was during the communal trouble which followed partition between India and Pakistan. Bernard was on his way to Lahul, valley lying north of the Punjab to which access is obtained over the Rohtang Pass (14,000 ft.) at the head of the Kulu valley. He spent the night at Koksar, a bungalow to the north of the pass, and the next day hearing a commotion outside, came out to see what it was. It turned out to be a party of Lahoulis (Buddhists) marching down to Kulu to avenge Hindus who had been massacred by Muslems [sic]. They were excited and drunk. Bernard had a beard, and they mistook him for a Musselman. Before he could explain, their leader (whom I know personally) shot him. Finding out after that he was an American, they buried him stealthily and tried to hush the matter up.[16]

To the members of the club and others,[17] this sounded conclusive, but there were still problems with the account, not the least of which was the fate of the young Tibetan monk, Senge. But these concerns could do nothing to change the situation in which Helen and Glen found themselves.

By 1953, Helen finally prevailed and convinced Glen that it was time they accepted the reality of the situation and have Theos declared legally dead and the dictates of his will acted upon. Citing the official New Delhi U.S. embassy report issued in 1950, stating that Theos had been presumed killed on September 1, 1947, Helen began the procedure. Filing an official deposition of her account of the events of August and September 1947 as Theos's "secretary," Helen cited the American embassy reports and the testimony of Prince Peter in support of her belief that Theos was dead. Glen petitioned the court to have himself declared "sole heir at law and joint tenet owner of personal property with the said Theos Casimir Bernard,"[18] thereby avoiding probate court and expediting the process. As a result, on November 27, 1953, Theos Casimir Bernard was officially declared dead by a Los Angeles court. The final verdict was: shot by bandits in the vicinity of Koksar (Lahoul)—body not recovered. But the will was not yet in effect; it would take another four years for his estate to be released to his father.

Back on the East Coast, the effects of Chinese and Soviet expansionism were playing out on a personal level following World War II. Annexed as part of the Russian revolution in the middle of World War I, the Mongolian region of Central Asia near the Caspian Sea had been collectivized into the Kalmyk Soviet Socialistic Republic. When German forces invaded Russian territory during World War II, the Kalmyks sided with them against the Soviets, but when the German forces were defeated, Stalin exacted his revenge on the Kalmyk Mongolians for their collaboration. Although they had numbered slightly more than 200,000 in their homeland, only 700 Mongolians managed to escape to DP (displaced persons) camps in Europe. Granted asylum in America, like so many before them, the Mongolian refugees arrived at Ellis Island in New York Harbor, passing under the shadow of the Statue of Liberty. Although other immigrants to America had simply made their home in one or more of the five boroughs of New York City, the Mongolians traveled slightly farther afield and settled across the Hudson River, inland in the small community of Freewood Acres, New Jersey, on lands donated to them by Countess Tolstoy.

It was a cold day in early February 1955 when the ocean liner *Liberté* made her way through the ice-filled Hudson River to dock at a New York pier. On board was a man who was no stranger to extreme cold or international travel, and though invited to America many years before, he was only then arriving. Wearing a heavy Tibetan-style brown fur-lined *puk-sha* with a bright orange sash, Geshe Wangyal stood on the deck of the French liner, waiting to set foot on American soil. Although he had returned to Tibet after Theos had last seen him, when the Chinese invaded in 1951, Geshe Wangyal went south once more to Kalimpong, leaving Drepung Monastery and Lhasa behind for the last time. Now, four years later, through the efforts of his old teacher, the Dilowa Hutukhtu,[19] Geshe Wangyal had been brought to America to help serve the religious needs of the Mongolian community in New Jersey.

Learning of his presence in New Jersey, Thubten Norbu, the Dalai Lama's older brother, who was living in New Jersey at the time, also came to Geshe Wangyal's aid. Through his influence, Geshe Wangyal was given a job teaching languages at Columbia University in New York, in the Indo-Iranian Languages and Cultures Department. But Columbia was not the

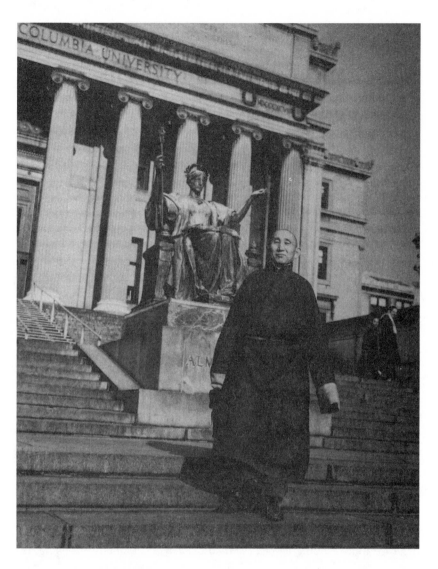

Figure 13.2 Geshe Wangyal at Columbia University, ca. 1958 (CUA)

only organization looking to take advantage of Geshe Wangyal's skills. With the end of the Korean War a few years earlier, Tibet was back on the priority list for the U.S. government. Acting along the lines of one of the suggestions made by Eleanor Roosevelt years earlier, the CIA decided to train and arm Tibetan fighters from Kham (Eastern Tibet), who had already gained notoriety for their fighting against the Chinese. Geshe Wangyal would soon be recruited to participate in the training of covert operatives who could be airdropped into Tibet, since by all accounts, the situation there was worsening drastically.

Thus, while Geshe Wangyal was settling into his new life in America, major events were transpiring on the other side of the world. Although with the "Seventeen-Point Agreement"—signed under coercion by Tibetan representatives in Beijing a few years earlier—Tibet was formally declared to be part of China, the Tibetans as a people and their culture were far from safe.

Back in Kalimpong, Tharchin was hard at work publishing his newspaper. What had begun as a personal vision and occasional medium for Christian propaganda going into Tibet and had later morphed into a chronicle of world events, by the 1950s was now a vehicle in the fight for Tibetan freedom from the Chinese invasion and occupation, with Tharchin now placing Buddhism on par with Christianity, even citing Buddhist scriptures in some of his articles.[20] A major hub for communications, Kalimpong, and Tharchin's newspaper offices in particular, became a clearinghouse for information about the ongoing Chinese aggression. He was receiving handwritten accounts of military occupations and aerial bombardments of monasteries and villages in eastern Tibet. After years of fighting during the Chinese civil war, Mao's Red Army was given free rein to exact vengeance on the Tibetans who spurned them during the Long March. Even in crude cartoon form, the picture Tharchin painted for his audience of events transpiring in eastern Tibet was sobering and hard to believe, and the accounts would only get worse.

Meanwhile, just as Theos was being declared legally dead, fascination with Buddhism and Tibet was on the rise, from genuine interest by the Beats to Tibet's growth into the icon of the exotic, typified by the image of Grace Kelly reading *Beyond the High Himalayas*.[21] Rights were being negotiated for a French translation of Theos's *Haṭha Yoga*—published as *Tout le Hatha Yoga*—and Spanish translation, followed by requests to translate *Heaven Lies Within Us* into French and German for European audiences, and Spanish for South American ones. In academic circles, his *Philosophical Foundations of India* book had been getting mixed reviews, reprinted under the somewhat more accurate title of *Hindu Philosophy*. Karl Potter, while claiming that none of the survey books on Indian philosophy then available on the market offered "new facts or new connections," noted that they all were, in his opinion, "improvements on Bernard's work," since

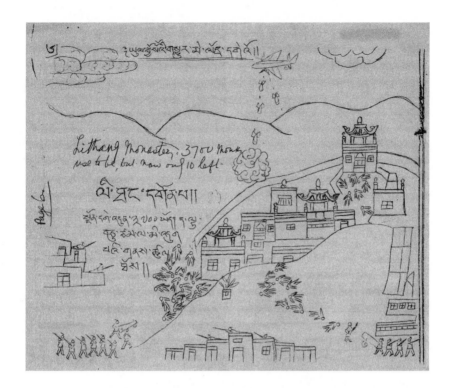

Figure 13.3 Eyewitness account of Chinese attacks on Tibetan monasteries (from Tharchin's *Mirror* newspaper, Dec. 10, 1956)

"Bernard's account of the purposes of the various systems can hardly be termed profound."[22]

Others alluded to Theos in less than flattering terms.[23] Nonetheless, between *Haṭha Yoga* and *Heaven Lies Within Us*, his works continued to have popular appeal and continued to inspire subsequent generations of readers to travel to India and pursue the study of yoga and Buddhism. Allen Ginsberg, having read *Penthouse of the Gods*, made his way to Gangtok and Dharamsala in search of tantric empowerments.[24] Philip Glass had read Theos Bernard's books as a young man and was so inspired by them that he traveled to Darjeeling and Kalimpong to meet Tharchin himself. Throughout the 1960s and '70s, many more would follow in their footsteps, as Theos came to be seen as the man who blazed the trail for young Americans seeking authentic Indian religion.

Back in California, with Theos's will finally in effect, Glen inherited the remainder of his trust fund from Viola and his stocks, but could not gain access to Theos's 1947 India acquisitions in storage in Los Angeles because Helen claimed the contents of the storage locker for herself, asserting that she had paid for its contents, and even threatened a lawsuit. Resolving the dispute, they agreed to have the entire collection cataloged and contacted Ferdinand Lessing at the University of California at Berkeley. Lessing agreed to help and sent his graduate student, Alex Wayman, down to Glen's house outside of Los Angeles to catalog Theos's library and collection of Tibetan art and artifacts.[25] With this new accounting, Glen and Helen divided the collection between themselves based on Helen's receipts and the inventory packing lists from Kalimpong ten years earlier. Helen managed to keep possession of the personal books and manuscripts that he had had in India with her. She had a bookplate stamp made for herself similar to Theos's original one and proceeded to stamp the remaining books as hers.

Glen immediately offered his share of Theos's books for sale, and the Harvard-Yenching Library quickly bought Lord Tsarong's personal copy of the Derge Kangyur and Tengyur, while the State Library in West Berlin purchased both copies of the Lhasa Kangyur.[26] A few years later, Wesley E. Needham negotiated with Eleanore Murray to buy close to four hundred Tibetan books for the Yale Library.[27] Although Glen and Eleanore also tried to sell many of the artifacts Theos had acquired in Tibet, no museum seemed interested in them.

Thus, while in America, Glen and Eleanore could find no one interested in purchasing their Tibetan artifacts, in Chinese-occupied Tibet, such items were being actively destroyed. Even more troubling, word was slowly coming out of Tibet that the high-ranking lamas and the abbots of monasteries were being "invited" to Beijing and were not returning. Consequently, a plan was devised by the Rockefeller Foundation, with the assistance of the CIA, to bring a small number of high-ranking Tibetan lamas out of Tibet along with their families and place them at major institutions around the world—London, Paris, Rome, Copenhagen, Leiden, Munich, Tokyo—wherever there seemed to be facilities and scholars eager for the opportunity to study. Dezhung Rinpoche, from the same Sakya lineage that Theos had visited in Tibet, was placed at the CIA's main language research center at the University of Washington in Seattle, and soon began to draw students interested more in religion than in language and politics.[28] Similarly, on the East Coast, although Theos had envisioned a school "something along the line of the training of the Lamas at Drepung monastery" as the ideal model for a school in either "Beverly Hills or Hollywood," when Geshe Wangyal set up precisely such a school, it ended up in the somewhat less scenic northern New Jersey. Still, students came,[29] and Geshe Wangyal oversaw a strict but genuinely compassionate environment. With Geshe Wangyal on the East Coast and Dezhung Rinpoche on the West Coast, Tibetan studies in America had officially begun.

Although these few were lucky enough to escape Tibet, many others were not. In 1958, the new Panchen Lama, only a few years younger than the Dalai Lama, went to China and did not return. In a secret meeting of the Tibetan cabinet, it was decided that the young Fourteenth Dalai Lama should be secreted out of Tibet since it was clear that the Chinese Communist forces would be coming for him next, and they began coordinating efforts to get him safely to India.

Although Lord Tsarong and his family had since moved to Kalimpong, when he heard that the escape of the Fourteenth Dalai Lama was being planned, Lord Tsarong himself returned to Tibet to help with the effort. By March 1959, the stage was set, but the situation in Lhasa was tense. The city was overcrowded, not only by the Chinese military but also by thousands of refugees from eastern Tibet fleeing the persecution and violence being unleashed there. The young Dalai Lama was at the Norbu Lingka, the summer palace, when the Chinese general in charge of Lhasa "invited" him to come to the military camp alone and without his bodyguards. Hearing the news, the people of Lhasa flooded into the streets and surrounded the summer palace, but the Chinese threatened to bombard the palace if the Dalai Lama did not emerge immediately. When word of the threat got out, monks in the surrounding monasteries headed into town and broke into the weapons caches left by the British to fight the Chinese in defense of their leader, and on March 10, 1959, the Tibetan Uprising against the Chinese occupation of Lhasa began. Having led the rearguard action to secure the safety of the Thirteenth Dalai Lama in 1909, Lord Tsarong took his place in Lhasa once more to do the same thing again, and at the age of seventy-four, led the fighting in the streets against the Chinese, this time on behalf of the Fourteenth Dalai Lama.

While the Chinese were bombarding the summer palace with mortar shells in an attempt to kill or drive out the Dalai Lama and his entourage, unbeknownst to all but a few, His Holiness had snuck out of the palace grounds the night before, disguised as a common guard, and was already on his way south toward India. In Lhasa, the Tibetans were no match for the modern Chinese weaponry they faced. Many were killed and others, including Lord Tsarong, were captured. Others, mostly monks, were pursued out of the city into the mountains and back to their monasteries. One monk from the Go-mang College at Drepung remembered hearing the fighting and the sounds of artillery. Packing a few books and some food into a bag, he headed out the back gate of Drepung and started climbing the mountain behind the monastery. Looking back as he got to the top of the hill, he saw a mortar shell fly in and strike his college. Knowing that he was witnessing the end of an era, he turned, crossed the peak, and began his own long walk to India and into exile. Not all were so lucky. With many Tibetans dead or taken prisoner, the last few fighters took refuge in the astro-medical college on the peak of Chakpori hill opposite the Potala Palace, where they had the advantage of elevation. Backing off from the mountain, the Chinese artillery opened fire on the peak, completely destroying the college, and continued firing until they had obliterated the upper fifty feet of the mountain as well.

The Chinese, however, had failed in their ultimate goal, and weeks later, the Fourteenth Dalai Lama reached the safety of India, where he and eventually thousands of Tibetan refugees who would follow were granted asylum by Prime Minister Nehru. But his escape had come at a terrible cost. Three months later, sitting in Kalimpong, Tharchin would hear a report that struck him personally: Lord Tsarong was dead. A true nobleman in every sense of the word, Lord Tsarong had made the ultimate sacrifice for his country, for his people, and for their leader.

Printing a picture of him in full uniform from his military days, Tharchin published his obituary in *The Mirror*.[30] As with many of the articles that Tharchin authored for his paper, the report had a personal touch:

Some extremely sad news: Recently, on the 14th day of June, under the power of unbearably bad conditions, Lord Tsarong, supreme and great lord of the earth, passed away in Lhasa. When I heard this unpleasant news, I fell into a state of deep sadness.

About the supreme Lord Tsarong: His pure actions and intentions were always in accordance with those of both incarnations of the Powerful Conqueror [the Dalai Lama]—indeed, any actions or plans, peaceful or wrathful, of the supreme government—and he was a man whose deeds were carried out in service at the feet of the Precious Conqueror with heroism, skillfulness, and good character. Not only that, but earlier, on the occasion of the conflict with the British in the Wood Dragon year

[1904], for the great purposes of [preserving] the Buddha's Teachings and the government, at that time he guarded His Holiness [the Dalai Lama] on his journeys in Mongolia and China, having entered into service at the feet of the Precious Conqueror at a young age. Also, in the Water Mouse year[31] on the occasion of the arrival of the Chinese army under Liu-chung, having once more entered into his service on this journey, while His Holiness was en route to India, without any regard for his own life or his own well-being, he protected the life of His Holiness through fierce fighting against the Chinese army at Chaksam Ferry. After exercising his might in this way, he joined His Holiness in India.

Later, in connection with his status as Commander-in-Chief, having returned to Tibet, once again he put an end to the Chinese army, driving them out and sending them away. Since he cast out those who remained from the plateau of Tibet, in accordance with the Department of Defense, he was made General of the Lhasa Army and Protector of the Teachings of the Land of Snows. From the very start, in connection with training and instruction in occasional military exercises and so forth, he established a new military administration for all of Tibet, a military barracks, and so on. In connection with his activities in the Department of Public Security, he was made a Minister (*bka' blon*) of the Tibetan Cabinet (*bka' shag*). Furthermore, he established the new Trapshi Electric Power Plant, and established a new mint, post office, secretariat, telegraph office, and so forth. By building a new textile factory and court-system, for example, through his virtue he benefited both the government and the common people. In short, he set a high and respectable mark in whatever he did at the highest levels or the most mundane. Since this produced a pure image of him in the minds of all the nobles, common people, his opponents, and others, he came to be a worthy object of praise. Recently, because of the severe repression by the Red Chinese, he suddenly passed away. This supreme venerable lord, in his previous actions, in his radiance, in his knowledge, and in his unrestrained courage, completed his final thought at the age of seventy-four.

As a result, unbearable anguish arose in the hearts of his relatives, his circle of friends, and his dependents, indeed, in all the people of Tibet, great or small. His sons, daughters, relatives, and circle of friends, without giving way to feelings of sadness, for the sake of this very venerable lord and for the purpose of engaging in virtuous activities, have made this earnest and heartfelt prayer, I beg of you to take responsibility for the general well-being of the government and the Teachings of the Buddha in a manner equal to the previous deeds of this very venerable man.

The body of the supreme Lord Tsarong has gone far away from us, but his good deeds will never depart but always stay in our hearts.

This I write in a state of deep sadness.

It was not his first obituary for someone that he knew, and it would not be Tharchin's last. Over the years that followed, the events unfolding in Tibet and in the rest of central Asia would take their toll in very human terms, and even those who escaped Tibet were not immune from their effects.

Back in the 1940s, after the Fourteenth Dalai Lama had been identified and the young boy and his family relocated to Lhasa, Reting Rinpoche, still acting as Regent, was under pressure from various quarters to step down. As Regent, he was responsible for conferring monk's vows upon the young Dalai Lama. It was common knowledge, however, that he had long since broken his own vows—specifically his vow of celibacy, in dalliances with men and women—and was therefore incapable of conferring vows upon anyone. Should he go through with the ceremony, it would be a sham and the new Dalai Lama would not receive a valid "transmission." Agreeing to step down—temporarily—as Regent, Reting had appointed his old teacher, Taktra Rinpoche,[32] in his stead. When years later he attempted to regain his former position in the government through force, his efforts only landed him in prison, where he would die under uncertain circumstances.

Following his final fall, his personal papers were searched and in them, correspondence between himself and Namkye Tsedrön was found—letters in which Reting had confessed his love for her and pleaded with her to leave her husband, the Gyantse fort commander. To expose "the corruption" of the Regent, the letters were posted on the walls in the streets of Lhasa for all to see, but the real effect was that Namkye Tsedrön was humiliated. Living in Gyantse, close to the Indian border, it was easy for Chokte and his wife to escape to India when the time came to flee the Chinese. They arrived like so many others in Kalimpong, though eventually moved to the Kulu Valley. But after a short time, Namkye Tsedrön found that life in exile was proving unbearable, and less than a year later, the women regarded by many as one of the most beautiful in Tibet took her own life with an overdose of sleeping pills. Once again Tharchin would be forced to write a heartfelt obituary for someone he had known and who had befriended him.

VERY UNPLEASANT NEWS

A while ago, the lord, former treasurer, the governor, Chokte [together with his] spouse, were staying in the area of Kulu and were engaged with uninterrupted effort in wholesome virtuous practices. Suddenly, the supreme consort's health slightly worsened, and in this way her hold on this life was no more. When I heard this, immediately and all at once, I fell into a state of deep sorrow. About this venerable consort: since the time of her childhood, she had a good nature and not only did she have respect and great love for her supreme lord [Chokte], but she also cared for [her] servants and those under her like [a mother] warming her own children. She had virtuous disposition being protectful, skillful, and more.

The lord Chokte, many years ago having retired from government service, saw all the marvelous things that are possible in this world to be without an essence, and so in order to make this life of leisure and fortune meaningful, on White Skull Mountain at Shuksep Hermitage, together with his honorable spouse engaged in retreat practices in consultation over many years at the feet of Ma-chig Je-tsun Rigdzin Chönyi Wangmo,[33] and so on. Later, in many holy places in regions of Tibet, Sikkim, and Bhutan, they did retreats countless times. They also came to India in connection with medical treatment and on pilgrimage, and just last year they were engaged in retreat practices at the Ḍākīnī's Abode in Kulita (or Kulu). Thus, although the venerable consort's hold on this life has come to an end, we ask those who were looked after by the great lady, her relatives, and her circle of friends not to give way to feelings of sadness. For, although we are parted from this supreme great lady, for the sake of this venerable consort, make offerings and worship in the various holy places in India and various monasteries. Thank you.

Now, without giving way to feelings of sadness, please take up virtuous deeds and do not be lowly. For, as it says in the *Categorical Sayings:*[34]

From that very first moment, the night
One enters the womb,

A person cannot remain and moves on, and
From where one has gone, one cannot return.

In the morning one sees many people,
But in the evening some will not be seen.
In the evening we see many people,
But in the morning some will not be seen.

When many men and women
Die even at a young age,
In saying "this person is young,"
Why is there such fierce confidence in their staying alive?

The end of all accumulation is exhaustion;
The end of erecting is falling down.
The end of meeting is separation;
The end of living is death.

All of us, ourselves and others, sooner or later and without exception, will be without any means whatsoever of avoiding the karmic predispositions of this path. Thus, I ask that henceforth, may we concentrate our strength on pure, virtuous actions as provisions for the road ahead.[35]

Not without his own problems—financial troubles that never seemed to end—two years later, Tharchin ceased publication of his newspaper, despite being offered a substantial sum of money and guaranteed subscriptions by the Chinese authorities if he would publish pro-Chinese articles. With the Tibetan exile community growing and Tibetan-language newspapers such as *Freedom* and others beginning to be published, Tharchin decided to put his efforts instead into the orphanage that he and his wife had established years earlier.

Back in America, still depressed over the death of his son, Glen took the passage of time hard. Often, he would spend his evenings with his small 16-mm film projector, watching Theos in his 1937 films of Tibet over and over again until the films were scorched and destroyed. Eventually the emotional weight of it all caught up with him, and one afternoon Eleanore came home to find Glen standing alone in the backyard of their home, crying and dumping box and after box of Theos's letters and papers into a blazing fire in a large metal drum. Dousing the fire and salvaging what she could, Eleanore tried to convince Glen that Theos's legacy was worth saving. Just the same, Glen made a point of systematically destroying all record of their activities together that he could, shredding and excising his son's letters to him discussing sexual yogas and the specific ayurvedic compounds they were obtaining and ingesting.

As time went on, Glen saw his brothers pass on, one by one: P.A. in 1955, then Irven and Ray. Transferring ownership of the house to Eleanore, Glen drafted his own will, leaving everything to Eleanore and his last surviving brother, Clyde, and declaring that if they should predecease him, his estate was to be split between the "Benieke Rare Book & Manuscript Library" at Yale University and the University of Washington at Seattle. "It is my desire," he wrote, "that the two foregoing charitable gifts be devoted to the use of translation of Tibetan [*sic*] literature by worthy, needy, qualified scholars who are devotees of the Buddhist philosophy. It is my further desire that said charitable gifts be maintained by the respective universities as a memorial to the memory of my son, Dr. Theos C. Bernard." As for the personal papers that remained, Glen left his final instructions to Eleanore: "Do not burden yourself with a lot of useless papers, destroy everything."

But in his final years, Glen began to slowly go blind. Writing to Viola in the early 1970s, he expressed his despondency over the way fate had judged them all. He told Viola that he was being held prisoner by an insane woman and, feeling that his brother Clyde was near death, he had every intention of leaving Eleanore to move into his brother's house as soon as possible afterward. But it never happened. Spending his last years completely blind, Glen died in 1976, at the age of ninety-two, still under Eleanore's care.

Unbeknownst to Glen, in 1966 an unidentified man came forth claiming to have information about the death of Theos and sought out Tharchin in Kalimpong. Tharchin passed the new information on to the American embassy in New Delhi, and thence to the U.S. State Department who wrote to Theos's youngest brother, Marvene, at the time a J.A.G. officer in Georgia. The letter read:

I am writing in reference to the 1947 disappearance of your brother, Dr. Theos Bernard, in the Kulu Valley, India. The American Embassy at New Delhi has received a communication from a G. Tharchin in New Delhi.

Mr. Tharchin states that he was Dr. Bernard's interpreter during his visit to Tibet in 1937 and that he sent one of his servants with Dr. Bernard on his fateful trip to Lahouli-Spiti in August 1947. The writer further declares that he has received information from a friend concerning the fate of Dr. Bernard, namely, that this friend can identify the man who murdered Dr. Bernard. Mr. Tharchin states, however, that this person, who has requested him to write to the United States Government about this, expects some reward for his information.

The Embassy has referred Mr. Tharchin's letter to the Department for guidance, particularly with respect to the question of a reward. As you will appreciate, the Indian police are the appropriate authorities to investigate a matter of this type but it is conceivable that the offer of a reward might produce some significant information. The Department would appreciate being advised regarding whether you have a personal interest in the above information in order that a decision may be made as to how to respond to Mr. Tharchin.

Offended at the suggestion that they should have to bribe someone in India to obtain such information, neither Marvene nor anyone else in the family ever responded.

As for Viola, after founding the Childrens' Psychiatric program at Columbia Presbyterian Hospital in New York, testifying before congressional committees, and being an active member in the American Psychiatric Association, she retired in the 1980s. Deciding to spend the remaining years of her life compiling her personal papers and those of both Pierre Bernard and Blanche DeVries, which she had inherited, she hired assistants to help, gave interviews to various individuals, and collaborated with members of the Arizona Historical Society in Tucson, who were compiling an archive on Theos. However, she was more than slightly disturbed when she received a letter from Eleanore Murray, introducing herself and claiming she "felt I know you" from having lived with Glen and having read all of Viola's letters to Theos and his to her.

Replying to Eleanore, Viola arranged to visit her in California. Arriving at Glen's old home, Viola found Eleanore living in the house with the walls and shelves filled with Tibetan art and artifacts, books and ephemera, the collateral remnants of Theos's life. Although they had a relatively pleasant meeting, Viola found Eleanore to be confused, alternately claiming that Glen had been her "guru" and that he had abused her and kept her "in hypnosis" all those years. Doing her best not to comment, the only sentiment Viola expressed was her regret over never obtaining a copy of the films from her trip with Theos around the world, and that if those still survived, she would be interested in seeing them again.

She did not hear from Eleanore afterward, and only from a mutual acquaintance learned that Eleanore had flown into a paranoid rage after Viola left, claiming that she was trying to steal Theos's materials from her. Lamenting the sad state of affairs in California, Viola dismissed the possibility of working with Eleanore to preserve these things, telling a friend she hoped that eventually Theos's materials would find a safe home befitting their value instead of remaining "in the depths of that woman's madness."

Eleanore continued to utilize what Theos had brought back from Tibet to her own ends. As individuals from time to time would "discover" Theos Bernard (a distant relative or yoga aficionado), they would contact Viola, while the more resourceful ones would find Eleanore. One such man contacted her, and she became convinced that he was the reincarnation of Theos Bernard come back to seek out the details of his former life and even gave him some of Theos's old possessions, disposing of the materials as she saw fit.[36]

Helen, following her retirement, had resumed her dream journal and gotten more and more interested in dream theory. For many years, she remained committed to the vision of life that Theos had instilled in her and even kept their portraits on her bedside table. In the 1970s, Helen encouraged her niece to pursue an interest in Tibet and Tibetan Buddhism, even funding her travel to India to study. In her later years, however, Helen became disillusioned with Theos, deciding that he had "only been using her" as a tantric consort.

By the late 1990s, all three women, the de facto curators of Theos Bernard's legacy, had died. Viola had organized, researched, and censored every aspect of Theos's life and the life of his uncle Pierre that she could, leaving the rest for posterity. Helen's collection of Theos's materials was almost lost when a dispute arose over her niece's inheritance, but was saved in the end and a private foundation established to care for it. Eleanore, however, had done far more damage than good to her portion of the collection over the years. When she died intestate in 1998, the same week as Viola, the house and its contents were seized by the State of California. Suffering from mildew, dry rot, and insect infestation, what remained of

Theos's effects were offered up for bidding to various institutions. Eventually the collection was donated to the University of California at Berkeley, where after preliminary cataloging, its contents were distributed as raw materials acquisitions to seven different divisions of the university, none of which had ever heard of Theos. Such was the final resting place of the legacy of Theos Bernard.

FOURTEEN

Postscript

The View from Ki, Sixty Years Later

I went in search of astral America, not social and cultural America, but
the America of the empty, absolute freedom of the freeways, not the deep
America of mores and mentalities, but the America of desert speed . . . a
fractal, interstitial culture, born of a rift with the Old World.

— JEAN BAUDRILLARD[1]

IN 1972, A NEWSPAPER REPORTER in Arizona, stumbling across the
story of Theos Bernard, wrote an article declaring: "The 'White Lama' Must
Be Dead, Most Agree Now."

> Even the most optimistic now agree that Theos Casimir Bernard, possi-
> bly the only white man in modern history to be made a lama of Tibetan
> Buddhism is dead.
>
> This is the 25th anniversary of the disappearance of this colorful, ro-
> mantic, handsome Tucsonan into the forbidding, and forbidden moun-
> tains of Tibet. The report that he was shot to death by angry hillmen in
> a case of mistaken identity must be true.

But not all would agree. Already by the late 1950s there were stories
circulating in India of a white man, a yogi, who from time to time would
be spotted in the mountains. One story told of an obviously Anglo yogi
seen near a mountain spring in a Himalayan vale, attended by three native women; some went so far as to identify him as Theos Bernard. It was
a story that Helen (and her astrologer) considered at least plausible. But
this was just one story.

In the northwest corner of India, just over the mountain ranges from the Kulu Valley and Lahoul, lay Khunu, birthplace of Tharchin. There, the venerated abbot known as Khunu Lama—like many others in the 1970s and 1980s—had begun to welcome Western students to his teachings . . . and he had an interesting story to tell.

According to Khunu Lama, in the late 1940s an American from California was attacked in the Lahoul–Spiti area. Escaping his captors, the man made his way to a Buddhist monastery, where he joined a group of monks traveling to eastern Tibet. After they arrived at Dzokchen Monastery, the man received teachings on the Nyingma tantric practice of the "Great Perfection" and entered into retreat in the upstairs room of a Tibetan house. After three years of intensive retreat, the lama further reported, he achieved full enlightenment in the form of a "rainbow body." The moral of the story, Khunu Lama reiterated to his students, was that as benighted as Americans were, *even an American* could achieve enlightenment—so *they* had no excuse.

The idea that enlightenment was a possibility for all was not a unique declaration by Tibetan lamas in exile in the 1970s and beyond. Lama Yeshe and Lama Zopa, who founded the Foundation for the Preservation of the Mahayana Tradition, were strong advocates of meditative retreats and the realistic possibility of enlightenment—even if they did not cite prior examples. In America, much as yoga had been popularized in the 1930s, Zen Buddhism in the 1950s, and Hinduism and Vedanta in the 1960s, after the fall from popular opinion of several Hindu gurus, by the 1970s and early 1980s Tibetan Buddhism seemed to be gaining ground and about to have its turn.

In popular music, references to Tibet and Tibetan Buddhism were beginning to be heard across the airwaves, from intimations of the doctrine of emptiness and the exhortation to bodhisattvas to the murmuring of the Heart Sūtra and the personal mantra of the Sixteenth Karmapa.[2] For several years in the 1970s, television viewers could watch the exploits of a Chinese Buddhist monk in the nineteenth-century American West fighting evildoers and defending the rights of the helpless.[3] In movies as well, there was an observable trend, with the popular comedian Bill Murray at the forefront of high-profile actors making repeated explicit and implicit references to Tibet and Buddhist themes in his films—from comedic claims of having served as a golf caddie for the Dalai Lama in Tibet to the trials of a man trapped in a cyclic existence,[4] even remaking the Theos Bernard dramatization, *The Razor's Edge*.[5]

With the bestowal of the Nobel Peace Prize upon His Holiness the Fourteenth Dalai Lama in 1989, Tibet and Tibetan Buddhism became securely planted as fixtures of Western culture, despite the fact that he had been authoring books for Western audiences for many years before. It was, in fact, one of those books that had aroused my interest in Tibetan Buddhist philosophy and ultimately led to my researching the life of Theos Bernard.

Coming to the field of Tibetan and Buddhist studies with a background in the "hard" sciences, I was dismayed when informed that the academic literature of Tibetan Buddhism—certainly in English, though to a lesser extent in Tibetan as well—was a far cry from a more or less homogeneous and unified, concerted effort by an academic community to explicate a single coherent subject. Instead, I learned, scholars in "the humanities" division of academia resembled more a fractious and contentious coalition born of necessity than a community united by a single purpose or agenda.

Attempting to grapple with the extant literature, I discovered that the twentieth-century field of Tibetan studies was just sectarian as medieval Tibet and was populated by proponents of various intellectual lineages (or "methodological disciplines"), each claiming the moral high ground of "objectivity" and "legitimate research," spanning the spectrum from Marx and Jung to Chogyam Trungpa and Dezhung Rinpoche. Only superficially aware of the choice I had made in picking a graduate school program, I found that I was studying in the lineage of Geshe Wangyal.

Having committed myself to this new career choice, I began as I had been taught to do as a young student in the sciences, by compiling—as completely and comprehensively as possible—a collection of the existing literature on my subject of interest in order to assess its content, its consistency with other analyses, and its agreement with the source literature in Tibetan and Sanskrit. In the process of amassing such a Tibetan and Buddhist studies library in the late 1990s, I stumbled upon a slightly worn first-edition copy of Theos Bernard's *Penthouse of the Gods* in a used bookstore in central Virginia.

Subtitled "A Pilgrimage into the Heart of Tibet and the Sacred City of Lhasa," the book appeared to be yet another pseudo-Orientalist travelogue. Though amused, I was also confused by the wealth of exquisitely detailed photographs and the seemingly accurate knowledge of the city of Lhasa in the mid-twentieth century contained within it. I decided to purchase the book for my personal reference library for the scant six dollars being asked. Only later that evening, as I sat down to catalogue the day's acquisitions, did I discover that the author was a strange individual who seemed to have passed unnoticed into the dustbin of American religious history. Over the months and years that followed, I dug deeper into the life of Theos Bernard, tracking down numerous primary source materials that revealed the life of a relatively unknown and forgotten American pioneer of Tibetan Buddhism.

Entering the Ph.D. program in religion at Columbia University a few years later, I happened to be present during the two hundred and fiftieth anniversary of the founding of the university. Responding to a solicitation for contributions, I constructed a series of Web pages for the celebratory project.[6] Bringing all the material that I had amassed together, I constructed my first coherent narrative of the life of Theos Bernard. As I consolidated and organized my resources for this task, I realized that Bernard and I shared three hometowns (Tucson, Arizona; Taos, New Mexico; and New York City), two *alma maters* (the University of Arizona and Columbia University), and the same (*param-*)*guru* (Geshe Wangyal). When I showed what I had produced to my advisor, he suggested that I write Bernard's biography,[7] so I took the project on as a distraction/procrastination from my main research, a translation and study of the works of the ninth-century Buddhist tantric master Buddhaśrījñānapāda.

As the time approached for me to begin writing my dissertation, as a diversion, every few weeks I would spend a couple of days working on the Bernard project. When it came time to embark on fieldwork for my dissertation, however, I found that the only funding opportunities available were related to my ongoing research on Theos Bernard. So, having already processed Helen's archive, I accepted a position as archivist for the Theos Bernard Papers at U.C. Berkeley and after discussions with my advisor, made Theos Bernard my new dissertation subject, and my research shifted from ninth-century Indian tantra to twentieth-century American religious history.

From reading her transcribed interviews, I learned that from time to time Viola Bernard had been contacted by distant relatives of Theos's family who discovered and became intrigued by stories about their cousin. I soon began to experience a similar phenomenon; however, I was contacted not by Theos's relatives but by his admirers and even individuals claiming to be his reincarnation. While many people were simply intrigued by the man, wanting to know more about him, others were more serious in their commitment to what they perceived as his "agenda." What additional information had I learned about Bernard's tantric lineage? What additional details on tantric practices had I uncovered in his unpublished papers? and similar such questions soon became a fairly regular part of my Internet "presence." One person, believing himself to be Theos Bernard's reincarnation, was more persistent and soon began to dog my footsteps, even contacting my friends and colleagues, attempting to obtain copies of my research in service of his own agenda.

Though they were acting out of what I can only assume were good intentions, it seemed that the involvement of these individuals in the struggle over the identity of Theos Bernard—in his previous life or this presumed one—was yet another symptom of the larger obsession of some Americans with the more glamorous aspects of Tibetan Buddhist culture, including the mystique of reincarnation. While it could have been a relatively harmless amusement, it seemed to me more of an attempt by some to perpetuate the myths of Tibet as well as the myths of America—an attempt that could only take place and succeed through denying the realities of Tibet, both political and religious, and masking the genuine accomplishments of that society with fantasies about Tibet and, for those attempting to participate in it, fantasies about themselves.

Given my familiarity with the geographic regions that Bernard inhabited, the subjects he studied, and the languages of the cultures with which he interacted, I realized that I was in a unique position to produce an academically responsible assessment of his life and work. Determined to do this to the best of my abilities and detail the truths behind Bernard's claims—his fabrications as well as his genuine accomplishments—given the amount of work I had done, initially only incidentally as a distraction, I felt that the responsibility to tell his story had circumstantially fallen upon my shoulders. With no vested interest in the outcome, I hoped to reconstruct the actual events of his life. Having done all I could with the primary resources at my disposal, I had only one task remaining before me—besides transforming my notes into a single narrative—to retrace Bernard's 1937 and 1947 trips to India and Tibet and gather whatever information existed there, even if only impressionistically.

I had been to India a number of times before and could remember quite vividly the experience of arriving in the "land of the Āryas." Indeed, everything was just as I had remembered: a sense of slight disorientation, the queasy stomach, and all-around strange, yet somehow familiar smells and sounds mixed together with the sights of privation and suffering—the kinds that are deftly masked in America—that impact a person on a deep, visceral level. With each visit, I was becoming more emotionally comfortable with the subcontinent. Even if at times it was not a physically comfortable experience, daily life in India was, on some level, honest—and it was something I had always appreciated and admired about the country.

Making my way from New Delhi eastward, I visited Calcutta, Kalimpong, and Darjeeling for the first time. Having organized and studied Bernard's more than 9,000 photographs taken in 1936–37, even 70 years later, I could still easily recognize many places in Kalimpong and Darjeeling. There was a quaint, almost nostalgic feel to Kalimpong, a town that still evinced its colonial heritage. From the bazaar and markets on the same streets that Bernard had walked through—remarkably similar to the photographs I had seen—to Tharchin's *Tibet Mirror Press* headquarters, boarded shut for many years, dusty, rusting, and abandoned, it all left me with a sort of *faux déjà vu*. Even the Himalayan Hotel conveyed—to my imagination at least—the feeling of old British India, with its high oak-beam ceilings and a verandah on which I spent many hours drinking tea and looking out over the hills in the distance at the snow-capped Himalayan peaks, just as Bernard had done so many years before. In Darjeeling, I found many signs of the past, including Jinorasa's YMBA—now an elementary school—and even a few remnants of Gedun Chöpel's activities.[8]

It was in Tibet, however, that my time would be both most rewarding and most frustrating. After a series of tedious and typically Chinese bureaucratic obstacles, I finally reached Lhasa. Passing Lord Tsarong's iron Trisam bridge, like Bernard and presumably so many others, I too felt a certain degree of awe and charge of excitement at my first glimpse of the Potala Palace. But before our taxi from the airport had even reached the Western Gate, it was clear that the Lhasa *I* knew, the Lhasa I had studied pictures of, read about, and anticipated seeing, was gone. The Potala Palace, which had marked the western edge of the city, was now at the center of the sort of concrete and cinder-block sprawl that passed for a city back in China, here transplanted and grafted (in all senses of the word) onto the austere landscape of Tibet.

It had taken Bernard months to travel around Tibet, and soon I learned that it could easily take me months as well, given the restrictions and

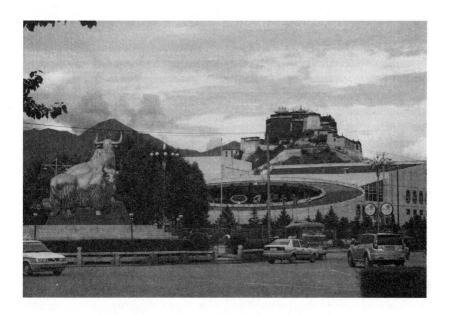

Figure 14.1 Lhasa under Chinese governance (photo by the author)

paranoia of Tibet's Chinese colonial overlords. Nonetheless, I was determined to make the best of the situation. The Jokhang and Ramoche temples seemed like the first places to start and although it was claimed otherwise, the buddhas housed there appeared substantially different from Bernard's photos taken prior to their confiscation and presumable destruction by the Chinese Red Guard during Mao's reign of terror, the Cultural Revolution. The Potala Palace, now run by the Chinese government as a tourist attraction, was rather depressing. With many walls stripped bare and other areas—like the Namgyal College—forbidden to access, I found enjoyment where I could, from talking with an old geshe from Tsang whose dialect was so close to that of my Tibetan teacher in America that it immediately cheered me up, to a kitten sleeping in a basket among the gold *stūpa*s of former Dalai Lamas, peaceful and oblivious as the iconic cat at the *parinirvāṇa* of the Buddha. Even in the absence of any obvious Chinese presence, there were the ubiquitous obnoxious, clueless reporters—the only kind the Chinese authorities tried to allow in.

Walking through the Potala two days after July 3, 2006—the date of the arrival of the first train on the completed Qinghai–Tibet railway and its attendant propaganda and fanfare—I became forcibly aware of this fact.

Postscript: The View from Ki, Sixty Years Later

In addition to ferrying Chinese passengers and officials, the train carried more than fifty foreign journalists to cover the event, chosen, presumably (based on my experiences with those I met) for their lack of knowledge of any and all aspects of Tibetan language, culture, religion, and history, and therefore the perfect vacuous vehicles for conveying Chinese propaganda about Tibet to the outside world.[9] Encountering an American journalist speaking Chinese to a Tibetan monk in one of the shrine rooms, I interrupted her to speak to the monk in his own language; the sorts of questions she subsequently asked me revealed her utter ignorance about where she was and the dynamics of the situation the Tibetan people were in. Did I know of any Tibetans who had pictures of the Dalai Lama in their homes? she asked—foolishly unaware, apparently, that such photographs were illegal. I found myself taking pains to explain that I did not and could not visit Tibetans in their homes since it would open them to scrutiny by the Chinese secret police and could make life difficult for, if not endanger them. She seemed to find this incredulous, as if Lhasa were no different from a Connecticut suburb. My contempt for her clearly marginal qualifications as an educated and informed journalist—which I only half-heartedly attempted to mask—led me to apologize to the monk for the embarrassing stupidity of my fellow American before taking my leave.

Wandering the streets of Lhasa looking for various landmarks was no less frustrating. I had more or less memorized Peter Aufschnaiter's map of Lhasa, but the old streets were now crowded by Chinese shops. Even the tourist maps being sold in front of the Jokhang were of no use—available only in Chinese or English translations of the Chinese, which rendered street and place names in an absurd sinified caricature of the Tibetan language, something the Chinese government called "Tibetan Pinyin." Left to my own devices, I hoped to spot something not obliterated beyond recognition. Exploring on my own was a little dangerous, but fortunately I had a cover story.

A few months before leaving for India and Tibet, I had attended a family gathering and, talking with relatives about my research, I gave the brief version of Theos Bernard's life. One of them told me something that if I had known, I had forgotten: my great-grandfather's last name was Bernard. Immediately I had a sinking feeling. Although I had taken the fact that Bernard and I had shared *alma maters* and interests as nothing more that a strange synchronicity, now there was the possibility that I was researching not just an intellectual predecessor but "cousin Theos." In all truth, the thought sent a shiver down my spine. Still, I realized that having neither confirmed nor disproven any actual biological relation to the man, I could conveniently and honestly make the claim either way.

Consequently, when asked—and I was—what I was doing running around the Lhasa Valley with photos from the 1930s, a camera, and a notepad, I could reply that a relative of mine had visited Lhasa seventy years earlier, and I was trying to retrace his steps and see what he had seen. It was an answer that appeared to satisfy most people. Soon, however, I realized that I knew more about twentieth-century Tibet than most Tibetans living in Lhasa, at least those of the younger generation. A notable example was the fact that contemporary Chinese education and Tibetan-language documents were engaged in what could only be an attempt to erase the name of Tsarong from history,[10] and with the complicity of some Western scholars, to go so far as to wipe Tibet, literally, "from the map."[11] Wandering through the streets south of the Jokhang, with great difficulty I located the Tsarong estate, eventually finding an elderly Tibetan woman who, without stopping, informed me under her breath that I was *on* the grounds of the estate. Hoping to see the old home of this great man, I learned that as an act of revenge against the man who had thwarted Chinese machinations in Tibet not once or twice, but three times in a row, the Chinese had incorporated the bulk of Tsarong's estate (and the adjacent prime minister's estate) within a sealed military compound, and had even begun demolishing his house, smashing the walls and roof and leaving it open to the elements. In typical Chinese overcompensation, the same held true at Chaksam Ferry, where the Chinese had been defeated by Lord Tsarong in 1909. The site was now a large Chinese military establishment that I was advised not to go near.

At the three great monastic universities of Drepung, Sera, and Ganden, the destruction by the Chinese was still quite evident despite the attempt to rebuild Ganden in particular, and all three were still crawling with Chinese "political re-education" squads, whom I was also told to avoid, even though I had a valid tourist pass. Even Reting Monastery, which had been built in 1075 in a secluded valley, had been razed to the ground, leaving only the *stūpas* and a small courtyard, presided over by a small boy—and his Chinese handlers—being groomed as a Chinese puppet to "pick" the next Dalai Lama when the time came. Back in Lhasa, Reting's famous personal residence with its glass wall and gardens had also been destroyed by the Chinese during the Cultural Revolution, and no trace of it remained. Worse yet, I learned that the destruction was continuing. At Dra-yer-pa, the site of Bernard's only actual empowerment in Tibet, ten years earlier the entire monastery and retreat caves had been torn down and rebuilt to conform with Chinese notions of suitable tourist structures.

South and west, the situation was not that much better. At Gyantse, large sections of the monastery had been obliterated, and the old administrative fort was vacant, except for absurd dioramas depicting Tibet's "degenerate" past. In garbage heaps scattered around the hill, I even found loose manuscript pages of the fourteenth-century handwritten Kangyur and Tengyur that had once been housed at the monastery and were now being sold for ten dollars a page by Chinese curio shops in Lhasa. All points south of Gyantse—Phari, Gautse, Yatung—were off limits and inaccessible to all foreigners other than the Chinese themselves. Although the Chinese presence in Gyantse was not as noticeable as in Lhasa, the situation in Shigatse was much worse. The old fort there, which had rivaled the Potala in size, had been bombarded by Chinese artillery until only the foundations remained; it was now being rebuilt—on the same eighteenth-century stone foundations—as a Chinese luxury hotel and casino. Likewise, sections of Tashilhunpo Monastery had been destroyed to make way for a sloping paved road so Chinese tour buses could easily reach the top of the hill, the altitude having proved difficult for lowland Chinese tourists walking up the extra two hundred feet.

For the next few days, I passed through small villages and clusters of Tibetan buildings, each—as mandated by Chinese law—flying the Chinese red flag, with patriotic slogans spray-painted in four-foot-high Chinese letters on the walls of all street-facing buildings. By the time I reached Sakya, I was feeling emotionally ill from everything I'd seen. Sakya, however, was far worse than anything that I could have imagined. In this secluded valley with a river running along one edge, where the hills once had been covered by temples and monks' residences, there were only ruined foundations and a single, desolate rebuilt temple. The main monastery in the middle of town remained with a minimal contingent of monks, but the city itself was effectively under martial law. Except for the route between the one hotel where non-Chinese foreigners could stay and the monastery, everything else was off limits. I had hoped to visit the Phuntsok Potrang, where Bernard had stayed as a guest of the Sakya Hierarch, but was told I could not go. I was also told not to even try to sneak out to see it, because the low elevation between the town proper and the former residence afforded no cover and I would be spotted by Chinese security cameras that scanned the city and the valley, monitoring the activities of everyone there.

Sitting in the middle of decimated land governed by leaders who enforced their rules through fear and intimidation and, occasionally, extreme violence and torture—ongoing even then—I remembered that back in 1997, when Chinese Premier Jiang Zemin visited the United States, he made several notable comments. Clearly believing himself to be educated about American history, he claimed that he was the Chinese equivalent of Abraham Lincoln "freeing the slaves" of Tibet, and the Chinese were "bringing civilization" to the Tibetans just as European settlers had done "to the Indians." Rather than vindicating himself and the actions of his country, as he likely thought he was, Jiang instead explicitly identified himself as a colonialist and his country as precisely the sort of imperialist power the controlling Communist Party routinely railed against.

In studying Bernard's time in Taos, New Mexico, I had discovered that Carl Jung had also visited Taos, although many years earlier. Meeting with the governor of the Taos Pueblo, Jung had experienced an epiphany that changed his formerly self-assured opinion of European cultures. As a result, Jung came away with a fresh perspective on European colonialism, even going so far as to observe that European countries were, in a disturbing way, much like the animals—the beasts of prey—on their coats of arms and other heraldry. Such an observation would seem, by Jiang's own admission, to likewise apply to modern China, which, like its dragon emblem, hoards and covets everything of value within range of its domain—and also, from time to time, demands human sacrifice.

Another American president, Thomas Jefferson, had lamented the consequences of a government abdicating any sense of ethical responsibility, as happened decades later with the barbarism of his fellow countrymen in their treatment of the original inhabitants of North America. If "God is truly just," he wrote, "I tremble for the fate of my country." Having seen firsthand the results of equal barbarism and what appeared to be a love of senseless violence and destruction on the part of the Chinese Communists in their treatment of Tibet and the Tibetan people, I felt I could just as easily say: if the functioning of the law of ethical causality (karma) is truly inexorable,[12] then I tremble for the fate of China.

With such thoughts running through my head, I went south and farther west, to Nepal and Kathmandu, and literally breathed a sigh of relief after crossing the Tibetan–Nepalese border. All in all, my experiences in Tibet left me with a certain amount of repressed rage—half at the Chinese themselves, and half at the numerous Western academics I had met over the years who, while I remained in America studying, had been visiting Tibet and would return to tell me that my notions of the place were misguided. It was not the repressed society that I had been led to believe; the Chinese had simply modernized Tibet, paving roads and building social infrastructure. Over many years I had come to almost believe them myself. When I actually visited the country, however, I found it was precisely the opposite of what they had described and nearly exactly what I had initially believed. Tibet was, to all appearances, a country under military occupation, overrun (infested, one might say) by a particularly arrogant, violent, and poorly educated Chinese migrant population[13] that took credit for anything notable and blamed the Tibetans themselves for the rampant destruction all around them.[14]

Walking the streets of Kathmandu, I sometimes felt like I was recovering from a traumatic experience. I even felt shock and fear when I spotted a picture of His Holiness the Fourteenth Dalai Lama in a bookstore window in Thamel, until I realized that, unlike in Tibet, such a photo here was not illegal. But all of this was but the prequel to the last stage of my trip: retracing the final journey of Theos Bernard.

Traveling to the Kulu valley, I arrived in late August, just as had Bernard had done some sixty years earlier. I could understand why, at the time of the Partition of British India into India and Pakistan, no European felt any compulsion to leave. Kulu was beautiful: a narrow valley carved from the Himalayan foothills by a wide, slow-moving river; the scenery punctuated by springs of water jutting out of the valley walls and falling hundreds of feet to the river below. When British attempts to rear horses there in the early nineteenth century had failed, the settlers turned to agriculture, so the valley was filled with apple orchards and walnut groves, all dominated by the snow-capped Himalayas towering above, and I could sit in the late summer Indian sunlight, drinking my afternoon Darjeeling tea and eating fresh-baked apple crumble made from apples and walnuts that had been on the trees only four hours earlier.

My time in Kulu was a much-needed rest and recovery from the oppressive atmosphere of Chinese-occupied Tibet, but I was there to finish my research. For several days, I traveled up and down the valley, talking with those of the older generations I could find who remembered the Partition or their parents' stories of those times. When I explained who I was and my reasons for being there, ironically one of the first questions I was repeatedly asked was whether I was one of Bernard's relatives. What had been a convenient cover story in Tibet was in Kulu the exact opposite, as I realized that many people feared that I was there on a blood vendetta, seeking revenge on the family of the men who had murdered Bernard. This time, with equal honesty—I had no proof that I *was* Bernard's relative—I explained that he had been a graduate student at my university many years earlier, and my interest was purely academic, only trying to write his biography for my dissertation.

Initially I only received the same response, "I remember my parents talking about this, but I don't know any details," and similar comments. Slowly, as I gained the confidence of some residents in the valley, I began to hear more, but even then I was asked not to repeat or publish many of the specifics. Although the story, it turned out, was well known even as far away as Tashilhunpo Monastery in Shigatse, the whole incident was an embarrassment to the people of the region. The descendants of Bernard's killers—innocent themselves—still lived in the area, and no one cared to perpetuate the stigma of such a crime.

Hoping to recover at least some physical trace of Bernard's presence in the valley—I had even brought a copy of his dental records with me—I had optimistically hoped to find his Leica camera and lenses, whose serial numbers I had safely recorded from his insurance documents. Although everyone I talked to assured me that such items would have disappeared long ago, at one point I was asked if Bernard had owned a gold Rolex watch. Although I had no record of this, it occurred to me that he probably did have a watch, and if so, in keeping with what I knew about his personal habits, it would be a Rolex since, I thought, he *would* be just the sort of jerk to wear a gold Rolex on an expedition to India. But was I enough of one to spend a couple thousand dollars to try to recover it, no questions asked, based on a hunch? Fortunately, the limits of my graduate student funding prevented me from having to answer the question. Having found the answers to the *rest* of my questions about Bernard—even the name of the man who killed him—I had only one thing left to do: retrace the path of his final trip.

Although I was told that I could purchase a bus ticket for the equivalent of two dollars and seventy-five cents that would take me from the last major city, Manali, at the northern limit of Kulu, to Ki Monastery, or close enough at least, I was also told that it would not be a pleasant journey. With time running out on my research trip—I had already delayed my return to New York once—and knowing I would want to make a few detours, I decided to hire a jeep instead.

As my jeep began winding up the road north toward the Rohtang Pass, I was suddenly overcome by a strange feeling. Initially I thought it was because I had left my computer equipment behind, safely locked away at my guest house; I was "going analog," as my friends in Silicon Valley called it, something that always left me with an uneasy feeling. But as the hours passed, I realized that there was something more to it as well.

After four months, thousands of miles, hundreds of people, and fifteen thousand photographs, I was embarking on the last leg of my journey. Strangest of all, it seemed, was that the trip, I knew in advance, had almost no academic value. It was solely for the sake of retracing the footsteps of a man I had never met and I had not even known existed ten years earlier. Regardless of these facts, I felt an obligation to make the trip nonetheless. Certainly on an aesthetic level, the trip was worthwhile, since each turn in the road in the valley revealed yet another scenic vista. Each corner, each side valley offered its own variation of jagged rocks, trees, and wisps of mist lilting and cascading down its slopes.

As we started to climb into the mountains, the terrain rapidly disappeared into the clouds except for erratic, tantalizing glimpses of tiny streams running through the cliffs, turning into waterfalls 20 to 80 feet in length, and then becoming streams again. But all was not to be smooth. An hour or so into the journey, we had to stop. The summer monsoons were still active and a mudslide had reduced one switchback to a muddy stream clogged with backed-up trucks, buses, and cars. By the time the mudslide had been cleared, a good hour had passed, if not more, and we continued the last 10 miles or so up to the Rohtang Pass. Reaching the summit and crossing the pass, I immediately understood the significance of the name of Kulu, an abbreviation, I was told, of *kulānthapiṭa*, "the end of the habitable world." Lahoul and Spiti were like Tibet—a stark contrast to the lushness of the Kulu Valley. Here, rocky outcrops and gravel rockslides dominated the landscape, broken only by the rivers at the bottom of the valleys—the Chandra in Lahoul and the Sutlej in Spiti—and the slowly diminishing glaciers visible from time to time between mountain peaks.

Later in the day, I only realized that we were crossing the Kunzom Pass into Spiti when we stopped to pay homage to what appeared initially to be

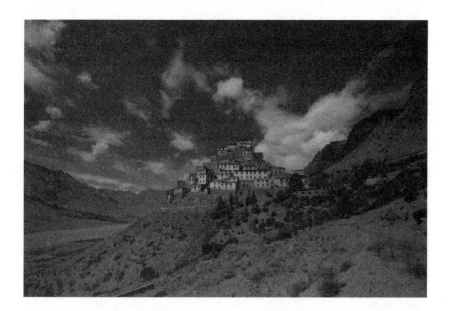

Figure 14.2 Ki Monastery, Spiti (photo by the author)

three, but upon closer inspection were four *stūpas* at the summit. Otherwise, to the naked eye, geographically there was little difference between Lahoul and the Spiti Valley to the east, where my destination lay. Where Lahoul's Chandra River meandered west toward Jammu and Kashmir, Spiti's Sutlej River carved sharp switchback canyons throughout the valley, winding its way ever east and south toward Kinnaur and the Gangetic Plain. After a few more hours, a short way into the valley, the monastery of Ki came into view. Immediately I recognized it, for the white specks of buildings atop a hill on the side of the valley were unmistakable, and I began taking pictures in earnest as we drew closer and closer.

Arriving at the monastery, I accosted an older monk walking nearby to confirm that I would be allowed to stay there. He directed me to the top of the monastery, and grabbing my pack, I began walking up, instructing my driver, who would stay in nearby Kaza, to return the day after next, between 7 and 8 a.m.

Entering the front gate into the monastery complex itself, I spied a sign, "Ki Monastery Office," and walked in to inquire about a room. Seated there were several monks, one of whom, I later learned, was the abbot. After an extended discussion of why I was there and a brief summary of

Bernard's life and death, I settled into a room in the northeast corner of the monastery, then returned downstairs in time for dinner in the kitchen with the staff, the abbot, and the older monks. Sitting there on a bench in the smoke-filled kitchen, I felt a sense of calm as I enjoyed the camaraderie of the monks. When I was handed a steaming hot bowl of Then-thuk, my favorite kind of Tibetan stew, the feeling only increased.

Returning to my room, I looked out over the valley and had a sense of comfort and contentment, as if I could easily remain there the rest of my life. Life in that monastery seemed uncomplicated, the obvious reflection in the mind from a superficial glance by an outsider; I was sure the abbot would give a different perspective, were I to ask. But nonetheless the feeling persisted. The next morning, I decided to spend the day at and around the monastery seeing the sights, taking in "the atmosphere," and of course, taking some photos. After my conversation the night before with the abbot and older monks, I knew—as I had suspected—that there would be no new information to add to the story. Ki was a "feeder" monastery, where young boys would be educated and the brighter students recommended for further study at one of the larger monastic universities in south India. Consequently, they offered me only discouraging news concerning any older monks who might remember Bernard. In response, I thought to contact the driver in Kaza and return to Kulu that day, but upon reflection I decided that a relaxed day in the monastery could only be a good thing.

My last night at Ki, I stood on the rooftop next to my room, looking out over the valley. To my right, a few buildings away, I noticed with a feeling of removed camaraderie the abbot, doing the same. As the hours passed and night came, he returned to his quarters, undoubtedly to continue attending to the never-ending obligations of his office, while I settled down in a corner as the temperature dropped, the winds picked up, and the stars in the night sky slowly came into view.

Struck with an idea, I retrieved my camera from my room and decided to take some night shots of the monastery. Trying out exposures with different constellations and monastery silhouettes, I finally decided to take a long exposure of Sagittarius—the heart of the Milky Way and direction of the center of the galaxy—just visible over the roof of the main temple and mountains to the south. As the camera sat a few feet away, its aperture wide open, I huddled next to a wall, staring southward at the same view juxtaposing monastic center and universe. At some point a meteorite shot along the southern limit of the constellation, just above the horizon. *A*

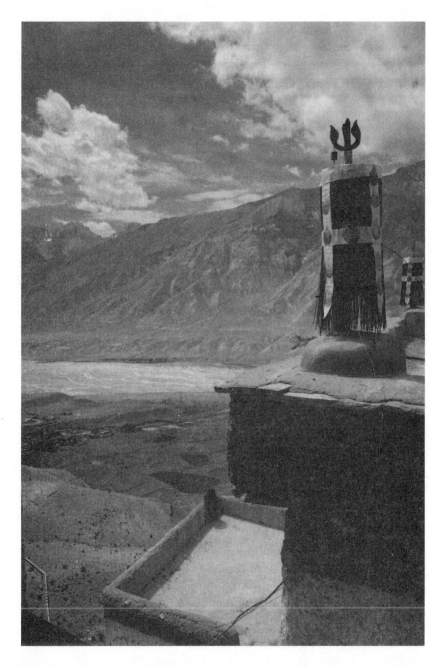

Figure 14.3 The abbot of Ki Monastery looks out over the Spiti Valley (photo by the author)

meteorite, I thought, *yes, but does it ultimately exist?* I laughed, for the thought seemed strange, a question formed from the juxtaposition of two world-views that seemed somehow incongruous.

On the one hand, I could describe—to a fairly accurate degree—the physical makeup of the universe, galaxy, and solar system (as understood in Western academic circles, at least), as well as our place within it, and even sketch the location of our sun in a spiral arm two thirds of the way out from galactic center . . . to anyone who cared, that is. Yet, on the other hand, I had been trained well by my Tibetan teachers and with airtight reasoning, I could also logically prove the lack of intrinsic existence and the epistemic contingency of it all. Reflecting for a moment, I understood intellectually that there was no reason the two perspectives should be con-tradictory and that the contradiction I was sensing was purely an emo-tional one on my part. The incommensurability of the two worldviews was not between them, but rather between my self-perceived identities over time—"who I was" when I had devoted myself to the study of each.

As I sat on the roof of a monastery founded by "the great translator," Rin-chen-sang-po, a man whose activities heralded the second great diffu-sion of Buddhism into Tibet, it struck me that this was precisely the pre-dicament I faced as a translator living in America: how to reconcile two apparently contradictory worldviews—the materialistic and the transcen-dent—and how to render the thoughts of one intelligible and accessible to the other, if indeed that was the purpose of my career. I wondered if that had been how Bernard had perceived the problem himself. Could his actions and writings be seen as a sort of "translation" between cultures?

Caught up in all these reflections, I had allowed my mind to wander; I had probably taken too long of an exposure, and the cold winds were blowing stronger and stronger down the valley. Unless I packed up quickly, I would spend the rest of my time in India in bed with a cold. Clicking off the remote shutter release on my camera, I glanced at the resulting photo. The ten-minute-long star trails of Sagittarius blended into a vivid orb of light at the center of the galaxy, broken only by the streaks of dark clouds of interstellar gases, all of it framed by the glowing parapets and blurry, windblown flags on the temple roof.

The next morning after a bowl of *tsampa*—roasted barley flour—washed down with hot buttered tea, I waited for my driver to arrive from Kaza. As we drove westward back to Lahoul and Kulu, we slowly accumulated more passengers—a mother and her children walking to a nearby village, a friend of the driver hoping to get back to Kulu—all of which, I found, reinforced the human element in the story. For better or worse, though I had satiated my curiosity about Bernard and his ultimate fate, my actions—what I said and did upon my return—would affect those I had met, just as assuredly as others' actions had affected Bernard. And so, I spent the better part of the day thinking about what I could and could not say when the time came to set the words down on paper.

So what happened to Theos Bernard? From the information I was able to gather, the primary sources at my disposal, and my hopefully correct inferences drawn from analyzing it all over several years, I had a consistent and plausible narrative in my head.

Sitting in Kalimpong in the spring of 1947, Theos Bernard was on a mission to compile enough raw materials for another sensationalistic return to America. While he and his father, and Helen as well, had ambitious plans for the future—a Tibetan language school, a yoga studio, perhaps even a retreat center—their ploy to fund it all with Ganna Walska's money had failed. To recruit students and attract benefactors, Bernard's return to America would have to make a big impression.

In 1947, if he could make it to Lhasa, he could try to meet the young Dalai Lama to receive his blessing; perhaps he could even secure the release of Gedun Chöpel from prison and bring him back to America. But Gould and Richardson had reserved the honor of conferring with His Holiness for themselves and were not about to let Theos anywhere near Lhasa, much less before the young ruler. Theos had fallback plans as well, so he petitioned Nepal for an entry visa. If he could not go to Lhasa, he could try to go to Sakya and western Tibet. But the British authorities were determined to keep him out—for reasons not that different from the ones that motivated Bernard—so that ploy also failed.

Bernard still had one last fallback plan—indeed, it had been part of his plan all along: an audience with a great lama or yogi and a great discovery as well. Although he had visited Ladakh and Hemis Monastery in 1936 with Viola and his father, he had not known then what he knew now, so he was determined to go back. For in the library of Hemis, he had discovered, lay the manuscript of the secret life of Jesus in India, and he, Theos Bernard, would be the one to bring that manuscript back to America.

In 1894, a Russian by the name of Nicholas Notovitch published a small book in Paris called *La Vie inconnu de Jésus-Christ*. Appearing in English translation later that same year, *The Secret Life of Jesus* detailed a trip that Notovitch claimed to have taken to Hemis Monastery in Leh, Ladakh. While there, Notovitch further claimed, he had seen a Tibetan translation of a manuscript written in the early years of the first millennium in India, detailing the activities of Jesus—"Issa," as he was called in Islamic sources—in India and Tibet, where he had "studied Pali and thoroughly read the Buddhist scriptures," proving once and for all that Christianity was not "a Jewish thing." Several scholars at the time took great exception to these ideas, while others attempted to confirm them and locate the manuscript themselves. Each concluded that Notovitch was a fraud and his account pure fiction.

In 1909, however, an aging "pioneer preacher" named Levi H. Dowling, who had served in the American Civil War, published his own book called *The Aquarian Gospel of Jesus the Christ*. In addition to announcing "The Age of Aquarius," he made similar claims about the life of Jesus in India. It was an interesting, if strange book, and Theos had read it.[15] But Dowling and Notovitch were not the only ones attesting to the truth of the narrative. In 1929, Swami Abhedananda published his own book in which he claimed to have retraced Notovitch's path to Hemis Monastery, found the same manuscript and more, and produced his own translation of the text.[16] Likewise, Nicholas Roerich was a firm believer, even plotting Jesus's journey from Jerusalem through Bactria, across India to Konarak, on to Varanasi and even up into Tibet to Lhasa. Calling him "Blessed Issa, the Prophet, who walked through these lands," Roerich had established that "Kulu and Mandi are the sacred lands Zahor, which so often are mentioned in ancient records. Here after the persecution of the impious King Landarma were hidden the most ancient books. Even the place of these hidden treasures is indicated approximately."[17]

When Theos Bernard came to Kulu in August 1947, he did so in preparation for a trip in search of the text of the life of Jesus in India, and specifically sought out Nicholas Roerich in hope of obtaining more clues that might enable him to locate the manuscript. It was Roerich who suggested that he try Ki Monastery, but the reasoning behind that recommendation is unclear.

Ki Monastery holds a unique place in the popular history of western Tibet. The monastery is situated in the heart of a landscape whose Buddhist roots can be traced at least as far back as the Fourth Buddhist Council of

King Kaniṣka (c. 125–152 C.E.). The actual structure, however, dates to the eleventh century and is held to be one of the four monasteries founded by the student of Atīśa, Drom-dön-pa (*'brom ston pa*). The missionary A. H. Francke also made several references to the monastery and its fame. But it is doubtful that Bernard (or Roerich, for that matter) had ever read Francke's account, since it would have mitigated against visiting the monastery in search of manuscripts:

> The Ki monastery was thoroughly ransacked in the petty wars between Kuḷū and Ladakh which preceded the Ḍōgrā war. And during the Ḍōgrā war itself it suffered even more severely. . . . But the Ki monastery has been restored since the turbulent times of the Ḍōgrā war. . . . As all the old books and idols had been destroyed by Ghulām Khān, the outfit of the Ki monastery is rather modern.[18]

Consequently, what Bernard found upon his arrival at Ki was likely only disappointment, for the simple reason that Ki did not *have* a library and Tabo, just down the valley, which did have one, was not in much better shape.[19]

Returning from Ki Monastery, Bernard and Senge made their way back through Spiti over the Kunzom Pass to Lahoul. Traversing the length of Lahoul, they approached the Rohtang Pass, but the storms that were sending torrential rains down on Helen and the others in the Kulu Valley were dumping massive amounts of snow on the mountains between Lahoul and Kulu. Attempting to cross the pass, Bernard and Senge were finally forced back by the weather. Still on the north side, they headed down the mountain from the pass and made their way farther west, toward the small village of Koksar, to seek food and shelter. After crossing the chain suspension bridge on their ponies, they encountered a group of men coming their way.

Days earlier, messages had come up from Kulu, both legitimate ones— the Banons' call for help in defending themselves—and fraudulent ones— from the same marauders who had engineered the slaughter of the Muslim population of the valley, claiming more Muslims were on the way seeking revenge. In southern Lahoul, their appeals were being answered.

Even at the time, the state of affairs in Lahoul was well known to both the British and American authorities in India.

The common talk in the [Kulu] valley regarding Lahoul is that there are four ruling families which at one time or another held power but are now merely land owners. Of these four, there is one who is ambitious for power and has organized residents in the form of gangs who roam the two entrances to the Lahoul Valley. While the northern part of the country is still under the domination of the monasteries, the southern part just over the Rotung Pass has been greatly influenced by Hinduism in the last fifty years or more, and the people are not considered as reliable or as peaceful as the northern Lahoulies.[20]

But regardless of feelings of allegiance, religious or ethnic, as one person I spoke to explained, most people would find it hard to kill. When the decision to send men to Kulu to support one or more of the factions there was made by local leaders in Lahoul, the appropriate men had to be found. Known for banditry in the area, the members of one family in particular were not strangers to killing, so they were chosen to lead the expedition. It was those men who approached Theos and Senge as they crossed the Koksar bridge.

One man raised his rifle and took aim. "Don't shoot! I'm not Muslim!" Bernard shouted out. But his cries fell on deaf ears, not because the man didn't speak English, but because he didn't care. A shot rang out and the bullet knocked Bernard off his pony to the ground. Senge quickly dismounted and ran to Theos's side as the men swarmed over them. But the shot had been fatal—Bernard was dead. Rifling through his clothes, the men took his possessions and threw his body into the river. But far from being disposed of, Bernard's body got caught in an eddy and became pinned against a rock only a few yards downstream.

But the men had an even bigger problem: Senge was still alive. He had seen it all and could identify them all. Although they were not Buddhists, the men were still hesitant to kill a monk. For some time they argued over what to do until finally they came to a decision. Grabbing Senge, they bound his hands and feet securely with rope and tossed him, still alive, into the Chandra River. Determined to conceal their crime, they then stripped the ponies of all their markings and pushed them into the river as well. It was a brutal series of murders that soon everyone in Lahoul would know about. Some, concerned for the future, found Senge's body farther downstream and, fishing it out of the river, buried it. As for the ultimate fate of Bernard's body, no one could say.

As the days and weeks went by, the significance of the men's actions became frighteningly clear to the people of Lahoul. In lands where an ordinary police officer was seldom seen, all of a sudden a Thanadar, a chief of police, had arrived, accompanied by a squad of Gurkhas and British officers, and the residents of the valley became truly terrified. Claiming to have no knowledge of anything they were asked about, they began an active campaign of disinformation. Bernard and Senge had never been anywhere near Koksar, or they had been spotted heading east toward the Hampta Pass.[21]

Although as time passed and the secret of Bernard's murder seemed to be safe, the stigma of the killings remained. With the murder of Bernard and Senge, two individuals innocent and unrelated to the events unfolding to the south in Kulu, the locals began to feel that the men who had killed them were cursed. Disgraced, they and their families were driven from the valley. Years later, a *stūpa* was constructed on the bank of the river at the site of the murders in the hope of expatiating the curse that some felt remained.

Fifty-nine years later, as the jeep driver and his friend were eating lunch, I walked down the same trail—now a road—that Bernard and Senge had ridden on their ponies. From the river's edge, the concrete mounts that had held the chains of the old bridge were still visible, though now a single-lane iron bridge served the needs of the area. Taking a few photos, I walked across the bridge, stopping midway to look down the valley at the water flowing westward toward Pakistan. Approaching the *stūpa* on the far side of the river, I took out a roll of incense that I had picked up at Ki and was carrying in my backpack. Lighting a stick of incense and placing it at the base of the *stūpa*, I stood back and contemplated the whole story that had culminated on the spot where I now stood.

After a few minutes, I returned to my driver and his friend at the road-side *dhaba*. Joining them at a small table, I sat there for some time, eating my mutton curry in silence. Perhaps I had been expecting something else, a greater sense of foreboding pervading the area surrounding the bridge, or some sort of dénouement to give the whole story a greater significance.

Our lunch finished, we got back in the jeep and began ascending the mountain toward the Rohtang Pass and the Kulu Valley. As I glanced back toward the bridge one last time, I could see the afternoon sun beginning to fill the valley with a slowly shifting golden light that glinted off the white *stūpa* by the river's edge. Turning again to face the road ahead, I thought about those events, and settling into my seat in the jeep—since there seemed nothing left to do—closed my eyes to rest for a while. Keeping my thoughts to myself, I could only hope that the villagers' prayers had been answered, and that the trauma of the deaths of Senge and of Bernard . . . of Theos, had truly been laid to rest.

NOTES

Preface

1. Entry dated June 26, 1937, Theos C. Bernard (TCB) Diary II. Given the extensive use of primary sources, letters, diaries, and so forth, only general citations have been provided for these materials. For precise page citations, see Hackett, "Barbarian Lands."

2. "Secret Rites I saw in Darkest Tibet," *Daily Mail* (UK), 13.

3. Following William McGovern in 1923 and Suydam Cutting in 1935, Bernard would be the last civilian American to set foot in Lhasa for over ten years.

4. Meinheit notes that the Library of Congress's collection was relatively small; having been established by the gifts and purchases of William Woodville Rockhill by 1942, it consisted of 68 titles and one copy of the *Sde-dge Bka'-'gyur* in 110 volumes. Similarly, Yale University's collection of Tibetan texts was minimal at best prior to the Bernard acquisitions in the early 1960s, consisting of assorted donations and one copy of the Lhasa *Bka'-'gyur*, while the British Library's collection of Tibetan texts was composed predominantly of Dunhuang manuscripts and acquisitions from the borderlands of Tibet. Meinheit, "The Rockhill Tibetan Collection at the Library of Congress."

5. See Jackson, *A Saint in Seattle*.

6. Among his other accomplishments, Bernard also seems to have earned the dubious distinction of documentably being the first American in modern history to have his "significant other" walk out on him the moment he became seriously interested in Tibetan Buddhism—a very "in joke" in Western Tibetan Buddhist circles. Claim to this "title" could be made for Colonel Henry Olcott, who broke with Madame Helena

Blavatsky over his interest in Buddhism, although Olcott maintained (adamantly) that he and Blavatsky were never in a romantic relationship.

7. See Prothero, *The White Buddhist*.

8. "Only a Hindoo Monk: Vive Kananda Believes Not in the Tricks of the Yogis," *Washington Post*, 6; T. Walter Williams, "M. M. Mizzle Quits His Lamasery, Pursued by Sable Amazon on Yak," *New York Times*, 41.

9. Lopez, *Prisoners of Shangri-La*, 6.

10. Hilton's book was so popular that it holds the distinction of being the first novel ever published in paperback form. Read even by the sitting U.S. President, Franklin Roosevelt, the book inspired him to name his presidential retreat center Shangri-La (now Camp David). The book would go on to win the Hawthornden Prize for Imaginative Literature in 1934. Hilton, *Lost Horizon*; "Wins Hawthornden Prize," *New York Times*, 21.

11. Although the U.S. Congress approved the sale of 3.2 percent beer on April 6, 1933, the ratification of the Twenty-First Amendment to the U.S. Constitution, repealing the Eighteenth Amendment, did not take place until December 5, 1933.

12. Since the fall of Aśoka's Mauryan Empire (ca. 322–185 B.C.E.) in India.

1. Life in the Desert

1. Yogananda, *Autobiography of a Yogi*, 341–343.

2. "Only a Hindoo Monk," *Washington Post*, 6.

3. Both opinions have been advanced by scholars both in India and abroad. See Marshall, *The British Discovery of Hinduism*.

4. Harry Emerson Fosdick, "Introduction," in Thomas, *Hinduism Invades America*, 9.

5. Given the plethora of individuals named "Bernard" in this story—Theos Casimir Bernard, Viola Wertheim Bernard, Glen Agassiz Bernard, and Pierre Arnold Bernard—I have chosen to use their personal, or preferred, names (Theos, Viola, Glen, and "P.A.") rather than their full names or infelicitous abbreviations (TCB, VWB, GAB, PAB), although the latter are utilized in the footnotes (as well as HGP for Helen Graham Park and GW for Madame Ganna Walska).

6. Graduating from Tombstone High School in 1921—just a few years before Theos—a neighborhood girl named Lorna Lockwood would go on to become an Arizona Supreme Court Justice (1960) and later, the first woman in the United States to head a state Supreme Court (1965).

7. See Hughes, *Tombstone Story*.

8. Later, TCB would claim that he was visited by a yogi during this period who introduced him to yoga: "A visit which was to have lasted a couple of hours continued through the night; I left him at the break of dawn. He was a rather elderly man, of heavy stature and sensitive features, radiating spiritual strength. His eyes gleamed, and his voice rang like a bell. It was enough for me merely to sit in his presence and listen to the sounds issuing forth from his lips, sounds whose literal meaning I

scarcely comprehended. Nevertheless they conveyed their own meaning to me, of a nature difficult here to define."

Years later, as she attempted to make sense of his life and her own, TCB's first wife, Viola, remarked that there were a number of problems with the stories of his early life; after compiling her personal papers for deposit at the Columbia University archives, she stated, "The discrepancy about early influences [on TCB vis á vis yoga] cannot be resolved from the materials here available." Furthermore, in his diaries written during his visit to Tibet, on one occasion (1937) TCB refers to the mental development he has experienced as a result of meditation and yoga, remarking that "during this last fifteen years, I have been steadily building up a consciousness that will absorb all there is to be offered." The lower limit that he gives for the start of his "training" (1922) corresponds not to the time of his illness (1927) nor even to when he met his father in L.A. (ca. 1932), but to some otherwise unidentified event at the age of thirteen. Bernard, *Heaven Lies Within Us*, 10; VWB Archive #9.1, entry dated June 16, 1937. TCB Diary I; see also chapter 9, note 21.

9. The Dwight B. Heard Scholarship, 1930–31. Since he had a C-average GPA, the scholarship was most likely awarded through the efforts of his uncle.

10. His University of Arizona transcript shows that in the spring of 1932 TCB took two courses, one in logic and the other in elementary psychology, for each of which he received a grade of B.

11. How or why Hamati came to be in Lincoln, Nebraska in the 1890s is unclear. Some have speculated that he might have come to America to work in a circus act as part of a traveling carnival. Little information about his identity is known. He was self-described as the son of a French woman and Persian man, born in Palestine and raised in India in the tantric yoga traditions of Bengal. See Love, *The Great Oom*.

12. Bernard, *Vira Sadhana*.

13. Glen states that he left home at the age of nineteen in 1903, at which point he appears to have joined his brother, Pierre, who introduced him to yoga and his guru, Hamati. By 1906, Glen appears to have been fully ensconced in his brother's organiza- tion, even filing a patent application for their publications in his own name. United States Patent Office, *Official Gazette of the United States Patent Office*, 669.

14. For a more detailed chronology of these events and the life of Glen's older brother, see Love, *The Great Oom*.

15. Glen Bernard recorded that he and Aura Crable were united (*yuj*) ["L.G.—G.B.— yoga March 18 1907."]/"married" on March 18, 1907. I have been unable to locate a marriage certificate, but there are other problems with this date as well. March 1907 is more than a year before Aura officially left her job as Postmaster of Tombstone (March 8, 1908), turning over the position to her brother, Francis D. Crable. Were this date a conscious fabrication on Glen's part to deceive Theos, since March 18, 1908 was just 39 weeks prior to TCB's birth (December 10, 1908) and only 10 days after the ter- mination of her position with the postal service, it would be far more in keeping with expectations. In either case, Francis Crable (Postmaster, 1908–12) appears to have performed the duties of the position in her absence for some time before her official

departure. Aura Crable maintained that religious training was her reason for going to New York City as a young woman. Of the different seminaries in New York at the time, the most likely for a young woman to attend would have been the Bible Teachers' Training School (later known as the New York Theological Seminary) founded in 1903 across the Hudson River in Patterson, NJ; it moved to New York City in 1905. The archives of the NYTS are currently housed at the General Theological Union in Manhattan, but I have yet to locate any reference to her attendance at any school in New York. Glen Bernard, "Notes," Theos Bernard Papers; "Arizona Statehood Post Offices & Postmasters, 1912–1979, Part XIII," 30.

16. Eleanore Murray reported that Paramahansa Yogananda visited Glen on numerous occasions. Her association with Glen Bernard did not begin until the early 1950s, close to the time of Yogananda's death, so it is unclear whether she was actually present at any of these meetings or was merely reporting what she had been told by Glen.

17. Theos's younger brother Dugald remembered that Theos would stand on his head often. One time, he recounted, when they were together in the Dragoon Mountains, Theos was standing in the middle of a small circle he had drawn on the ground. "What is the difference between doing this here and up there?" he said to his brothers, pointing at a cliff ledge on Sheepshead Mountain. "The difference," he said, "would be in the mind, the thought of danger, of fear, that we might fall, whereas here we don't have this fear." According to Dugald, to illustrate his point, Theos climbed up Sheepshead Mountain—visible from both the Gordon house and the cabin—and stood on his head on the cliff edge.

18. Bernard, *Heaven Lies Within Us*, 45.

19. It is possible that this was J. Lawrence Kulp, a member of the Department of Geology, but there are chronological problems with this identification.

20. "Evolution," *Fortune* Magazine, 4.

2. New York and New Mexico

1. TCB to VWB, August 5, 1935, VWB Archive #9.6.

2. When Viola's father, Jacob Wertheim, the founder and president of the General Tobacco Company, died in 1920, *The New York Times* reported that he left an estate worth in excess of $6 million, of which Viola and Diana each received trust funds of $750,000, yielding $35–40,000 a year. By 1938, the *Times* estimated his estate to be worth $9 million, which was divided among Viola, her two brothers, two sisters, mother, and six aunts. "Miss Wertheim Wed at Country Home," *New York Times*, May 31, 1929, 26; "Jacob Wertheim Estate: Tobacco Manufacturer Leaves $6,038,284 Net to 38 Beneficiaries," *New York Times*, December 24, 1921, 8; "$20,000 Yearly for Girls," *New York Times*, June 16, 1922, 13; "Wertheim Estate put at $9,324,243; Accounting Covers Trusts Set Up by Investment House Head," *New York Times*, May 24, 1938, 16.

3. More than an idle fear, in the 1930s the scandals of the "white slave trade" and the perfidious activities of "swamis" remained a staple of the tabloid newspapers and

constant fodder for Broadway plays and Hollywood thrillers. Sexual seduction and the New York–Barbary Coast slave trade were featured prominently in Mae West's hit Broadway play *Diamond Lil*, later remade as the heavily bowdlerized film *She Done Him Wrong*, the latest in a series of movies beginning in the late 1910s—some perhaps inspired by PAB himself—portraying the horrors of "Oriental" cult seductions. The titles of most of these—often featuring only an otherwise nameless "swami"—speak for themselves: *The Love Girl* (1916), *Upside Down* (1919), *Thirteen Women* (1932), *Sinister Hands* (1932), *Sucker Money* (a.k.a. *Victims of the Beyond*, 1933), *The Mind Reader* (1933), *Secrets of Chinatown* (1935), and *Moonlight Murder* (1936), to name a few. Not until the 1940s did the figure of the less sinister, con man "swami" begin to appear as a comic foil, with such characters as Zero Mostel's "Rami the Swami" (*Du Barry Was a Lady*, 1943) and Boris Karloff's "Swami Talpur" (*Abbott and Costello Meet the Killer*, 1949).

4. Née Dace Shannon. Harkening back to the historic foundations of New Amsterdam, in the early twentieth century in New York, a Dutch-sounding name was still preferable to an obviously Irish one in certain social circles.

5. The well-known film critic for *The New York Times*, Andre Sennwald, in reviewing W. C. Fields's most recent film, had remarked just a week earlier that Fields himself was "the omnipotent oom of one of the screen's most devoted cults." Andre Sennwald, "The Old-Fashioned Way," *New York Times*, July 14, 1934, 16, col. 5.

6. Despite the precautions she took—"leaking" false information to the telephone operators in Nyack about a planned August 3 wedding—the tabloid newspapers still found out about the marriage; lacking photo evidence, they were forced to run stock photos of PAB.

7. Over the course of the ten weeks that they were apart—from June through August 1935—Theos wrote over sixty letters to Viola, most three or more pages long, in addition to cablegrams and frequent phone calls. Theos appears to have routinely destroyed his received correspondence. He remarked to Viola, having not heard from her in a while, "guess what I did; something that is almost impossible for me to do . . . today I found myself rereading some of your letters . . . which I luckily failed to destroy." TCB to VWB, June 24, 1935, VWB Archive #9.6.

8. Quite conscious of his need to practice his narrative skills, he wrote to Viola, "Now to get it all down on paper. . . . My papers may be rotten, but [Columbia professor] Randall doesn't turn me down so I can satisfy or qualify now and then; so let's see if I can satisfy the government. I am so glad to get this experience for I am now able to practice on others so that when the day comes when I want to get something for myself that may be worthwhile I do not have to let it slip by because I have not had the experience." TCB to VWB, June 21, 1935, 2, VWB Archive #9.6.

9. Theos does not seem to have attempted to climb Taos Mountain as he claimed he would. Taking the sanctity of the mountain quite seriously, the members of the Pueblo consider it their duty to safeguard it as the location of a "Sipapu," or portal into the earth where refuge is sought at the time of great destruction. Even seventy years later, the town of Taos made publicly known to visitors that to set foot on Taos Mountain was to invite death from the Pueblo's mountain patrols.

10. The Taos Pueblo governor at the time appears to have been a remarkable individual. Carl Jung, during his visit to Taos in the 1920s, had occasion to meet the man as well, and claimed that the encounter resulted in deep insights into his own culture. Jung, *Memories, Dreams, Reflections.*

11. Theos on one occasion insisted that they take horses through the fresh snow on Mount Wheeler—resulting in one of the horses falling fifty feet down a snowy embankment.

12. A Spanish pejorative; the community prefers the name Tohono O'odham.

13. Ansel Adams recalled that it was his meeting in Taos with Paul Strand, who showed him his recent photos of the area, that prompted him to pursue the photographic style for which he became famous. Phillips, "Adams and Stieglitz: A Friendship."

3. Two Parallel Paths (I)

1. Bernard, "Introduction to Tantrik Ritual," 20.

2. William Duncan Strong to Commissioner of Indian Affairs, October 26, 1935, 5–7, The Papers of William Duncan Strong, Box 47, "[Correspondence] Bureau of Indian Affairs, 1934–1937."

3. Upon leaving the Bureau of Indian Affairs, Collier chose to retire to Taos, New Mexico and pursued his own research on the Taos Pueblo, resulting in several publications.

4. Collier, "Office of Indian Affairs," in *Annual Report of the Department of the Interior,* 164–165.

5. G. B. Spotorno, *Memorials of Columbus.* (London, 1823), 224, quoted in Balmer, *Blessed Assurance,* 46, 122n7.

6. This move to scriptural literalism under the guise of interpretation was solidified in America by the publication of the Scofield Reference Bible (1909) and a series of pamphlets published between 1911 and 1915 called "The Fundamentals," from which "Fundamentalist" Christianity draws its name.

7. Tappan, *Discourses through the Mediumship of Cora L. V. Tappan,* 8. Thanks to Erika Dyson for this reference.

8. Franz Boas (1858–1942) himself characterized the orthodox state of anthropology as "painstaking attempts at reconstruction of historical connections based on studies of distribution of special features and supplemented by archeological evidence." Boas, "Introduction" to Benedict, *Patterns of Culture,* xii.

9. Schneider, *Philosophy Will Never Be a Science,* 3.

10. Bernard, *Philosophical Foundations,* 10–11.

11. This and subsequent otherwise unidentified quotes in this chapter are from Bernard, "Introduction to Tantrik Ritual," 1–6, 18–26, 34–35.

12. Taken by most people at the time—Theos Bernard included—as a pseudonym of Sir John Woodroffe. Recent scholarship has shown that the appellation is more aptly applied to Atal Behari Ghosh. Woodroffe himself implies as much in the first

volume published, *The Principles of Tantra*, where the author is described as an "Indian Pandit." Taylor, "Arthur Avalon, the Creation of a Legendary Orientalist,"144–63.

13. Bhattacharyya was under the impression that all Buddhas were the same individual. Bhattacharyya, *An Introduction to Buddhist Esotericism*, 8.

14. Bhattacharyya, *Sādhanamālā*, 2:xix.

15. Theos noted that Woodroffe, in his *Principles of Tantra*, identified references to "the founder of the Kuchbehar Rāja, which was established within that time" within the Yoginī Tantra. Avalon, *Principles of Tantra*, xxxvii.

16. Avalon, *Principles of Tantra*, 1:lxx, cited in Bernard, "Introduction to Tantrik Ritual," 19.

17. Avalon, *Principles of Tantra*, 1:lxxi.

18. The draft version of his thesis and the final submission version show so few differences that any changes suggested by his committee must have been merely cosmetic, grammatical, or bibliographic.

4. Two Parallel Paths (II)

1. GAB to VWB, February 11, 1935, VWB Archive #11.11.

2. "Indian Melodies Charm Denizens of the Jungle," *San Francisco Examiner*, May 25, 1914, 19.

3. Section 13 of the Criminal Code of the United States, cited in Jacobsen v. United States, 7th Circuit Court of Appeals, 272 F. 399.

4. "Bernstorff Active in Irish Plots Here," *New York Times*, January 10, 1921, 3.

5. Advertisement, *San Francisco Chronicle*, October 1, 1922, C-1.

6. Swami Kebalananda, a.k.a. Ashutosh Chatterjee, 1863–1931.

7. Taylor points out that Woodroffe himself remarked early on that

in his preface to *Śakti and Śākta*, the first of the Tantric books to come out under his own name, Woodroffe explained that it was not his own identity that was referred to by "Arthur Avalon". His previous books had come out under that name "to denote that they have been written with the direct cooperation of others and in particular with the assistance of one of my friends who will not permit me to mention his name. I do not desire sole credit for what is as much their work as mine." (second edition, p. x). We have already seen that Woodroffe was not concerned to conceal his interest in Tantra. The person who wanted to keep his involvement secret was someone else. The pseudonym did not only refer to a team of collaborators—the named editors of the individual volumes of *Tantrik Texts*, for example—but especially to one person in particular.

It was only later that he seemed to accept its attribution to himself, though Taylor suggests that "Arthur Avalon" should be thought of as the mutual creation of both men. Taylor, "Arthur Avalon," 155–156.

8. Though the documents are unidentified in her research, Kathleen Taylor remarks that the letters to Ghosh from Glen and others "express a flood of personal feelings and reflections, as well as showing how they looked up to Ghose as a teacher" and implied a relationship "closer to that of guru and disciple, or at least of teacher and pupil." Taylor, *Sir John Woodroffe, Tantra and Bengal*, 209.

9. A reference to Woodroffe's remarks in his *Sakti and Shâkta*:

> The English-educated people of this country were formerly almost exclusively, and later to a considerable extent, under the sway of their English educators. In fact they were in a sense their creation. They were, and some of them still are, the Manasaputra of the English. For them what was English and Western was the mode. Hindu religion, philosophy and art were only, it was supposed, for the so-called "uneducated" women and peasants and for native Pandits who, though learned in their futile way, had not received the illuminating advantages of a Western training. (33–34)

10. As early as 1928, Glen was supplying ayurvedic medicines to doctors in California—some of whom were more than a little suspicious—and by 1930 Glen came to identify himself as a "salesman" working in the "Home Medical Supply" industry. U.S. Bureau of the Census, 1930, Los Angeles, California, roll 148, page 14, enumeration district 19–423, line 33, April 14, 1930.

11. "Oxonised"—a variant of "oxonianize"—was a term of derogatory slang derived from the medieval name for the county of Oxfordshire, Oxon, home to Oxford University. It referred to a person educated there who, in the words of a Socialist detractor, underwent a certain "process":

> The process of converting a human being into an "Oxford man" takes at a moderate estimate some twenty-five years. To be entirely successful, it must begin before the boy is born. His father must actually enter his name on the college list before the boy sees the light of day. The early youth of the candidate for initiation must be spent in the preparatory atmosphere of Eton or Rugby. Even then, so recalcitrant and naturally free are some youths, the process sometimes fails, and the boy, to the horror of his pastors and masters (the operating magicians, you understand) grows into mere manhood without acquiring the Oxford "tone." But such cases are comparatively rare. Ninety-nine out of every hundred succumb to the "training" and become Oxonised and dehumanised. (R.M., "The Magic of Oxford," 261)

12. In the early 1920s, Woodroffe published a series of small books under the collective title "The World as Power" with such subtitles as "Reality," "Power as Life," "Power as Matter," etc. Woodroffe's collaborator, P. N. Mukherji, a.k.a. P. N. Mukhyopādhyāya, was coauthor of "The World As Power: Power As Matter" (Madras: Ganesh & Co., 1923). Kathleen Taylor, private communication.

13. The *Sāradā-tilaka*, attributed to Laksmaṇa (dates unknown), was described by "Arthur Avalon" as comprising twenty-five chapters, the first twenty-four of which correspond to the Samkhya *tattvas*, while the twenty-fifth discusses yoga. Avalon, *Sāradā-tilaka*.

14. Of the few letters that survive of GAB's own personal correspondence from this time, one letter from a student of Glen's, identified simply as "Bob" and a follower of Rosicrucian (AMORC) teachings, presents a cryptic window into GAB's activities during these years. In 1930, "Bob" wrote,

Glen dear: —
 This my last letter to you for the present . . . on Sat. 31*st* I leave on S.S. Yale [from San Francisco] for L.A., and Mr. Poland or someone at 1040, will meet me at P.E. and take me out to the house and my old room . . . I want to keep your name unknown, as I apparently have, so far. . . .
 I am going into experienced danger, in order to open up what lies between you and me and complete it to the higher development of each of us, if possible. There is no subtlety behind any terms of endearment, nothing to discover, nothing to dread, from me. There is a definite goal and I am aware of my inexperience and weaknesses, which naturally prevents expression of latent higher forces—it all depends on how they are attacked + guided + as far as I have ever known, you have the ability, if the will and the courage. . . .
 It would not be conducive to the best interests of either of us if always forced to meet in public. You should be able to call on me quietly and without questions. I cannot endure the masks and hypocrisy and camouflage of modern life. In any café, hall, park, +c. the vibrations of the world would destroy confidential talk by intrusions of various kinds breaking the continuity. I am sure you know what it is to be so. In a way I am to talk to you as to a Father Confessor—a Priest—and you know it means a holy place—a Sacrament. One who is as close to another's soul as I am to yours Glen, stands close to the borderland—sometimes I feel something of me that is etheric—sort of a floating away, that does not all come back—it is not mental—it is a vibration—You will know, you will steady it whatever it is. I need a guide, a teacher. Oh Glen, have I the wisdom, the strength? Yet go on I must. Sounds crazy but it is very vivid—it hurts, yet I know I am on the path, and cannot retrace.

Yours—
Bob

"Bob" to GAB, May 25, 1930, Theos Bernard Papers.

15. Von Koerber, *Morphology of the Tibetan Language*.

16. Glen, taking the dictates of his Vedic horoscope quite seriously, expected to die sometime in 1940–41. He would, in fact, outlive all of his brothers, as well as his own son, living for another forty years.

17. It is unclear exactly how many students Glen Bernard had, although he did instruct several in tantric yoga. One of them, Helena Zak, who had studied on and

off with him for more than five years, had taken to writing directly to Atal Behari Ghosh as much as a year earlier, both in praise of Glen and concerning her own religious practices. She wrote, "Glen Bernard has been (these last five years) my only companion.... The best I can do each day is a little study and my practices.... So he will be with you—happy as I am that he has been able to go to India—his leaving left me lonely indeed. He has been fine to me during these years—karma has placed us at a cross-road in our pathway." Helena Hopkins Zak to Atal B. Ghosh (incomplete), undated (ca. March 8, 1934), British Library; copy courtesy of Kathleen Taylor.

5. On Holy Ground

1. Kuvalayananda, *Asanas*, 32.

2. Alter, *Yoga in Modern India*, 83.

3. Yogananda, who was visiting his teacher Śrī Yukteśwar (1855–1936) just prior to his death (on March 9), gave a copy of his latest book to Glen while in Calcutta, inscribing it: "To brother Bernard with very best wishes, S. Yogananda. With these whispers mingle your whispers and after these with God. Yours, Jan 10th, 1936." Yogananda, *Whispers from Eternity*, Theos Bernard Papers.

4. Glen established a working correspondence with Prakash Dev, who was just then publishing related treatises (which he sent to Glen): *Yoga as the System of Physical Culture* and *Yogic System of Exercise (Full Course)*; he promised that another book, *Pranayama*, would be forthcoming. Prakash Dev to GAB, November 29, 1935, and June 2, 1936, Theos Bernard Papers.

5. A photo and brief identification of Swami Syamānanda is given by Evans-Wentz in the opening of his *Tibetan Yoga and Secret Doctrines*, ii, xviii.

6. Swami Syamānanda briefly mentions their time together during the nine years that Kawaguchi spent in Varanasi. Brahmachary, *Truth Revealed*, 178.

7. It is likely that Jinorasa was referring to Dro-mo Geshe Nga-wang-kel-sang (*gro mo dge bshes ngag dbang skal bzang*, 1866–1936) of Dung-kar Monastery near Yatung, who was revered throughout the Chumbi Valley and Sikkim.

8. Several newspapers around the world carried the story of one such high-profile case in early 1938, a "mystic youth-maker," the yogi Tapsi Bishanj Das Udasi—reputed to be 172 years old—when he treated a 77-year-old associate of Gandhi, Pandit Mohan Malaviya, after which it was claimed he had "discarded his spectacles, lost the wrinkles of an aged man and noted the approach of a third set of teeth." "Yogi 'Turns Back Years' For Follower of Gandhi," *New York Herald Tribune*, February 27, 1938; also cited on the same day in several other newspapers.

9. For several years, Glen had been at work on a manual of advice, which he called "The Rationale of Sex." While he was certain that this practice was connected to it, "For reasons poorly understood," he wrote, "these teachers suggest that the sexual act be prolonged without allowing it to result in the loss of semen, by which performance some 'magic result' is said or supposed, to be effected.... We are not given a rational notion of what is transmuted into what, nor why indulgence in amorous play

without consummation effects this transmutation." Glen Bernard, "The Rationale of Sex," undated ms. (ch. 5, "Strengthening the Life Principle"), Theos Bernard Papers.

6. Pretense and Pretext: Studies in India

1. TCB Diary I,18(r), Theos Bernard Papers; second draft, 58, VWB Archive.

2. Ruth Fuller Everett—later Ruth Fuller Sasaki, wife of Sokei-an. She would later introduce her son-in-law Alan Watts to both Pierre Bernard and Sokei-an; the latter then accepted Watts as his student. Ruth spent lengthy periods of time at Pierre Bernard's country club throughout the 1930s. Fields, *How the Swans Came to the Lake*, 187–188.

3. Later that year Ruth Everett would be in Nyack with "a Chinese monk . . . helping her to translate some Chinese and Japanese Buddhistic stuff." PAB to VWB, August 21, 1936, VWB Archive #17.15.

4. "U.A. Student to Study Primitive Indian Folk," *Arizona Daily Star*, July 10, 1936, 3.

5. His childhood friend Dan Hughes remarked, "I remember a time when I was out working in my garden. Up pulls a big limousine with a negro chauffeur. Theos stepped out." "Interview with Daniel Hughes," VWB Archive #16.23.

6. Melville, *Moby Dick*, 152.

7. Such disturbances were not unknown throughout China. In addition to being in an effective state of civil war, it was also on the brink of war with Japan, and the *New York Times* considered the whole region to be in a state of chaos:

In the south, large forces of Nanking troops exchange raids with forces from the Provinces of Kwangtung and Kwangsi. In the northeast and Inner Mongolia, Japanese military preparations and demonstrations grow more ominous. In Outer Mongolia, a mutual assistance pact has recently been concluded with the Soviet Union. To the northwest and the west the great regions of Sinkiang and Tibet are subject to foreign control and are in the throes of political unrest. ("Tragedy in China," *New York Times*, July 1, 1936, 24)

In this atmosphere, railroad highjackings in particular were a quite reasonable fear, and there were known to be "pirates and trouble along the railroad from Chengsha to Canton." Although the dangers were perhaps not as dramatic as portrayed in von Sternberg's *Shanghai Express* (1932), nonetheless when the film was first released, it was banned in China for the negative portrayal of the country and its ongoing political troubles, presumably for being not too far from the truth:

"Can you tell me what's wrong now!?!"
"You're in China now sir, where time and life have no value." (*Shanghai Express*, Paramount Studios, 1932)

8. The Thirteenth Dalai Lama left Tibet on only two notable occasions in the twentieth century: from 1904 to 1909, to Mongolia and China following the British

invasion of Tibet led by Francis Younghusband, and from 1910 to 1912 to India following the Chinese invasion of Tibet engineered by Chao Erh-feng. There is no indication that he ever visited Shanghai during either period. It is possible that the Ninth Panchen Lama may have visited Shanghai, but the details of his activities in China are hazy and difficult to confirm.

9. Forman recounted his adventures first in a short excerpted article for *Harper's* and later in a full-length book. Forman, "I See the King of Hell," *Harper's Magazine*, 14–25; Forman, *Through Forbidden Tibet*.

10. Goldenweiser, *History, Psychology, and Culture*, 164.

11. TCB's contact print boards are now part of the photographic collection at the Hearst Museum. Theos Bernard Collection, Phoebe A. Hearst Anthropological Museum, University of California at Berkeley.

12. The only luxury hotel in Rangoon at the time, described as "the finest hostelry east of Suez," the late-Victorian era Strand boasted thirty-two suites outfitted with polished teak, chandeliers, and ceiling fans. *A Handbook for Travelers in India Burma & Ceylon* (1910); "The Hotels," *The Rangoon Gazette*, September 10, 1936, 7.

13. Woodroffe, *Garland of Letters*, viii–ix.

14. One of only a handful of luxury hotels, along with the Windamere and the Planter's Club, the Mount Everest Hotel was considered one of the finest places to stay in Darjeeling.

15. At the time of my research (2007), Mr. Espenschied (age 94) could no longer recall any details about these events.

16. Wangchuk Dorji (a.k.a. "Willie," 1902–63). Rhodes, *S.W. Laden La*, 89.

17. Henry Albert Carpenter was yet another individual, emblematic of the growth of counterculture American religion in the early twentieth century. He maintained his interests privately, only occasionally discussing them among friends and colleagues, although was a well-known figure at the Windamere Hotel and a friend of the Laden La family. Since he died in March 1937, and in the absence of any evidence to the contrary, it is unlikely that Theos and Viola met him.

18. Viola records in her diary that they purchased two human skull cups and a thigh-bone trumpet.

19. Theos did manage to acquire the two phonograph records available at the time: Gramophone records nos. 16622 and 16623, which included chants from "Muru Monastery" and performances by the "Lhasa Orchestra" and "Kyumu Lunga troupe." Ironically, both were broken in his luggage on his return from India. The records, however, still exist and the recordings have recently been recovered digitally thanks to the efforts of the author, the Phoebe Apperson Hearst Museum, and Lawrence Berkeley Laboratories.

20. In her later years, seeking to protect the reputations of both PAB and DeVries, Viola destroyed these diary entries, leaving a gap in her India trip journal from September 26 until October 12, 1936.

21. An early twentieth-century movement in America that asserted decidedly testosterone-fueled notions of Christian social ethics. Alter, "Yoga at the Fin de Siècle: Muscular Christianity with a 'Hindu' Twist," 759–776; Rodrigues, *The Householder Yogi*.

7. A Well-Trodden Path: Studies in Darjeeling and Sikkim

1. Aśvaghoṣa and Covill, *Handsome Nanda*, 135.

2. Defined as the suppression (*stambha*) of the elemental force of water (*jala*), allowing one to float for any length of time.

3. *Kumbhaka*, the aspect of *prāṇāyāma* related to breath retention.

4. Van Manen's Chinese butler, Twan Yang, commented on his master's fluency in Tibetan. Yang, *Houseboy*, 123.

5. See Richardus, *The Dutch Orientalist*.

6. Yang, *Houseboy*, 179.

7. Richardus, *The Dutch Orientalist*, 33.

8. Jung, "The Dreamlike World of India," in *Civilization in Transition*, 516.

9. The book was sent to David Macdonald to review, who subsequently vouched for its accuracy, having been the one who saved Schary's life. See Schary, *In Search of the Mahatmas of Tibet*.

10. Bowles had completed a similar survey two years earlier in eastern Tibet and western China (Szechuan). See Bowles, *The People of Asia*.

11. Lachen Gomchen (the great meditator at Lachen), as the locals called him.

12. From the Tibetan *mda' gling* meaning "realm of the arrow" and the pan-Indian (though properly speaking, Kannada) word for "fort," *kote*, after an old Bhutanese fort that stood in the southeast part of the town until the British–Bhutanese War of 1864–65. *Darjeeling District Gazetteer*, 181, 214.

13. *bka' blon spung*. See *Darjeeling District Gazetteer*, 215.

14. *spu*. A small village, little known, frequented more by missionaries than scholars or explorers, with only Sven Hedin briefly passing through on one of his returns (in 1906) to mark it on the map.

15. D. Tharchin, "Brief Biography of the Editor of the Tibetan Newspaper 'Yulchhog-so-soi sangyur melong' Printed and Published at Kalimpong, District Darjeeling," undated typescript (ca. 1945), Gergan Dorje Tharchin Papers, Starr East Asian Library, Special Collections, Columbia University.

16. At this point in time, the British capital of India was Calcutta; it was only changed to Delhi following the proclamation of King George V on December 12, 1911, along with other redistricting measures.

17. That is, the Coronation Day in honor of the British King, George V and Queen Mary. More significantly for India, it was on this day—December 12, 1911—that King George V would be made Emperor of India.

18. Karma Sumdhon Paul repudiated his Christian conversion in 1920, though he continued to act as headmaster for the school for another three years. After his dismissal by the missionary authorities, he was left with little means of support. With the help of Johan van Manen, he was able to obtain an appointment at Calcutta University as a Lecturer in Tibetan. He went on to work closely with the Young Men's Buddhist Association and the Sri Ramakrishna Vedanta Ashram in Darjeeling, supporting their promotion of Tibetan and Buddhist culture for several decades afterward.

19. By the early 1960s, Tharchin's primers had been adopted and used by Tibetan school systems across north India from Leh (Ladakh) to Sikkim. Given Tharchin's self-described inadequacies in his command of the Tibetan language and his highly idiosyncratic Tibetan writing style, this is more than a little ironic. In later years, Tharchin would reprint copies of his primers; these reveal the grammar to be based entirely on indigenous Tibetan mnemonic "Thirty Letters" (*sum cu pa*) textbooks.

20. Manuel, *A Gladdening River*, 160.

21. Tharchin notes that Do-ring Theji (*mdo ring tha'i ji*) and "Kung Kusho" [Chang-lo-chen, So-nam-gyal-po] (*gung sku zhabs; lcang lo can bsod nams rgyal po*), Tibetan military officers from Lhasa, came down to Gyantse to study English and Hindustani, since the latter was the medium through which they were receiving their military training. D. Tharchin, "Brief Biography of the Editor."

22. In the short term, however, Tharchin noted that the Christian orientation of the school piqued the curiosity of the abbot of Palkor Chöde Monastery (*dpal 'khor chos sde*) in Gyantse, who, much to Tharchin's delight, borrowed his copy of the Tibetan Bible (New Testament), sharing it with members of the faculty there—many of whom would visit Tharchin from time to time to debate religious questions—before returning it some months later.

23. The school, according to Charles Bell, had been in the planning as early as the time of the Simla Convention of 1914 that officially recognized Tibetan sovereignty over the Tibetan Plateau, over the objections of the Chinese delegates. Macdonald notes that there were a number of reasons the school was closed, including "(i) the parents were opposed to sending their sons so far away from home; (ii) the lamas were against the school because they reasoned that if there was a division in the use of the boys' time between English and Tibetan they would not learn either language properly; and (iii) the Tibetan government was unable to maintain regular payment of the Headmaster's salary." This latter point McKay attributes to the Lhasa government's representative, Lo-sang-jung-ne (*blo bzang 'byung gnas*), who was sent to oversee the school and forced to pay for its operation out of his own pocket. Others have cited the possible influence (i.e., bribery) of Chinese and pro-Chinese factions in Lhasa, who would later establish their own school in Lhasa ten years later. McKay, *Tibet and the British Raj*, 117.

24. Tharchin to Ch. Bell, July 25, 1937, Bell Papers, OIOC Mss Eur. F-80, fol. 130, British Library.

25. The Kashak (*bka' shag*) and the Tsongdu (*tshogs 'du*), respectively.

26. George Knight, who had attempted to reach Lhasa in 1922 (accompanied by William McGovern on *his* first attempt) had a distinctly hostile—and some consider false and slanderous, except for the charge of spying—opinion of Tharchin:

The native schoolmaster at Gyantse, who spoke English rather well, and taught little Tibetan boys and girls to sing Tibetan songs to the tune of "Auld Lang Syne," "Mother McCree," "Molly McIntyre," etc., was always on the *qui-vive,* and his reports to the Tibetan officials on our conduct in general were not couched in very favorable terms. This, however, did not trouble us greatly, since we afterwards learned that he never thought well of anyone outside of his own race, and his opinions of Mr. Macdonald, the British Trade Agent, and Major Bailey, the Political Officer, are unprintable. He was engaged to spy upon us during our month's stay in Gyantse, and he was candid enough to admit it while under the effects of a strong dose of Indian whisky, the worst in the world, which everyone is strictly forbidden to drink in Tibet, although all the Tibetan officials with whom we came into contact admired its flavor exceedingly much. (Knight, *Intimate Glimpses of Mysterious Tibet*, 60)

When questioned by the British Political Officer for Sikkim, F. M. Bailey, upon his arrival that year, Tharchin defended himself and his conduct, stating that no objection or opposition had arisen from any of the Tibetans themselves, lay or clerical—upon which Bailey approved Tharchin's request to accompany his students to Lhasa.

27. David Macdonald cited more personal difficulties for Tharchin as playing a significant role in his return. Macdonald writes that Tharchin "remained for some time in the capital, but found life there very trying, and not very remunerative, as living expenses for a person not of the country are high. Finally, he tried to augment his income by trading in a small way, but still found that he could not make ends meet. He is now with me in Kalimpong, where he is employed as a lay teacher by the Tibetan Mission in that place." Macdonald, *Twenty Years in Tibet*, 223–224.

28. *yul phyogs so so'i gsar 'gyur gyi me long*. D. Tharchin, "A Brief History of the Tibetan Newspaper."

29. The donation was a sum of money 200 times the advertised cover price of 1 anna 6 peonies. Tharchin, "A Brief History."

30. Tharchin notes that he was granted an audience with the Thirteenth Dalai Lama at 10 a.m. on December 5, 1927. Although they had a very pointed exchange concerning events in India, Tharchin also noted that the entire audience lasted five minutes. Tharchin, "A Brief History.".

31. The first issue produced on the new Litho Press was vol. 3, no. 5/6, dated September 14, 1928.

32. Tharchin reported that Rev. Knox was particularly obstructive and caused no end of problems, from attempting to prevent Tharchin from using the litho press to eventually charging him for its use while forcing him to return to his previous duties. As a result, Tharchin's publication of the newspaper would be sporadic over the ensuing five years. Tharchin, "A Brief History.".

33. As a result, the printed date of an issue was determined more by dictates of consistency than the actual date of release.

34. From the Greek *katekhistes* ("to teach by word of mouth"), the term refers to a Christian instructor who educates would-be converts prior to their participation in the requisite rituals.

35. Do-kar-wa Tse-ring-wang-gyel (*mdo khar ba tshe ring dbang rgyal*, 1697–1763), *bod rgya shan sbyar ngo mtshar nor bu'i do shal*; published as Bacot, *Dictionnaire tibétan-sanscrit*.

36. Bacot, *Une grammaire tibétaine du tibétain classique*.

37. *gdan sa gsum*, referring to the great monastic universities situated around Lhasa: Drepung (*'bras spungs*), Ganden (*dga' ldan*), and Sera (*se rwa*).

38. Sāṅkṛtyāyana says nothing of what transpired in Tibet on this first journey, only making passing remarks about the disregard in which Sanskrit manuscripts were held in Tibet. Sāṅkṛtyāyana, "Sanskrit Palm-Leaf Mss. in Tibet," 21.

39. Sāṅkṛtyāyana reports that his second trip lasted slightly more than six months, from April 4 to November 10, 1934. Sāṅkṛtyāyana, "Sanskrit Palm-leaf mss. in Tibet," 22.

40. *zur khang, rwa sgreng rin po che*, and *bka' blon bla ma*.

41. *bstan 'gyur*, the "Translated Treatises."

42. *bka' 'gyur*, the "Translated Words [of the Buddha]."

43. *rdo sbis dge bshes shes rab rgya mtsho* (1884–1968).

44. It is reported that Gedun Chöpel related the story that "Though [dGe-bshes] Shes-rab was supposed to be teaching me textbooks, [he] and I didn't get along at all. Whatever he taught I would only oppose and debate against. Apart from calling me 'madman,' [he] did not call [me by] my [real] name." Mengele, *dGe-'dun-chos-'phel*, 52.

45. *dge 'dun chos 'phel* (1903–1951).

46. *dge bshes chos [kyi] grags [pa]*.

47. A complete list of his acquisitions in Lhasa, at Kundeling (*kun bde gling*), Pö-kang-tsok-pa (*spos khang tshogs pa*), Ngor (*ngor*), and Shalu (*zhwa lu*) is given in Sāṅkṛtyāyana, "Sanskrit Palm-leaf mss. in Tibet."

48. Gedun Chöpel remarks early in his "White Annals" (*deb ther dkar po*) that he had read a number of original Tun-huang manuscripts; this appears to have been when he had the opportunity to do so. Gedun Chöpel (*dge 'dun chos 'phel*), *Bod chen po'i srid lugs dang 'brel ba'i rgyal rabs deb ther dkar po* (Dharamsala: Sherig Parkhang, 1993), 28; Choephel and Norboo, *The White Annals*, 33.

49. TCB reported that he had put Tharchin on a salary as opposed to paying for individual lessons.

50. Although it is certain that Glen was regularly ingesting mercury compounds, it is unclear to what extent Theos and Viola were.

51. A single mention in a single sentence, which sixty years later Viola would still find worth remarking on. "Notes re Letters from Theos Bernard from India and Tibet to VWB dictated July/August 1996 by VWB," VWB Archives #1.4.

52. McGovern, *To Lhasa in Disguise*, 281.

53. The manuscript, Jang-lung Paṇḍita's "Assorted Scripts and Diagrams," appears to have been one of many resources that Tharchin kept on hand for his own reference. Jang-lung Ārya Paṇḍita Nga-wang-lo-sang-ten-pay-gyel-tsen (*lcang lung ārya paṇḍi ta ngag dbang blo bzang bstan pa'i rgyal mtshan*, 1770–1845), *rgya dkar nag rgya ser ka smi ra bal bod hor gyi yi ge dang dpe ris rnam grangs mang ba*.

54. One of the practices central to the *vajroli-mudra*.

55. TCB's referral to Viola in the third person is confusing here, as the rest of the letter clearly indicates that the person he is writing to is Viola herself.

56. A hat popularized by the British King Edward VII. Pallis, *Peaks and Lamas*, 124.

57. A region of Russia that lies west of the Volga River and north of the Caspian Sea. Some have maintained that the Kalmyks took their name from the Mongolian word *kalimak*, meaning "beyond the shore," although this appears to be a false etymology. Others, citing Islamic sources, offer a different etymology of the name, claiming that "Kalmyk" comes from the Turkic word *qalmaq*, meaning "to remain," and designates those peoples of Central Asia who did *not* convert to Islam, but rather *remained* Buddhists. This too may be a false etymology, since the Turkic word *qalmaq* means to (physically) remain somewhere or to settle down, and may simply refer to a group of Mongols who did not return to Mongolia but remained behind in the Uzbek/Khazak area.

58. The most prominent member of the group ca. 1918 was Sergey Stepanovich Borisov, a Russian Turk disguised as a Mongolian monk. Charged with opening diplomatic relations with Tibet, he was to bring guns and ammunition as an offering to the Tibetan government.

59. Something that was eventually done to Kham, and Amdo to the north, following the second Chinese invasion of Tibet in the twentieth century, in 1950.

60. A Lhasa-born half-Tibetan, half-Chinese Muslim who worked for China's Mongolian and Tibetan Affairs Commission, Liu Manqing does not seem to have been present at Geshe Wangyal's New Year's party. Upon meeting her a few weeks later in Calcutta, TCB described her to VWB as "a Tibetan Woman Ambassador going to China (Nanking) and . . . one of the most forceful, impressive personalities that I have seen in a long time."

61. Drawn from "sngags chen bdar ba ho thog thu blo bzang bstan 'dzin 'jigs med dbang phyug gi rnam thar rags bsdus," *bod kyi lo rgyus rig gnas dpyad gzhi'i rgyu cha bdams bsgrigs*, 80–91.

62. The vast majority of sūtras and tantras contained in the Tibetan canon never reached China, and the Tibetans therefore always viewed Chinese Buddhism as an inferior, partial transmission. In addition, it was widely believed in the Lhasa governmental circles that Geshe Sherap Gyatso had strong pro-Communist leanings. Whether this was true or not, his political opinions would ultimately prove unacceptable to both sides of the Tibetan–Chinese conflict, and he would be tortured to death by Chinese Communists during the Cultural Revolution.

63. Kipling, *Kim*, 259.

64. Other notable figures who appeared in *Kim* were Sir Charles Macgregor ("Colonel Creighton"), Quartermaster-General of the Indian army and head of the Intelligence Department, and Captain Charles Christie ("Mahbub Ali"), who "traversed Baluchistan dressed up as a Tartar horse dealer." French, *Younghusband*, 35.

65. In Kipling's book (and subsequent movie adaptations), the character of the Tibetan Lama is an absurd caricature of an elderly monk, and is one count on which the charges of Orientalist fantasy seem well grounded.

66. Das, *Narrative of a Journey to Lhasa in 1881-82*, 1, 31; Das, *Narrative of a Journey Round Lake Yamdo (Palti) and in Lhoka, Yarlung, and Sakya in 1882*.

67. Candler, *The Unveiling of Lhasa*, 203. Landon gives a different set of numbers in one appendix to his rendition of the events. He listed the company as comprised of:

91 British officers, 11 British warrant officers, 521 British N.C.O. and men, 32 Native officers, 5 Native warrant officers, 1,961 Native N.C.O. and men, 1,450 Followers, and 3,451 mules and ponies. Landon, *The Opening of Tibet*, 455–459.

68. Early reports had stated the opposing Tibetan force as "some 2,600 Tibetan soldiers . . . occupying the heights and passes along a line running between Phari and Shigatse. 1,000 rifles manufactured at Lhasa have been issued to the Lhasa Command, and 500 each to the Phari and Shigatse Commands." When the military confrontation finally occurred at Gyantse, the battle was decidedly one-sided. "Political Diary of the Tibet Frontier Commission," in *The British Invasion of Tibet: Colonel Younghusband, 1904*, 122ff.

69. Sir Francis Younghusband, "Speech at Clifton College," Younghusband Papers, Oriental and India Office Collection, British Library Mss. Eur 197, f. 510, quoted in French, *Younghusband*, 10.

70. *gtsang pa blo bzang rgyal mtshan* (b. 1840). The post of Ganden Tri-pa (*dga' ldan khri pa*) is a rotating appointment typically of three to six years' duration. The Ganden Tri-pa is the official head of the Gelukpa (*dge lugs pa*) lineage and technically the man to whom both the Dalai and Paṇchen lamas are subordinate.

71. Younghusband, "An Explorer's Religion," 652–53. Younghusband would continue his speculations on topics of "natural philosophy," going so far as to suggest the existence of other forms of life on other worlds, and possibly on this one as well. These would be beings, "possessed of subtly delicate sense-organs . . . on a plane where they are profoundly conscious of the Spirit of the World." It was, in Younghusband's opinion, precisely this *esprit de corps* that was the religious and spiritual motivation inherent in all beings, and something to be venerated and encouraged. Younghusband, *Life in the Stars*, 131–134.

72. Amiruddin, "World Congress of Faiths," *Star of India* (Calcutta), March 8, 1937, 4, col. 4.

73. Younghusband's decoration as K.C.B. (Knight Commander of the Bath) was blocked by the political enemies of Lord Curzon and he received only a K.C.I.E. (Knight Commander of the Order of the Indian Empire), but years later (1917) he would be decorated as K.C.S.I. (Knight Commander of the Star of India). French, *Younghusband*, 307.

74. Since he was not one to pass up such an opportunity, it is surprising that no photo of this gathering exists in Theos Bernard's papers. It is possible that photos were taken, since the roll of film corresponding to this period of time contains only six photos of Ngak-chen Rinpoche and his attendant; the remainer of the roll may have received the wrong exposure in inexperienced hands. The negatives for this roll of film (D-XXIII) are currently undergoing conservation and may in the future reveal prints recoverable by new means. Another possibility is that the lack of photos was the result of a mechanical failure. TCB, in fact, remarked to VWB that he was experiencing problems with his Leica, and "in several very critical instances film has jammed on me and the camera has failed to work completely." One can imagine such a gathering as easily meeting the description of a "critical instance."

75. Heather Stoddard notes that during this time in Calcutta, one of the conversations going on was between Gedun Chöpel and Geshe Sherap Gyatso, in which Gedun

Chöpel attempted to convince his teacher that the shape of the Earth was, in fact, round. Whether he succeeded or not is unclear, but rather than admit the slightest defeat, he took the conversation as an inspiration to write a short, if somewhat inflammatory article for Tharchin's *Mirror* newspaper, entitled simply, "The Earth: Round or Spherical." Stoddard, *Le Mendiant de l'Amdo*, 178; "drang po dharma" (a.k.a. Gedun Chöpel), "'jig rten ril mo 'am zlum po," *Mirror*, vol. 10, no. 1 (June 28, 1938), 11.

76. An article in Calcutta's *Star of India* newspaper reported that "Mr. An Chhin Huthoktu Ta Lama Rimpochhe . . . popularly known as 'Bara Lama' . . . after a stay of nine days in Calcutta . . . will visit China in connection with some important work relating to the Governments of both the countries (China and Tibet) and is expected to return to Lhasa after three years." Given the romanization of the Chinese pronunciation of Ngak-chen Rinpoche's name, it is likely that the information was relayed by one of the Chinese officials accompanying the entourage. It is also interesting to note the discrepancy between the apparent Chinese perspective on events ("to return . . . after three years") and Ngak-chen Rinpoche's own intention, expressed to TCB, to return to Shigatse the following September. "Bara Lama," *Star of India* (Calcutta), February 26, 1937, 3 col. 5.

77. *Religions of the World*, 1:16–17, 64, 72.

78. Well informed of movements afoot in China, the Chinese Republican government had intended to forcibly return the Panchen Lama to Tibet with a Chinese military escort, and "in mid-August the Panchen and his party moved to the La-hsiu monastery on the Tsinghai-Tibet border." When the 1937 war between Japan and China began, however, the Nanking government wired Jyekundo suggesting a postponement of the Panchen Lama's return to Tibet, which was then forwarded to the monastery. After debating the measure for more than a month, in October 1937, the Panchen Lama and his entourage began their return journey to Jyekundo, but he developed a cold and became seriously ill; he would die in Jyekundo on December 1, 1937. Boorman and Howard, *Biographical Dictionary of Republican China*, 3:60–61.

79. This same timetable for a return to Tibet by the Panchen Lama was reported by Tharchin to Charles Bell at the time. D. Tharchin to Charles Bell, February 16, 1937, OIOC Eur. Mss. F-80, fol. 130.

80. Berg, *Lindbergh*, 364; "Still Modest," *New York Times*, March 5, 1937, 20.

81. Indeed, the fact that Lindbergh was even visiting India and attending the conference was kept secret. Newswire reports made papers around the world, tracking Lindbergh's flight to an "unknown destination," "their movements shrouded in secrecy," and his arrival in Calcutta "on the fifth anniversary" of the kidnapping and death of his son. French, *Younghusband*, 368. "Lindberghs Still Missing," *Star of India*, February 24, 1937, 1; "Lindbergh's Movements," *Star of India*, February 25, 1937, 1; "Colonel Lindbergh," *Star of India*, February 27, 1937, 4; "Lindberghs at Calcutta," *New York Times*, March 1, 1937, 9.

82. "dge ba'i bshes gnyen shes rab rgya mtsho," *Mirror*, vol. 8, no. 12 (March 13, 1937), 7 col. 3.

83. Dr. Morgan later told TCB that such occurrences were not uncommon. Given the problems of the British empire,

sending men to such outposts as this [Lhasa] and the one at Gyantse . . . seems to be causing them considerable grief, for the loneliness of the place makes it almost impossible to leave a man there for longer than 2 years even by offering him a little change by an occasional tour down to Yatung to make an inspection. It seems that some official in India that doesn't have the slightest idea where Tibet is located was trying to urge them to send someone up for five years which meant, of course, certain insanity, for they report that the two year stay doesn't seem to help any of their men. (TCB Diary II)

84. Whether this is true or not, Chapman does seem to have struggled with "manic-depressive tendencies" for a large part of his life. Barker, *One Man's Jungle*, 128.

85. The translation would be completed by Tharchin, typed, and later sent on to TCB in America.

86. Gould and Richardson, *Tibetan Word Book*. When it was finally published in 1943, Gould thanked a number of individuals, including David Macdonald and Tharchin, though for reasons that will become obvious later, not TCB.

87. Macdonald, *Touring in Sikkim and Tibet*, 32.

88. "a mi ri ka'i sa heb," *Mirror*, vol. 8, no. 12 (March 13, 1937), 4 col. 2.

89. "gsar 'gyu do dam pa'i sger zhu," *Mirror*, vol. 9, no. 1 (May 11, 1937), 6 col. 3.

90. *spom mda' tshang*. Hailing from Kham (Eastern Tibet), the patriarch of the Pang-datsang family was considered the richest Tibetan trader, having secured a position as an Agent of the Tibetan Government in India. His import-export company had a major branch in Kalimpong with agents "all over Tibet and in China and in India." *Who's Who in Tibet*, 53.

91. Telling VWB of his dislike for the phrase "Roof of the World," TCB suggested this as his alternate metaphor.

8. Tibet, Tantrikas, and the Hero of Chaksam Ferry

1. TCB Diary #1, 23(r), Theos Bernard Papers; second draft, 74–75, VWB Archive.

2. Attributed to Tourgiit Jentsen, a Kalmyk Mongolian scholar at Urga Monastery in Ulaanbaatar. Joshua Cutler, "Preface to the New Edition," in Geshe Wangyal, *Door of Liberation*, xxi.

3. Although staying at the British Regency in Gangtok as a guest of Gould, TCB took Gould's draft manuscript back to the dak bungalow after Tharchin had arrived. Although TCB was able to make organizational suggestions, it was Tharchin who made many of the content suggestions and corrections to Gould's books, though he allowed TCB to present them as his own. Years later, when Gould finally published his books, having discovered the actual state of TCB's knowledge of the Tibetan language, he thanked Tharchin in his preface, omitting any mention of TCB, while Richardson went so far as to omit TCB's name from his list of foreign visitors to Tibet up through the 1940s. Gould and Richardson, *Tibetan Word Book*; Richardson, "Foreigners in Tibet," in *High Peaks, Pure Earth*, 409–419.

4. Although in his later works, Gould speaks of the Indian heritage of Tibet, he never so much as mentions the word "tantra," positively or negatively. Gould, *The Jewel in the Lotus.*

5. In addition to recycling material from his letters to VWB, there are points scattered throughout the "diaries" where TCB is clearly making observations and references addressed specifically to the reader of the documents, often speaking self-consciously in the first person plural or making references that only VWB would understand, including code words from their cablegrams, even ending one entry (May 18) with "nothing else of any consequence, so goodnight everyone." It is clear that TCB envisioned his composition first and foremost as a book draft and less as an actual diary per se. He states as much, at one point (May 20) expressing his concern that his account might "be read by someone else who will offer me criticism of misunderstanding rather than the consideration of a faith."

6. Although the "-la" suffix means "mountain pass" in Tibetan, to differentiate rest stops from passes, I have added the redundant "Pass" to these place names.

7. Dro-mo (*gro mo*) is the Tibetan name for the same locale called Yatung by the Indians. According to TCB, the monastery lay five miles south of the town proper at the lower end of the valley.

8. *Gom-pa* (*dgon pa*), literally meaning "[place in the] wilderness" (*araṇyaka*), is the word usually translated in English as "monastery."

9. Strictly speaking the term "yak" only applies to the male of the species, "dri" being the female. Hence, although generally accepted in the day-to-day usage of foreigners, the notion of "yak milk" or "yak cheese" is often a source of amusement to most Tibetans. Nonetheless, since TCB uses such phrases throughout his diaries and letters, I repeat them here as well.

10. A *khata* (*kha btags*), a traditional sign of respect.

11. *rgyud 'bum.*

12. *klong chen rab byams pa* (1308–64). His "Seven Treasuries" (*mdzod bdun*) are held to explicate the Nyingma tantric worldview.

13. *dung dkar dgon pa.*

14. Geshe Nga-wang-kel-sang (*ngag dbang skal bzang*), a.k.a. Dro-mo Geshe (*gro mo dge bshes*).

15. *dud sna.*

16. Chapman and his guide Pasang alone attempted to reach the summit by taking advantage of a clearance in the weather, but close to the top they were caught in a blizzard. Although they eventually succeeded, they nearly died in a fall of several hundred feet on their way down. Barker, *One Man's Jungle*, 139–156.

17. A light midday meal.

18. Although Hugh Richardson was the actual British Trade Agent in Gyantse, the Escort Commander, Gordon E.P. Cable, was acting in his stead until Richardson was permanently transferred to Lhasa, at which point Captain Keith Battye took up the post. Gould, *Jewel in the Lotus*, 204; Williamson, *Memoirs of a Political Officer's Wife*, 190.

19. "sa zla'i dus bzang," *Mirror* 9, no. 2 (June 9, 1937), 3 col.

20. *rdo rje dbang rgyal*; a.k.a. *lcog bkras*; also "Choktepa" (*lcog bkras pa*).

8. Tibet, Tantrikas, and the Hero of Chaksam Ferry

21. His younger brother, Sidkeong Tulku, an incarnate lama who had been educated at Oxford, succeeded to the throne instead, but was murdered less than a year later—it was thought that his reforms were resented by the Sikkimese landlords—and Taring Raja's half-brother, Chögyal Tashi Namgyal, succeeded to the throne. Taring, *Daughter of Tibet*, 106.

22. Rinchen Dolma and Jigme Taring were married in 1930, at the same time as their respective younger siblings, Changchub Dolma ("Daisy") Tsarong and Chime Taring. Tibetan family politics, especially among the aristocracy, were notoriously complex, and the history of the Taring and Tsarong families is no exception. A more detailed chronology is given in Taring, *Daughter of Tibet*.

23. Although such affairs would later cause considerable trouble for Reting, at the time he remained powerful and highly influential.

24. Theos attempted to document the meal as best he could in his diary, noting everything from stewed mutton in gravy with onion and carrots, herrings, peaches, and tinned pineapple slices to Mongolian ham, yak tongue, and various beef dishes, all washed down with a continuous supply of *chang* (Tibetan barley beer)—all of which, he soon learned, was merely the appetizers leading into all manner of soups and dumplings.

25. Ernst Schäfer, leader of the German expedition two years later, would remark at length on her beauty as well.

26. An apparent reference to the macro lenses that enabled TCB to photograph books and prints.

27. Over the summer of 1937, TCB would personally be responsible for more print runs of Tibetan stamps than any other visitor in the existence of the Tibetan postal system, and likewise for the vast majority of Tibetan stamps that made their way to America.

28. Determined to maintain friendly relations with Cable as well as preserve his image in the Gyantse community, Theos accompanied him only to photograph gazelle—none of which they encountered anyway.

29. Although such statements could appear to be racially motivated, there is reason to believe that they were not. As the months in Tibet passed, TCB began writing more and more about the "beautiful" Tibetan women he was meeting. Being fully conscious of VWB as the primary audience of his "diaries," he remained careful to follow every mention with some caveat ("without being of your own kind, which of course is the best," or "objectively speaking," and "don't get the wrong idea," etc.).

30. This observation about the equitable relationships in Tibetan families was something TCB would return to, seeing the same pattern of shared responsibility in the Tsarong household as well, where Lady Tsarong—"the Lacham"—"in business affairs . . . runs the household . . . and even to this day, she handles the books to a certain extent." It was striking to Theos that in Tibetan society the women "play a much more important role then does the Indian wife, who apparently has only one reason for being."

31. Chokte and Namkye Tsedrön appeared to have had a rather unique relationship in this regard, even within Tibet, though it was not without certain problems.

They were both students of the famous Lo-chen Rinpoche, a female incarnate lama in the Nyingma tradition who lived in a hermitage in the hills above Lhasa. As tantric practitioners, they engaged in sexual yogas, but this appears to have been a problem for Chokte since, despite being married to a woman regarded as the most beautiful in Tibet, Chokte appears not to have been sexually attracted to women. The leader of the German expedition to Lhasa a few years later, Ernst Schäfer, noted in his diary Chokte's request for the medicine "Okasa," a male sexual stimulant being produced in Germany, which had gained popularity and a certain notoriety in Lhasa. This appears to have been the use—tantric consort practice—to which Chokte intended to put the medication. "mi snyan pa'i gnas tshul," *Mirror*, 27 no. 8/9 (May–June 1961), 5–6; Isrun Engelhardt, private communication; for a detailed biography of Lo-chen Rinpoche and discussion of her age, see Havnevik, "The Life of Jetsun Lo-chen Rinpoche (1865–1951)."

32. TCB consistently makes the mistake of referring to these as being associated with the "Kargyupa" (*bka' brgyud pa*) sect.

33. TCB states that the back of the *thangka* has "an inscription of the Lama who had it created with the seal of both of his hands on the back." It is "a large painting of Guru Rinpoche, or Padma Sambhava seated on his lotus with his yidam (protector) on the left and the revealer of his teachings on the other, . . . In the upper right corner is a figure representing the founder of the Kargyupa sect and a devotee in the opposite corner." This may be the ca. eighteenth- to nineteenth-century *thangka* of Padmasambhava now housed in the Berkeley Art Museum (provisional catalog number B-17); during my tenure at UC Berkeley, I was unable to obtain any further information about the items in the Bernard collection from the staff at the Berkeley Art Museum to make a firm identification.

34. TCB notes that on one occasion he managed to purchase a beautiful silk embroidery and on another, was able to get some tutoring in spoken Tibetan from Kyipup Wang-di-nor-bu, the assistant Tibetan Trade Agent, who had studied English and engineering as a young boy in London twenty years earlier. "Kyi-pup II," *Who's Who in Tibet*, 36.

35. TCB records that his countryman William Caesar Smacky had made a short-lived attempt to cross into Tibet on his quest to meet his "1,700 year old yogi near Gyantse," a German fellow "who had similar ambitions" had made it as far as crossing a first pass before being apprehended, and finally "Cedar Bloom," a Swedish woman, had deceived all the guards disguised "as a coolie-woman with a heavy load on her back" and had even made it as far as Yatung; she escaped capture once in Pedong, only to be rounded up by the border guards.

36. Bell, "Pious Tibet Searches for a Little Child," *New York Times Magazine*, May 23, 1937, 12–13, 28.

37. Dundul Namgyal Tsarong further recounts,

The most important were the relics of the Lord Buddha, given to my father at Benares by His Holiness the Thirteenth Dalai Lama. This was by far the most sacred room of the house. It was a sad moment when I was told that during the

Chinese Cultural Revolution in the late 1960s, Red Guards entered our house and the three life-size images were thrown out of the window and smashed. Nobody knows what happened to the precious ornaments with which they were adorned.

According to the account, Lord Tsarong was in Varanasi (Benares) and saw British officers breaking open a Buddhist *stūpa* and extracting fragments of bones, manuscripts and other items. Approaching one of the Indian workers, Lord Tsarong gave the man all the money he had on him in exchange for some of the relics when the British officials were not looking. After presenting them to the Thirteenth Dalai Lama, Lord Tsarong was honored in return, being given some of them back for his own personal altar. Tsarong, *In the Service*, 72.

38. Tsarong, *In the Service*, 71–73.

39. Tsarong was educated at the Phalai school, housed at the Dalai Lama's summer palace, the Norbu Lingka. Although much of the education system in Tibet was housed in the monasteries and open only to monks, there were numerous private schools in Lhasa run, typically, by former government officials of the secretarial office (*drung yig*). There were two larger schools for administrative training—the Tse school and the Tsikhang (*rtsis khang*)—and close to fifty private, nongovernmental day schools that provided free education to Tibetan children. Dundul Namgyal Tsarong, interview; Taring, *Daughter of Tibet*, 46–47.

40. As his son, Dundul Namgyal Tsarong, notes,

The name Chen-tsel . . . was only used when referring to the rare few who were designated as close associates. The literal translation of this name is "clear eyes" and it means "as seen through the clear eyes of His Holiness." Later on it became a nickname for Father; everyone called him Chen-tsel. Many people have since misinterpreted this name, regarding the "clear eyes" to be those of Tsarong. However, this name actually referred to the eyes of the Dalai Lama, which were able to clearly perceive who were to be the trusted favorites. (Tsarong, *In the Service*, 21)

41. While visiting the Chinese "sacred mountain" of Wu Tai Shan, William Woodville Rockhill came to pay his respects to the entourage; this was "the first official contact between Tibet and the United States of America." Tsarong, *In the Service*, 21.

42. Mullin notes that Chao was notorious for beheading any and all who opposed him at whim. David Macdonald speculated at the time that the capture and assassination of the Thirteenth Dalai Lama may have been the intent of the Chinese government all along. He remarked:

It must be remembered that the present Dalai Lama is the first during the past century of the pope-kings of Tibet to reach and pass his majority. Very many of his predecessors failed to reach governing age, probably owing to the machinations of the Chinese, working through the Tibetan regents, who had no desire to hand over their powers to a young ruling prince. Even after he had reached Lhasa, and was among his own people, the Dalai Lama still did not feel safe, and when he heard through spies that a force of two thousand Chinese troops had been dispatched from Peking immediately after his own departure from that city, and that they were hard on his heels, he made all preparations for immediate flight should such a course become necessary. These troops had been sent to Tibet ostensibly to reinforce the Chinese garrisons in that country, and to police the Trade Marts. Their real objective was, however, undoubtedly the capture, and possibly the assassination, of the Dalai Lama, and the strengthening of the Chinese hold over Tibet. The advance party of these troops arrived in Lhasa at the end of January 1909, marking their entry into the city by firing on the crowd of Tibetan onlookers gathered to witness their arrival. (Mullin, *Path of the Bodhisattva Warrior*, 75; Macdonald, *Twenty Years*, 60–61; see also Teichman, *Travels of a Consular Officer in Eastern Tibet*, 28ff.)

43. Macdonald's full account of their meeting is recounted in his memoirs. Macdonald, *Twenty Years*, 65–67.

44. Macdonald likewise recounts the actual border crossing by the Great Thirteenth and his entourage: a portent of his life—and the life of his successor—to come.

The party arrived at Gnatong, the first village in Sikkim, after nightfall, in a snowstorm. I had telephoned to the two British military telegraphists who were posted there to keep a look-out for His Holiness, and to report his arrival. I quote the actual words of one of these typical pre-war British Tommies, in describing the arrival of the Grand Lama of Tibet in Gnatong.

"Me an' Tubby," reported this military telegraphist, "was sittin' in front of the office fire abart eight pip emma, when we 'ears someone knockin' at the door.

"''Oo's thet?' I shouts, an' gets no arnswer.

"Arter a bit we 'ears another knock on the door, an' I gets up an' opens it. I sees seven Tibs standin' there. ' An' 'oo the 'ell er you?' I asks.

"'I'm the Dally Larmer!' one of 'em says.

"'Ho! Yus!' I arnswers, 'yer the Dally Larmer, are yer? I've 'eard abart you! Come in an' 'ave er cup er tea!'

"An' 'e comes in an' sits darn in front er the fire an' 'as a nice 'ot cup er tea. The other coves stands up rarnd the walls, an' wouldn't sit darn! The ole bloke made us bring our rifles in an' keep 'em in a corner, while 'e dossed darn in front er the fire! We gave 'im what grub we 'ad, but it wern't much. 'E left early next mornin'!"

And so the priest-king of Tibet, a fugitive from his country, was watched over by two British Tommies, who took his arrival as a matter of course in the duties of the day. How he and they managed to understand each other passes my comprehension, but it takes a lot to defeat the British soldier. (Macdonald, *Twenty Years*, 71–72)

45. During this time, many individuals—even within his own entourage—had unprecedented access to the man. Laden La, the chief of police in Darjeeling, related his own experiences to Walter Evans-Wentz some years later:

Once when he was traveling with the late Dalai Lama in India, he had occasion to inspect the preparations for His Holiness's bath and stepped into the bathroom. Unexpectedly the Dalai Lama appeared naked except for a towel around his middle ready for the bath and S. W. Laden La saw his bare back, and that at the places where the two extra arms of Chenrasi are supposed to be joined to the body, observed two small fleshy protuberances like elongated warts and dark curved marks beneath them. He is convinced that the Dalai Lama is really an incarnation of Chenrasi. ("Notes on the late Dalai Lama from Sardar Bahadur Laden La" in Gray Notebook, Evans-Wentz notebooks, Evans-Wentz Papers, M0278, Box 5, Dept. of Special Collections, Stanford University)

46. For a detailed account of the retaking of Tibet, see Tsarong, *In the Service*, 36ff.
47. *tshongs 'du*. Taring, *Daughter of Tibet*, 30, 36.
48. Handed a humiliating defeat a second time by Dasang Damdul, the official Chinese chroniclers could only compensate as they had in the past—by rewriting history. In their account of events in Tibet, Chinese sources claimed:

The Chinese revolution that began in October 1911 caused the newly asserted Chinese control over Tibet to collapse. The Chinese military garrison at Lhasa revolted, killed its officers, and turned to looting the city. After the overthrow of the Ch'ing dynasty, the Dalai left Kalimpong in June 1912 to return to Tibet. He was unable to enter Lhasa, however, because Chinese troops still occupied the city. In July 1912 Yuan Shih-k'ai's government at Peking ordered a new expedition from Szechwan for the relief of the Lhasa garrison troops. It was only through British intervention at Peking that the Chinese occupation of Tibet was terminated and that Chinese forces were repatriated through India.

Given the radical divergence from eyewitness accounts, it seems clear that Chinese Nationalist historical materials about Tibet are just as unreliable as Communist period documents—which at the present are attempting to remove all mention of Dasang Damdul from history. Howard and Howard, *Biographical Dictionary*, 2:3–4. For the "disappearance" of Lord Tsarong from contemporary accounts of Tibetan history see, for example: Ding-ja Tse-ring-dor-je (*sding bya tshe ring rdo rje*), "nye rabs kyi bod dmag dang bod ljongs dmag spyi khang gi skor sogs 'brel yod 'ga' zhig," and Sek-shing Lo-sang-don-drup (*sreg shing blo bzang don grub*), "de snga'i bod dmag ka dang sku srung dmag sgar gyi sgrig srol dang, rang nyid sku srung ru dpon byed mus su 1949 lo'i zing 'khrug langs pa'i 'brel yod gnad don 'ga' zhig," both in *bod kyi lo rgyus rig gnas dpyad gzhi'i rgyu cha bdams bsgrigs* 8:149–180 and 250–271.

49. *dza sag* and *zhabs pad*, respectively.

50. Part of the problem that the Tibetan government experienced was related to the undervaluing of the Tibetan *trangka* and *srang* against the Indian rupee. Minted in pure gold and silver, these Tibetan coins had a metal value that exceeded their exchange rate; consequently, there was a thriving industry in currency exchange at the Tibetan–Indian border by profiteers who melted down the Tibetan currency, sold the raw metal at a profit, and leveraged the capital into more currency exchanges. Consequently, Tibetan *trangka* and *srang* remain rare in the numismatic world. See also note 73, below.

51. It is reported that 8,000 people died of the disease in a short span of time before the epidemic was brought under control. Macdonald-Bayne, *Yoga of the Christ*, 17.

52. Goldstein notes that Lord Tsarong reorganized the existing military system and "raised an additional 1,000 troops by requiring that every two military fields in Ü, and every four in Tsang Province, provide one soldier." The resulting "4,000 troops were placed under the command of a Commander-in-Chief's Office headed by Tsarong and were formed into five regiments." Goldstein, *History of Modern Tibet*, 1:66–67.

53. *rtsis dpon lung shar.*

54. Mullin, *Bodhisattva Warrior*, 271–272.

55. *ka shod pa.*

56. In addition to this punishment, it was decreed that all subsequent generations of Lungshar's family would be prohibited from holding any post in the government. It was this last punishment that Lungshar himself felt to be unfair. The loss of his eyes, he later remarked, was just and nothing more than the workings of karma for as a young boy, he recalled, his favorite pastime had been shooting out the eyes of sheep with a slingshot. Although eventually released into the care of his family in May 1938, he did not live long after.

57. "P.A. got mad as hell," she wrote, "and tacked your formal letter of resignation (no sign of the personal one) on the bulletin board of the clubhouse," until DeVries removed it a few hours later. Confronting P.A. herself a few days later, Viola informed him that she had been under the impression that he valued discretion, and if he preferred otherwise, she would feel free to discuss all such matters with her friends at the club. "He sputtered about your thinking you didn't need anybody ever just because you got into Tibet, and had to show them no one should stick here whose heart wasn't in it etc. etc." The letter was still in the possession of VWB in the 1990s, though it appears to have been subsequently destroyed by her and not included in her archives.

58. Goldstein, *History*, 1:188.

8. Tibet, Tantrikas, and the Hero of Chaksam Ferry

59. Silön Lönchen (*srid blon blon chen*).

60. Petech, *Aristocracy and Government in Tibet: 1728-1959*, 24–25.

61. *Who's Who in Tibet*.

62. *glang chung ba spen pa (?) don grub*.

63. *bka' blon bla ma bkras khang zhabs pad thub bstan shakya*.

64. Petech, *Aristocracy and Government in Tibet: 1728-1959*, 109.

65. *bkras mthong zhabs pad* and *spo shod zhabs pad*, respectively.

66. TCB claimed that Tucci's "work" was nothing more than "buying out a monastery for Mussolini who furnishes him with all the money that he wants to spend so long as he brings back everything complete." As a scholar, TCB thought Tucci was a "puffed up" fraud, who "knows no more about the religion than I did twenty years ago."

67. D. Tharchin to Charles Bell, February 16, 1937, OIOC Eur. Mss. F-80, fol. 130.

68. This appears to have been one of the issues that infuriated Lungshar and inspired him to attempt his coup, believing that Reting Rinpoche was coerced by the Chinese representative into assenting out of his own weakness, youth, and inexperience. Goldstein, *History*, 189.

69. D. Tharchin to Charles Bell, July 1, 1937, OIOC Eur. Mss. F-80, fol. 130.

70. "Autonomy for Inner Mongolia," *Star of India* (Calcutta), Oct. 29, 1937, 1 col. 4; "New Autonomous Mongolian state," *Star of India* (Calcutta), Oct. 30, 1937, 1 col. 7.

71. D. Tharchin to Charles Bell, July 1, 1937, OIOC Eur. Mss. F-80, fol. 130.

72. Dundul Namgyal Tsarong noted that the Tsarong family helped many Mongolian monks get their geshe degrees. Because Lord Tsarong spoke some Mongolian, the monks would always come to their house.

73. Tharchin records receiving 75 "dotse" (*rdo tshad*) from Lord Tsarong, which he equated to slightly more than 900 Rs. at 12.5 Rs/Dotse. According to Das, one dotse was "a bar of silver bullion of about 4 pounds in weight," and according to Rockhill, it was "an ingot of silver weighing fifty Chinese ounces (*taels*), and also called *yambu* (from the Chinese *yuan-pao*), *tarmima* (*rta rmig ma*, also pronounced *tänpema*), or simply *do*." There appears to be a serious discrepancy in the actual figures here, since Tharchin's exchange rate of 12.5 Rs per dotse is off by a factor of more than ten (!) from the figure given by Das from 50 years earlier (160 Rs. per dotse). If true, it marks a substantial shift in currency values and may be the reason for the currency exchange problems mentioned above (see note 50 above). Das, *Tibetan-English Dictionary*; Das, *Journey to Lhasa and Central Tibet*, 51, also Rockhill, *The Land of the Lamas*, 51.

74. Tsarong notes that the Tibetan "sang" (*srang*) was "the main unit of Tibetan money . . . [which] was then broken down into smaller units; one sang equaled ten sho, one sho equaled ten kar, etc." For 1,250 monks, this amounted to 187.5 Rs., while the offerings at Ramoche a week later for 1,000 monks amounted to 150 Rs. Tsarong, *In the Service*, 52.

75. This appears to be the same text (*ārya-bhadrakalpikā-nāma-mahāyāna-sūtra; 'phags pa bskal pa bzang po shes bya ba theg pa chen po'i mdo*) currently held in the East Asian Library at the University of California at Berkeley.

76. Ganden Tri-pa (*dga' ldan khri pa*), Mi-nyak Ye-she-wang-den (*mi nyag ye shes dbang ldan*, r. 1933–1939).

77. Following the flight of the Paṇchen Lama in 1923, the Tibetan government ordered the seizure of the Paṇchen Lama's estates and sold off their contents to fund the new modernization efforts. TCB remarks that while many entrepreneurs—British and American—who purchased items for museums repeated claims that the *thangkas* and statues came from Drepung or other monasteries or temples, such claims were patently false, for such items would never be sold. Rather, Lord Tsarong informed him, all such items sold had come from the Paṇchen Lama's estate, with many still on the market in the late 1930s, while more came from the confiscated properties of Lungshar and other participants in the failed coup.

78. Responding to one of Bell's letters from Kalimpong a few months after his return, Tharchin wrote that in Tibet in monastic circles there was even support for the Japanese over China in the ongoing war since some felt that "if Japan comes to Tibet it is much better because they are Buddhist the same as our religion, and also the customs are almost the same," a view Tharchin felt was being propagated by Mongolian monks on behalf of Japan. The aristocrats—most notably, Lord Tsarong— felt "if we want to be [independent] we must prepare ourselves, and independent is the best thing for us." Tharchin to Charles Bell, December 11, 1937, OIOC Eur. Mss. F-80, fol. 130.

79. Within a few years of the war, in fact, Japanese spies were sent into Tibet via Mongolia and eventually to India. For one first-hand account, see Kimura, *Japanese Agent in Tibet.*

80. One of the tantric vows taken as part of initiation is a vow against discussing tantric teachings with the uninitiated.

81. Ironically, while TCB was trying to impress upon Fox the value of the Buddhist tradition, Tharchin was busy across town trying to locate artists who could be commissioned to create Tibetan Buddhist-themed "Christmas cards" for Theos and Viola to distribute to their friends the following winter as a follow-up to their enthusiastically received "Chinese Forbidden City" New Year's cards sent out months earlier.

82. The roasted barley flour that is the staple Tibetan food.

83. The books (possibly from Litang)—and book covers—appear to have survived the Chinese occupation intact and were still housed in Drepung as of 2006.

84. Although unmentioned by TCB, undoubtedly part of the fascination—if not confusion—on the part of the monks was TCB's odd changes from Tibetan aristocratic dress to monk's robes, with mixing and matching in between, *including* the incorporation of ritual deity headdress elements that would never be worn outside of an empowerment setting.

85. Following the destruction of Ganden Monastery during the Chinese Cultural Revolution, the *stūpa* containing Tsong-kha-pa's body remained an object of pilgrimage and veneration until it was desecrated by the Chinese in their attempts to undermine such activity. It was reported that in addition to destroying the *stūpa*, the Chinese had Tsong-kha-pa's body chopped up and thrown into the river, but that

some Tibetans managed to recover pieces, which were later carried to Dharamsala where they were reinterred.

86. Unbeknownst to Theos, one reason for the Ganden Tri-pa's slowness and "hands-on" blessing was that the man had been effectively blind for several years. The doctor attached to the British Mission, William Stanley Morgan, examined him only a few weeks later and diagnosed the Ganden Tri-pa with cataracts in both eyes— an operable condition—but unfortunately also progressively degenerative "keratitis" (an infection of the cornea), an inoperable condition often accompanied by a painful sensitivity to light, which could also explain the darkness of the throne. Morgan, *Amchi Sahib*, 190–191.

87. TCB does not give any details of this meeting (although he would make dubious claims about it later), stating that "The results of these discussions will perhaps appear at odd intervals in the diary, but they cannot be added until I have a chance of organizing the notes which were made—all of this is only for the purpose of my memory." Later, Tharchin would state to British authorities that TCB "went into the private sanctuary of the Tri-Rinpoche alone and was there for a couple of hours" but claimed ignorance as to what actually transpired.

88. "Tummo" (*gtum mo*).

89. TCB remarks that at one party Rai Bahadur Norbu informed the Chinese official in Lhasa about the recent attack on Nanking by Japanese forces, "whereupon the Chinaman went into a rage and commenced to drool and froth at the mouth and his armed escort drew their guns . . . you could hear him holler above the drone of the beating drum and all eyes were focused in our direction," requiring much negotiation through the official's Tibetan interpreter, for despite having "spent three years in this place as well as having received an English education—no one can understand his English or Tibetan."

90. TCB remarks that on one occasion, having gone to visit one of the "durzees" working on his silk book wraps, he noticed "his young daughter [who] had a few of her friends over—one of them being a young nun—possibly just entering the teens."

> She seemed filled with the vigour of youth and not having lost any of mine, we had a romping good time together for they were all out to be chased and frolic only as children can. The entire household looked on with amazement at the way I was running about with them . . . I will admit it is not in keeping with being a good Lama; however the better of them even have a good sense of humor, and I even have seen them run.

91. TCB knew well that Chapman was planning to publish a book on Lhasa based on his British Mission diaries, and was anxious to see "what sort of an imagination" Chapman had as a competitor on the book market who—just like TCB—while in Calcutta had "bought copies of Waddell, Bell and Macdonald on Tibet with the idea of getting his material out of them." He knew that Chapman was lying when he told the Calcutta press about his ability to speak Tibetan, but wrote, "I fully agree that he should keep right on for he is doing the right thing, but for personal information, I

have been anxious to ascertain the truth so that I might too, learn how to proceed in the face of such ways of doing things."

92. In the end, an entire herd of yaks would have to be slaughtered just to provide enough hides to cover his more than sixty boxes.

93. TCB appears to be mistaken here. Since Agniveśa's *Caraka Samhita* was not translated into Tibetan, more likely he was referring to Vagbhata's synthesis of the Caraka system, the *Condensed Essence of the Eight Branches [of Medicine]* (*aṣṭaṅga-hṛdaya-saṃhitā; yan lag brgyad pa'i snying po bsdus pa*).

94. About this time in Tibet, Tucci would write:

Others have gone to Gyantse before me and have described the land. I could not add new things. But I have discussed in this book the art monuments found along the roads and the reflections that can be made and the conclusions to be drawn for the study of the political, religious and artistic history of Tibet.

Lest anyone question the significance of Gyantse over any other locale—such as Lhasa—Tucci informed his readers that "geographical distance does not make a difference in culture" for "we are always faced by the same religious and artistic world and by the same spiritual unity." Nonetheless, if there were any shortcomings in his work, it could only be the fault of the Tibetan government, for

I will deem compensated for my labours if this investigation can be a guide for future researchers who follow my steps [and] will have more time and more funds to pursue further and deeper researches. This will be possible only when the Tibetan government will open the doors of its land. (Tucci, *Gyantse and Its Monasteries*, "Preface," 1:2–3)

95. Cutting likewise attended and filmed the dances in Lhasa, which his wife described as "very religious; very dull." "Tibet's 'Forbidden City' Penetrated by American Woman for First Time," *Journal-News* (Nyack, NY), Jan. 3, 1938.

96. When compared with another letter written by Reting to Adolph Hitler the letter addressed to U.S. President Roosevelt is striking given its lack of normal formal protocols between sovereign leaders. It remains possible that TCB's account of its genesis is not entirely truthful, its content possibly having been "suggested" by TCB himself.

97. *ngag dbang mthu stobs dbang phyug; sa skya khri chen*, 1900–1950.

9. "The Clipper Ship of the Imagination"

1. David-Neel, *Secret Oral Teachings*, 1.

2. Cosulich, "Bernard Would Trade Tibet's Yak Meat for Yankee Hot Dog," *Arizona Daily Star*, Sept. 27, 1937; "Religious Wealth In Tibet's Wilderness Seen By Bernard," *Arizona Daily Star*, Nov. 4, 1937; *Columbia Alumni News*, Nov. 5, 1937, 17.

3. Although he had arrived in Kalimpong *ten* months earlier and entered Tibet *five* months earlier, the article about "Mr. Theo. Bernard" read: "Eight Months In Tibet." *Calcutta Statesman*, Oct. 28, 1937, 21.

4. A newspaper for which Frank Perry also worked as an "outpost correspondent."

5. The reference was to the German writer Theodor Burang, who published under the pen name Theodore Illion and at the time, had recently authored such works as *In Secret Tibet* and *Darkness Over Tibet*. Capitalizing on Hilton's *Lost Horizon*, Illion revived the "hollow earth theory" and claimed to have visited Tibet and the now popularly famous "hidden valleys" (*sbas yul*). Miss M. N. Kennedy, Secretary, Royal Central Asian Society to "Mr. Rumbold," Nov. 19, 1937. OIOC, L/P&S/12/4203 Pol Ext Coll 36 File 31 25ff; CIT-5, fiche 376–377, item #7; see also Illion, *In Secret Tibet* and *Darkness Over Tibet*.

6. Maugham, *The Razor's Edge*, 2.

7. For Maugham, this was a far more flexible literary device than Bernard's actual story—of a child from a poor broken home who married into wealth and used it liberally in his pursuit of the religious life. Even so, years later when consulting on the set of the 1946 production of *The Razor's Edge*, Maugham encouraged director Edmund Goulding to cast a Theos Bernard look-alike, Tyrone Power, in the lead role. Maugham's Larry Darrell, despite trauma and difficulties, eventually finds a sense of peace, but such contentment seems to have escaped Bernard. In December 1946, as the film debuted across the country, Theos Bernard was already embarking on his final trip to India and Tibet.

8. "Tales of Tibetan Trip Told by Member Of Clarkstown Country Club on Return From Six Months Tour of Exploration," *The Journal-News* [Nyack, NY], Sat., Nov. 27, 1937.

9. "Tibetan New Year Greetings Here," *New York Sun*, Feb. 17, 1938; "Rocklanders Get New Year Greeting from Rocky Tibet," *Rockland County Herald*, Feb. 26, 1938, 1, 4.

10. So horrified, in fact, that even sixty years later she had difficulty speaking of it. Asked repeatedly about the break-up of her marriage to TCB during the last years of her life, she routinely answered that they had had "different visions for the future" or that their "careers had diverged" and they amicably split. Only in her last interview, after repeating her stock answer, did she pause and add, "and then, of course, there was the sexual thing."

11. Other Westerners before TCB had claimed similar "recognitions" of themselves as reincarnate lamas, but most did not take them seriously, interpreting them merely as a cultural politeness. If such statements were in fact made to TCB, it is unlikely that they were made with any seriousness. Bruce, *Assault on Mt. Everest*, 47.

12. Dominated by a Republican majority, the U.S. Congress refused to ratify the treaty—not because of its terms but because signing it would have automatically included the United States in the League of Nations, and the fear of a "one world government" remained linked in the minds of conservative Christian legislators with the so-called "Anti-Christ" described in the Book of Revelation in the Christian Bible.

13. "No Dalai Lama May Be Found," unidentified newspaper clipping, ca. April 1938. VWB Archive.

14. Giving them the benefit of the doubt at first, when she finally learned the truth, Viola would not speak to DeVries again for ten years.

15. TCB's childhood friend Dan Hughes reported that as a child Theos had a lisp when he spoke. Extant sound recordings of TCB's lectures display clear evidence of coached speaking.

16. Advertisement, "Theos Bernard: 'Penthouse of the Gods,'" *Reno Evening Gazette*, Mar. 18, 1939.

17. Orson Welles's production of H. G. Wells's *War of the Worlds* was broadcast on CBS radio, staged as the interruption of a music show on Sunday night, October 30, 1938. "Radio Listeners in Panic, Taking War Drama as Fact," *New York Times*, Monday, Oct. 31, 1938, 1.

18. Spiritualists, Zionists, and others who wanted to establish their presence at the fair were excluded as well. Todd, "Imagining the Future of American Religion at the New York World's Fair, 1939–40," 105–106, 110.

19. See figure 9.1. Although neither man appears to have been able to successfully and correctly bind the lower robe, TCB is nonetheless dressed meticulously, while Harrison Forman has only jokingly half-dressed in them with his hat on backward.

20. Indeed, a few years earlier, a student of Jiddu Krishnamurti had observed, "When I arrived in the United States in the autumn of 1934 I soon noticed that the disappointment and the growing mistrust of purely material salvation, resulting from the economic disasters of the last few years, had created in many people a hunger for things of the spirit." Landau, *God Is My Adventure*, 258.

21. Glen also claimed to have met an Indian yoga teacher as a teenager, and in his case, it was true. Like the vast majority of events recounted in *Heaven Lies Within Us*, this "meeting" between a teenage boy and an Indian guru refers to Glen Bernard and, presumably, Sylvais Hamati. See also chapter 1, note 8; Love, *The Great Oom*.

22. An apparent reference to Trivikram Swami of Bhurkunda, who died four days after Theos arrived in Calcutta.

23. Glen *did* participate in a tantric initiation in Calcutta in 1926, with the aid of an adoptive family—his "tantrik bother and sister"—and with "a friend of the family," presumably Sylvais Hamati, who had been living in India for some time. Theos states that when he met the Maharishi, "he was about to have his seventy-first birthday," which places his year of birth in 1865/6. If, once again, the account was of *Glen's* experiences, this would correspond exactly to the late Trivikram Swami, with whom Glen had done *his* retreat, and who was seventy-two years old. In the absence of any evidence to the contrary, I conclude that this is an account of Glen's initiation in 1926. The fact that the yantra reproduced on the title page of *Heaven Lies Within Us* is the one given not to Theos but to Glen, reinforces that the vast majority of events related reflect Glen's life, not Theos's. See Lilaboti Raye to GAB, May 2, 1936, Theos Bernard Papers; Dasgupta, *Kriya Yoga and Swami Sriyukteshvar*, 150–151; Bernard, "Haṭha Yoga: The Report of a Personal Experience," vii; International Congress of Free Christians and Other Religious Liberals, *New Pilgrimages of the Spirit*, 8; Bernard, *Heaven Lies Within Us*, 208, 218–220; Satyananda Giri, *Yoganand Sanga*; Bernard, *Penthouse of the Gods*, 30; Yogananda, *Autobiography of a Yogi*, 406.

24. Bernard, *Heaven Lies Within Us*, xiv.

25. The reporter went on to state that while TCB "lives in a modest little white cottage nestled against a hill in a quiet wooded canyon in Beverly Hills . . . instead of a solemn-faced prophet Bernard seems more like a college boy out for a lark, until he starts talking about the philosophy he has chosen." Others were somewhat more skeptical, reporting later in the same paper:

> Bernard, an American lama ("Penthouse of the Gods," a Tibetan volume) got himself some knowledge of yoga and went to India, where he indulged in the breath-holding, arm-withering and pin-pricking tricks of faakirs. His book is a manual of the art of living in the hereafter while the body stays squatted on the earth, loin-clothed and goat-smelling.

"Only White Lama of Tibet Finishing Book in Southland: Former American Lawyer Tells How He Came to Take Up Philosophy of Land of Shangri-La," *Los Angeles Times*, Aug. 13, 1939; W.N., "Yoga Studied First Hand," *Los Angeles Times*, Oct. 29, 1939, C-6.

26. W. Coulson Leigh, Inc., Promotional Flyers for 1939–1940. Pacific Geographic Society. Collection M-166 (box 6, folder 70; box 3, folder 27). Department of Special Collections, Stanford University.

27. Arnold, "Nazis and Fascists Are Filtering Into Tibet As a Key in World Drive, Expert Reports," *New York World-Telegraph*, Apr. 5, 1939.

28. An attempt to capitalize, perhaps, on an earlier book of a similar title, *Shrines of a Thousand Buddhas* (1936), detailing Tucci's expedition to western Tibet through Lahoul and Spiti. Indeed, TCB confused the two titles later himself.

29. Bernard, "I Become a Lama," *ASIA* (Apr. 1939):206–211.

30. Bernard, "The Peril of Tibet," *ASIA* (Sept. 1939):500–504.

31. Pointing out that he was the first American to live in Lhasa itself, not like the other white men, who must remain outside the city walls. The British, great respecters of other people's privacy, never attempted to violate the rule of going only when they were invited. Indeed, he further declared that the Tibetans themselves were of a noble character, and "do not show that sense of inferiority, of submission, which the English knock into every race with which they come into contact," while the British on the other hand, he thought, were pathetic.

> The English could be neighbors to this culture for the next ten thousand years and still be stewing in their ignorance, without once thinking to ask a question and forever making damn sure that every one passes them by with the proper greeting. (Bernard, *Penthouse of the Gods*, 127–28)

32. "American Became Only White Lama of Tibet," *Evening Standard* (UK), May 11, 1940; "Secrets of Tibet Were Revealed to Author" [Review of *Land of a Thousand Buddhas*], *Psychic News* (UK), June 8, 1940.

33. E. W. Fletcher to B. J. Gould, re: Theos Bernard, D.O. No.F-238-X/40, June 26,

1940. OIOC, British Library. CIT-5, "Travelers and Entry Control, 1905–1958." Fiche 376–377 (77–78).

34. Rai Bahadur Norbu to Basil Gould, Oct. 4, 1940. L/P&S/12/4203 Pol Ext Coll 36 File 31 25ff. OIOC, British Library. CIT-5, "Travelers and Entry Control, 1905–1958." Fiche 376–377 (77–78).

35. For example, it was literally true that "at no time was [TCB] seen associating with monks or carrying out religious Buddhist ceremonies," since no British officer was ever present at such ceremonies (though they knew full well that Theos was). Likewise, it was also true that "Bernard has not seen or witnessed a ceremony or Buddhist worship which has not also been open to the British personnel." That no British officers ever availed themselves of the opportunity to do any of the things that TCB did, and more often than not displayed a degree of contempt for such things, was quite noticeable to the Tibetan populace. With regard to the Cuttings, after TCB tried to get to Tibet in their company, they simply did not cross paths until the couple arrived a second time at the beginning of September, at which point they actually spent a fair amount of time together. As for TCB's Tibetan language skills, "proficiency" being a somewhat subjective term, as a native speaker, Norbu could easily disparage TCB's abilities. For most Tibetans, however, TCB had mastered the spoken language to a sufficient degree to make himself understood and to understand simple sentences spoken to him in response. Indeed, almost ten years later when Heinrich Harrer and Peter Aufschnaiter arrived in Lhasa (January 15, 1946), Harrer would write: "Every day people tell us that how very well we know to speak Tibetan. Apart from us only Bell and an American mastered Tibetan language so well. All the others only spoke it rather badly or not at all." Heinrich Harrer, diary entry for January 23, 1946. Thanks to Isrun Engelhardt for this reference.

36. For example, when inquiring about the appropriateness of hosting TCB at the Royal Asiatic Society, the society's secretary was informed that he was "not at all reliable" and sent a copy of Norbhu's letter, "for your strictly confidential information." "Miss M. N. Kennedy," Secretary, Royal Central Asian Society, to "Mr. G. E. Crombie," Nov. 1, 1940; also, a note in response, Crombie to Kennedy (handwritten), Nov. 5, 1940. OIOC, British Library. CIT-5, "Travelers and Entry Control, 1905–1958." Fiche 376–377 (77–78).

37. Unidentified newspaper clipping, *Johannesburg Star*, June 12, 1939. Theos Bernard Papers.

10. Yoga on Fifth Avenue

1. Jung, "Psychological Commentary on *The Tibetan Book of the Great Liberation*," lv–lvi.

2. Based on comparable "consumer price index" data for 1940 versus 2000, this would be the current equivalent of $300 per hour.

3. Talbot Mundy (a.k.a. William Lancaster Gribbon, 1879–1940), author of *King—of the Kyber Rifles*, became interested in Theosophy late in his life. He subsequently

began incorporating Theosophical doctrines and ideas about Tibet into his writings while living in the Roerich research institute in New York following his consultation with Evans-Wentz at Point Loma. Mundy, "Mystic India Speaks," 15–16, 63; Taves, *Talbot Mundy, Philosopher of Adventure*, 120, 172.

4. "Captain Spaulding, the African Explorer" (Groucho Marx), *Animal Crackers*. Paramount Pictures, 1930.

5. Robertson, "The White Lama on Yoga," 15.

6. GAB had been at work for some time on a treatise he called "The Art of Yoga," apparently intended as a response to and repudiation of his brother, P.A. In this work he claimed that "[p]retending Yogis and teachers of Yoga are daily gaining influence over the credulous, spreading their deceptions to the danger of intelligent men." Glen Bernard, "The Art of Yoga," 4–5. Theos Bernard Papers.

7. TCB even published a short article—substantially reduced from his 100-page manuscript—in Columbia University's *Review of Religion*. Bernard, "The Tibetan 'Wheel of Life.'"

8. For example, on October 5, 1939, GAB attended Claude Bragdon's lectures on "Yoga for the West" for *Psychic Forum* at the Hotel Iroquois in Manhattan, and obtained a copy of a transcript of the talk for Theos. Theos Bernard Papers.

9. See Jung, *The Kundalini Yoga*.

10. The subheadline read: "'White Lama' Theos Bernard Testifies That He Can't Sit on Water, Float in Air or Support Himself on One Finger and That It's Not His Fault If His Pupil Went Crazy So Strangely Like Barbara Rutherfurd, Fashionable Disciple of 'Omnipotent Oom' Bernard (Same Name, Same Game But No Relation)." "Wealthy Mrs. Donovan (Now in the Asylum) and Her Yogi Teacher," 3.

11. A twenty-foot piece of muslin cloth partly swallowed, then extracted in order to remove excess stomach acid.

12. Brest-Litovsk, Poland. Unless otherwise stated, the following account is drawn from Walska, *Always Room at the Top*, and Crawford, *Ganna Walska Lotusland*.

13. According to her official biography, "Madame was the customary title for well-known actresses and operatic singers in Europe, Ganna is a Russian form of Hanna and Walska reminiscent of the her favorite music, the waltz."

14. Even being convinced at one point that she was the reincarnation of the Comptesse de Castiglione, the celebrated singer who captivated Napoleon, Ganna went so far as to purchase the jewel-encrusted tiara once worn by the diva.

15. According to the Southern California Earthquake Data Center (SCEDC), a magnitude 5.5 earthquake struck 4 miles east-by-southeast of Santa Barbara at 11:51 p.m. on June 30, 1941.

11. Tibetland and the Penthouse of the Gods

1. TCB Diary II, Theos Bernard Papers, p.139(r), Bancroft Library.

2. This, and what follows, drawn from Walska, *Always Room at the Top*.

3. S. K. Jinorasa to TCB, Jan. 26, 1940. Theos Bernard Papers.

4. Alfred A. Hunnex (American Express Company) to Madame Ganna Walska, July 9, 1941. Theos Bernard Papers. Also, telegram, Phelan Beale to Madame Ganna Walska, Aug. 1, 1941. Theos Bernard Papers.

5. "Lama Geshe Chompell," *Journal of the Mahabodhi Society* 49, no. 8 (Aug. 1941): 3.

6. Telegram, GW to Phelan Beale, Oct. 23, 1941. Theos Bernard Papers.

7. Telegram, Phelan Beale to GW, Nov. 1, 1941. Theos Bernard Papers.

8. This Gedun Chöpel appears to have done, beginning with an otherwise unidentified "Tibetan Medical manuscript." The location of this translation is unknown; it is not to be found in either the HGPF or Theos Bernard Papers. TCB to GW, Feb. 7, 1942. Theos Bernard Papers.

9. "Lama Chophel" to TCB, Nov. 11, 1941. Theos Bernard Papers.

10. One writer, remarking on the lackluster season at the Met, commented that "the orchids will probably be scattered, but in recent years the emeralds in the horseshoe have been concentrated on Mme. Ganna Walska, the diva who finds it less toilsome to listen to opera from a box than to try to sing it from the stage." Robb, "The Old Met 'Opry' House 'Ain't What It Used to Be,'" *Washington Post*, Nov. 20, 1942, B-13.

11. Hedda Hopper, "Looking at Hollywood," *Chicago Daily Tribune*, Nov. 23, 1942, 20; the text was corrected when reprinted to read "High Lama": [Hedda Hopper], "Hedda Hopper's Hollywood," *Los Angeles Times*, Nov. 23, 1942, 14.

12. See Sinh, *Haṭha yoga Pradīpikā*.

13. Bernard, "Tantrik Yoga: A Clinical Report," 1–3. Theos Bernard Papers.

14. "Cycles of Psychism," *Theosophy* 31, no. 10 (Aug. 1943): 442–447.

15. It was the same era in which Edgar Cayce, "The Dreaming Prophet" was flourishing and beginning to make headlines in newspapers for his purported dream-state psychic abilities.

16. As time went on—her time with TCB, in particular—HGP would devote more and more portions of her dream journal to commentary, most directly related to her relationship with TCB, either in an attempt to psychoanalyze the situation or simply to "vent" her frustration.

17. HGP is apparently confusing the minimalist style of Japanese Zen with Tibetan, which cannot be described as either "simple" or "austere." HGP, Dream Journal, entry #1496, Aug. 16, 1944. HGPF Archive.

18. HGP, Dream Journal, entry #1504, Sept. 12, 1944. HGPF Archive.

19. On November 4, 1939, the U.S. government passed an amended Neutrality Act, making it illegal for any U.S. citizen "to travel to or in any area declared by Proclamation of the President to be a combat area." Many of the travel restrictions remained in effect well after World War II, as passage on commercial vessels was regulated to allow military and displaced persons travel privileges. Neutrality Act (40 Stat. 227; U.S.C., title 22, sec. 221).

20. Responding on behalf of his father, Dundul Namgyal ("George") Tsarong replied, "you hope someday we will be able to visit your country. We have now so many

friends in America, and we shall certainly be pleased to come as soon as the conditions become normal." George Tsarong to TCB, Dec. 17, 1944. Theos Bernard Papers.

21. The working draft of this book shows many embellishments of his story—some of which appeared in his *ASIA* article—such as lengthening his stay in Lhasa to a year and a half. Theos Bernard, "Tibetan Saga." Theos Bernard Papers.

22. Landon, "Review," 530.

23. First reviewed in the *Journal of Philosophy*, the journal cofounded by Wendall Bush, founding professor of religion and anthropology at Columbia University and advisor of Herbert Schneider (TCB's advisor), who was then the acting editor of the journal.

24. A reference to the *Kuṇḍalinī śakti*, which TCB described as "the Fountain of Knowledge."

25. Tibetan Text Society Minutes, October 30, 1945. Theos Bernard Papers.

26. Schlagintweit, *Buddhism in Tibet*, 65.

27. "Suit Discloses Fifth Ganna Walska Marriage," *Los Angeles Times*, May 26, 1946, A3.

28. "He Can't Work But He Stands on His Head For 3 Hours," *Gettysburg Times* (PA), July 13, 1946.

29. Answer of A. Bernard. "T. Bernard v. A. Bernard," Complaint for Separate Maintenance. Superior Court of California, County of Santa Barbara, case no. 38378, 4ff.

30. "Mme. Walska Fights Her Yogi Husband's Suit," *Chicago Daily Tribune*, July 9, 1946, 6.

31. "Ganna Walska Fights Mate's Support Suit," *Los Angeles Times*, July 9, 1946, A-1; "'Buddhist Monk' Sued By Singer," *Tucson Citizen*, July 9, 1946.

32. "Ganna Walska Is Freed," *New York Times*, July 14, 1946, 31.

33. "On the Aisle: Audience More Fun Than Opera at Met's Opening," *Chicago Daily Tribune*, Nov. 14, 1946, 29; "Lily Pons is Star of Opening Opera," *New York Times*, Nov. 12, 1946, 35.

12. To Climb the Highest Mountains

1. M. R. Jayakar, foreword to Swami Sambuddhananda, *The Message of the Himalayas*, 12–13.

2. One gossip columnist, poking fun at TCB and GW, wrote at the time:

Five or six years ago, a handsome, athletic young man who had just emerged into his thirties with several university degrees to his credit took the cultural-minded in the Bay Area by storm. While in San Francisco, Dr. Bernard was the house guest of Dr. and Mrs. William Palmer Lucas at their Pacific avenue residence. He was considerably wined, dined and feted.

. . . Ganna Walska, a woman to whom the gods of love and beauty have been more than generous, the muse of music on the other hand has given her a bad time. (Robbins, "From Where I Sit," *San Francisco Chronicle*, Aug. 11, 1946)

3. On August 13, TCB drafted his "Last Will and Testament" in New York, leaving everything to his father, or in case of *his* death, splitting it evenly between his surviving brothers, while his Tibetan library was to be donated to the Library of Congress. TCB to GAB, Aug. 26, 1946. Theos Bernard Papers.

4. TCB notes that although some of them had been sold, the new owners, in a tribute to Tibetan graciousness, even sought him out and returned them to him. TCB to GAB, Mar. 10, 1947. Theos Bernard Papers.

5. In actuality, "Dawa Sangpo" was a Japanese spy, Hisao Kimura, who had been posing as a Mongolian monk for more than eight years while conducting espionage in Tibet. See Kimura, *Japanese Agent in Tibet.*

6. Goldstein, *History*, 1:453.

7. Goldstein places Gedun Chöpel's arrival in the first week of January. Heinrich Harrer and Peter Aufschnaiter arrived on January 15, after twenty months walking on foot through the Himalayas following their escape from a British prison camp in India. Goldstein, *History*, 1:453; Harrer, *Seven Years in Tibet.*

8. Of all the early Russian Tibetologists, only Fyodor Stcherbatsky would escape "liquidation," though he would die in Kazakhstan only a few years later. Snelling, *Buddhism in Russia*, 247–249.

9. "a mi ri ka'i sbar na ṭe sa heb," *Mirror* 15, no. 2 (Dec. 1, 1946), 1.

10. Fearing Chinese incursions into Tibet, the Tibetan government was preparing to send official representatives to the Asian Relations Conference in Delhi—to the usual consternation of Chinese officials. Putting the best possible face on things, TCB told his would-be publisher, Dagobert Runes, that he was at the age where he "no longer fancie[d] the idea of trekking across fourteen thousand foot plateaus and crossing seventeen thousand foot passes" and so had decided to stay in Kalimpong. TCB to Dagobert Runes, Feb. 1, 1947. Theos Bernard Papers.

11. "dar mdo rin po che," *Mirror* 15, no. 4/5 (Feb./Mar. 1947), 4 col. 2.

12. See Vidyabhusana, *Bilingual index of Nyāya-bindu.*

13. Indeed, when this same text was translated some thirty years later by students of Geshe Wangyal in America, the compilation of a dictionary of terms and their philosophical definitions would be one of the by-products. Jeffrey Hopkins et al., "Tibetan-English Dictionary."

14. Lapierre and Collins, *Freedom at Midnight*, 130.

15. Kimura recounted that at least one Tibetan in Lhasa had recognized him as being Japanese, though had felt no need to reveal his secret. Dilowa Hutuktu had recognized him while passing through Kalimpong, and Geshe Wangyal and several others in Kalimpong suspected his ruse as well. Indeed, when they first met, Geshe Wangyal remarked "that I did not look like a Mongolian," but left it at that. Kimura, *Japanese Agent*, 146–147, 152–154.

16. A formal, polite request for a visit.

17. Having chosen to work with Roerich in lieu of TCB, Gedun Chöpel remained unhappy, and it has been argued that George Roerich, in particular, was the object of much resentment on Gedun Chöpel's part. See Bogin and Decleer, "Who was "this evil friend" ("the dog", "the fool", "the tyrant") in Gedun Chöpel's Sad Song?"

18. Roerich, "Remains," *The Mahabodhi Journal* 50, no. 2 (Feb. 1942): 60–63.

19. Enclosure to Restricted Dispatch No. 300. Howard Donovan to U.S. Secretary of State (Washington, DC), Sept. 29, 1947. RG-84, "India; New Delhi Mission; Confidential File, Classified General Records (1942–55)," Box 36, Folder 310, "Theos Bernard (1947)." National Archives and Records Administration.

20. In the early 1940s, Firoz Khan Noon was the High Commissioner for the Government of India; he would go on to become the seventh Prime Minister of Pakistan (1957–58).

21. Interview with Vicky Noon in Collins and Lapierre, *Freedom at Midnight*, 373–374.

22. Tessaldar = land revenue officer; Thanadar = chief of police.

23. Enclosure to Restricted Dispatch No. 300. Howard Donovan to U.S. Secretary of State (Washington, DC), Sept. 29, 1947. RG-84, "India; New Delhi Mission; Confidential File, Classified General Records (1942–55)," Box 36, Folder 310, "Theos Bernard (1947)." National Archives and Records Administration.

24. The Chinese delegation, as would be expected, protested vehemently over this. *Asian relations, being report of the proceedings and documentation of the First Asian Relations Conference, New Delhi, March-April, 1947.*

13. The Aftermath

1. Kipling, *Kim*, 353.

2. Not without a sense of humor, GAB appears to have given her this name in reference to a newspaper article he saved about a girl discovered in India, reputed to have been "raised by wolves." Unidentified newspaper clipping. Theos Bernard Papers.

3. Russel K. Haight, ex-Colorado policeman and insurance salesman, had seen extensive fighting in World War II as a commando during the invasion of France. Believed by his wife to have experienced difficulties in readjusting to civilian life, following the war, Haight had quit his job, abandoned his home, and flown to Afghanistan, where he made his way to Poonch and enlisted in the "Azad Kashmir Forces" in their fight for Kashmiri independence from both India and Pakistan. Newspaper reports from Lahore had identified him as being "given command of an important sector on the Barasula front," and he had even been spotted fighting "in cowboy boots and a big cowboy hat [leading] 400 Moslems into action against Indian troops" in Kashmir. Neither the Indian nor the Pakistani government was pleased about this, and demanded immediate action from the U.S. embassy. See assorted correspondence and newspaper clippings, RG-84, "India; New Delhi Mission; Confidential File, Classified General Records (1942–55)," Box 36, Folder 310 "Russel K. Haight (1947)." National Archives and Records Administration.

4. In the book-length account of their visit, Lowell Thomas Jr. qualifies this statement, identifying himself and his father as "the seventh and eighth to be received officially by the Tibetan ruler." Even this is problematic, since his usage of the phrase "received officially" is unclear. William McGovern and the members of the CBI crew were all "received officially" as well, so presumably he meant "granted prior permis-

sion to visit Lhasa," which (thus excluding McGovern) would make them the fifth and sixth Americans on that list. Thomas Jr., *Out of This World: To Forbidden Tibet*, 21.

5. Thomas and Thomas Jr., "Out of This World: A Journey to Lhasa," *Collier's* (Feb. 11, 1950):13–17, 70.

6. Story told by Helmut Hoffman to his students in Bloomington, Indiana. Isrun Engelhardt, who worked extensively on Schäfer's diaries and his life, was unfamiliar with it, however.

7. Mao Tse-tung, "Fight for a Fundamental Turn for the Better in the Nation's Financial and Economic Situation" (June 6, 1950) in *The Collected Works of Mao Tse-tung*, 5:26–31.

8. They were hosted by The Explorers Club, who described them as "somewhat bewildered" by New York City. A newspaper reporter went on to note that Captain Ilya Tolstoy, the OSS (now CIA) officer who had visited Tibet years earlier, served as their translator. Schurmacher, "They Try to Come Back Alive," *Los Angeles Times*, June 5, 1949, F-14-15, 27.

9. Loy Henderson (American Embassy, New Delhi) to Elbert Matthews (U.S. Dept. of State), Feb. 4, 1950. RG-84, "India; New Delhi Mission; Top Secret Subject Files (1944–50)," Box 2, Folder "Top Secret Subject Files (1950)." National Archives and Records Administration.

10. Krishna Menon (Ministry of External Affairs, India) to J. Graham Parsons (First Secretary and Consul, American Embassy), April 11, 1950. RG-84, "India; New Delhi Mission; Top Secret Subject Files (1944–50)," Box 2, Folder "Top Secret Subject Files (1950)." National Archives and Records Administration.

11. Top Secret Memo from [Eleanor] Roosevelt, undated [July 1950]. RG-84, "India; New Delhi Mission; Top Secret Subject Files (1944–50)," Box 2, Folder "Top Secret Subject Files (1950)." National Archives and Records Administration.

12. Bessac, "This Was the Trek to Tragedy," *Life*, Nov. 13, 1950, 130. See also Laird, *Into Tibet.*

13. *bka' blon bla ma thub bstan kun mkhyen.* Kalön Lama Rampa to Loy Henderson (U.S. Ambassador, New Delhi), dated 5th day of the 6th month, 924 A.K. (July 20, 1950). RG-84, "India; New Delhi Mission; Top Secret Subject Files (1944–50)," Box 2, Folder "Top Secret Subject Files (1950)." National Archives and Records Administration.

14. Top Secret Informal Statement, Sept. 3, 1950. RG-84, "India; New Delhi Mission; Top Secret Subject Files (1944–50)," Box 2, Folder "Top Secret Subject Files (1950)." National Archives and Records Administration.

15. Harrer, "Flight of the Dalai Lama," *Life*, Apr. 23, 1951, 130ff.

16. "Third Danish Expedition of Central Asia," *Explorer Journal* 28, no. 3 (Summer 1950).

17. The report was, in fact, repeated and published by the Circumnavigator's Club (to which TCB also belonged). Cotlow, "Farewell and Luck To You," *The Log of the Circumnavigator's Club* 38, no. 3 (Fall 1950): 8.

18. Commenting on this later, Theos's brother Marvene remarked that he felt that GAB never bothered to inform their family that Theos had been declared dead, and often acted as if he "ignores the fact that Theos has brothers."

19. The word "Hutukhtu" (*qutuy-tu*) is the Mongolian translation of the Tibetan word *'phags-pa* (in Sanskrit, *ārya*), meaning "noble" or "enlightened" one. It is one of the words—along with the Tibetan word "Tulku" (*sprul sku*), meaning "recognized reincarnate" lama (literally, the "emanation body" of an enlightened being)—from which the Chinese produce the English oxymoron "living buddha."

20. From the content of the article, Tharchin's understanding of Buddhism appears to have been limited to the Laṅkan tradition. "'jig rten bde ba gzhan bde 'dod las byung, 'jig rten sdug bsngal rang bde 'dod las byung," *Mirror* 18, no. 8 (July 1, 1950): 8.

21. Alfred Hitchcock, *Rear Window*, Universal Studios (1954).

22. Potter, *Philosophy East and West* 7, no. 3/4 (Oct. 1957–Jan. 1958): 147–148.

23. In 1939, just as TCB was beginning his teaching career, Carl Jung wrote, with apparent reference to both TCB's yoga studio in the Hotel Pierre just off Fifth Avenue and the sentiment expressed earlier by TCB concerning the ability of a person to practice yoga without the need to "sacrifice an iota of his religion":

> If the European could turn himself inside out and live as an Oriental, with all the social, moral, religious, intellectual, and aesthetic obligations which such a course would involve, he might be able to benefit by these teachings. But you cannot be a good Christian, either in your faith or in your morality or in your intellectual make-up, and practise genuine yoga at the same time. I have seen too many cases that have made me sceptical in the highest degree. The trouble is that Western man cannot get rid of his history as easily as his short-legged memory can. History, one might say, is written in the blood. I would not advise anyone to touch yoga without a careful analysis of his unconscious reactions. What is the use of imitating yoga if your dark side remains as good a medieval Christian as ever? If you can afford to seat yourself on a gazelle skin under a Bo-tree or in the cell of a *gompa* for the rest of your life without being troubled by politics or the collapse of your securities, I will look favourably upon your case. But yoga in Mayfair or Fifth Avenue, or in any other place which is on the telephone, is a spiritual fake. (Jung, "Psychological Commentary on *The Tibetan Book of the Great Liberation*," lv–lvi, reprinted in *Psychology and religion: West and East*, 499–500)

24. Ginsberg, *Indian Journals*, 25–27, 71.

25. Inspired by TCB, a few months later Wayman would write a follow-up to TCB's "Wheel of Life" article. Wayman, "The Concept of Poison in Buddhism," *Oriens* 10, no. 1 (1957): 107–109.

26. Claus Vogel, preface to Eimer, *Die Xerokopie des Lhasa-Kanjur*, 2–3.

27. About Yale's collection, see: "The Tibetan Collection at Yale," *Yale University Library Gazette* 34, no. 3 (Jan. 1960): 127–133; "Tibetan Books from a 'Peak Secretary,'" *Yale University Library Gazette* 35, no. 3 (Jan. 1961): 126–133; and "Edna Bryner Schwab, Tibetan Scholar and Yale Benefactor," *Yale University Library Gazette* 44, no. 1 (July 1969): 21–29.

28. Jackson, *A Saint in Seattle*, 286ff.

29. Illson, "Ex-Ivy Leaguers aim to be monks: Three Studying at Buddhist Monastery in Jersey," *New York Times*, December 15, 1963, 71 col.1.

30. "shin tu nas skyo ba'i gnas tshul," *Mirror* 26, no. 1 (June 1959): 5, col.3.

31. Tharchin is mistaken here. The "water-mouse year" (*chu byi*) would be 1912, the time of the expulsion of the Chinese. Tharchin presumably intended to say the "earth-rooster year" (*sa bya*), 1909.

32. *stag brag rin po che.*

33. Taring, *Daughter of Tibet*, 111; also Havnevik, "The Life of Jetsun Lochen Rinpoche (1865–1951)."

34. *udānavarga; ched du brjod pa'i tshoms.* Sde-dge Bka'-'gyur, MDO vol. SA fol. 209a1–253a7, ch.1 vss. 6–8, 22.

35. "mi snyan pa'i gnas tshul," *Mirror* 27, no. 8/9 (May/June 1961): 5–6.

36. I have been told that these materials have since been passed on to *yet another* individual claiming to be the reincarnation of Theos Bernard. At the time of this writing, I had a list of seven such self-proclaimed Bernard reincarnations.

14. Postscript: The View from Ki, Sixty Years Later

1. Baudrillard, *America*, 5.

2. John Lennon, following his experiences with meditation and studies with "Guru Deva" (the Maharishi Mahesh Yogi), alluded to "emptiness" (*śunyatā*, or "nothingness" as it was sometimes translated) in one song by cryptically telling his listeners that "nothing's gonna change my world," while the lines of another song declared "Bodhisattva, won't you take me by the hand? Can you show me the shine of your Japan, the sparkle of your China? Can you show me?" The Beatles, "Across the Universe," *Let It Be.* Apple Records (1970); Steely Dan, "Bodhisattva," *Countdown to Ecstasy.* ABC Records (1973); Shadowfax, "Brown Rice/Karmapa Chenno" *Shadowdance.* Windham Hill Records (1983).

3. "Kung Fu" (1972–1975). American Broadcasting Company (ABC).

4. *Caddyshack.* Orion Pictures/Warner Brothers (1980); *Groundhog Day.* Columbia Pictures (1993).

5. *The Razor's Edge.* Columbia Pictures (1984). In the 1946 production of the film, the protagonist is advised by a Hindu swami; in Murray's version of the film, the teacher is a Tibetan monk.

6. http://c250.columbia.edu/c250_celebrates/remarkable_columbians/theos_casimir_bernard.html

7. I learned only months later that he had not been entirely serious and had not expected me to follow his expressed advice.

8. For a brief account of some of my research activities in Darjeeling, see Hackett, "Looking for a Lost Gita," *Nāma-rūpa* 7 (Fall 2007): 41–45.

9. This is not to disparage all who came, and who subsequently proved themselves to be very competent and intelligent journalists. A notable example is the very

insightful and well-written article by Pankaj Misra—whom I wish I had had the good fortune to meet in Lhasa—the only account I have read that truly captured the feel of Tibet in those days. Misra, "The Train to Tibet," 82ff.

10. In contemporary publications, Tsarong is barely mentioned, while Richardson is vilified as being the influence upon the Tibetans and the sole reason they were incited to turn against the Chinese motherland. The tone of these articles is quite in keeping with the portrayal of Tibetans by the Chinese authorities as intellectual children easily swayed by "Western" corrupting influences, apparently considered a more plausible explanation than the alternative—that most Tibetans simply view the Chinese with contempt. Ka-shö Chö-gyel-nyi-ma (*ka shod chos rgyal nyi ma*), "lha sdod dbyin ji *ri car san* gyi bod kyi nang srid la the jus ngan skul byas te bzos pa'i don rkyen zhig dang ngos bka' blon gnas dbyung btang skor," in *Bod kyi lo rgyus rig gnas dpyad gzhi'i rgyu cha bdams bsgrigs* 8:232–238.

11. Joseph E. Schwartzberg, *A Historical Atlas of South Asia* (University of Minnesota Press, 1978) is a notable example. In this work Tibet has ceased to exist on all maps, and the lands north of India and Nepal bear the anachronistic identifications "Chinese Empire" and "Republic of China."

12. *las 'bras mi slu.*

13. When I walked into a Chinese-run (as are nearly *all* the stores in Lhasa) grocery store looking for something that I couldn't find—but for which I knew the Tibetan name—I asked a Chinese worker if she spoke Tibetan. Apparently, "pö gey kyen gyi yö bey?" was the *only* Tibetan phrase she could understand, and the girl began stamping her feet and jumping up and down, with her eyes closed, yelling "No, no, no, no, no!!!"

14. In this new Chinese-fostered mythology about Tibet, the only identifiable Chinese person in recorded history, the Chinese princess Wen-ching—bartered to the Tibetan king as a concubine in exchange for a cessation of hostilities after the Tibetan army defeated the Chinese in repeated battles in the seventh century—was now being credited with the construction of everything left standing in Tibet, including the Potala Palace. When I asked about the destruction still visible around the Lhasa Valley and in the countryside, I was similarly told that all of it was done by the Tibetans, who did not value their heritage—hence the necessity of the Chinese presence to preserve Tibetan culture.

15. Dowling's *Aquarian Gospel of Jesus the Christ* appears on inventory lists of TCB's library collection, dating from the late 1940s and onward.

16. Abhedananda, *Kasmira, Amaranatha, o Tibhata bhramana*. Translated as *Journey Into Kashmir and Tibet*.

17. See Roerich, *Shambhala*.

18. Francke, *Antiquities of Indian Tibet*, 1:45–46.

19. See Scherrer-Schaub and Steinkellner, *Tabo studies II: manuscripts, texts, inscriptions, and the arts*.

20. Enclosure to Restricted Dispatch No. 300. Howard Donovan to U.S. Secretary of State (Washington, DC), Sept. 29, 1947. RG-84, "India; New Delhi Mission; Confiden-

tial File, Classified General Records (1942–55)," Box 36, Folder 310, "Theos Bernard (1947)." National Archives and Records Administration.

21. Henry Banon, much to HGP's later anger, reported that he had received word from TCB that he would arrive the next day. It is difficult to interpret this statement, since it implies that Banon was aware of what had happened to TCB and either actively or (more likely) unwittingly was perpetuating the disinformation.

BIBLIOGRAPHY

Photo Credit Abbreviations

AZHS: Theos Casimir Bernard Papers. Fig. 1.1 (f35); courtesy of the Arizona Historical Society, Tucson.

BANC: Theos Bernard Papers. Figs. 4.1 and 4.2 (Box 2 f. 21), 5.1 and 5.2 (Box 6 f. 1), 5.3 (Box 5 f. 1), 9.1 (Box 1 f. 19), 10.1 and 10.2 (Box 1 f. 17), and 11.3 (Box 2 f. 1); courtesy of the Bancroft Library and the Regents of the University of California.

CUA: Fig. 13.2 (Geshe Wangyal, biographical files, image #2026); courtesy of University Archives, Columbia University in the City of New York.

CUHS: Viola W. Bernard Papers. Figs. 2.1 (OV-1 fol. 2), 2.2 (OV-1 fol. 3), 3.1 (Box 374 fol. 6), 6.1 and 6.2 (OV-2), and 6.3 (Box 374 fol. 43); courtesy of Viola W. Bernard Papers, Archives & Special Collections, Columbia University Health Sciences Library, New York, NY.

HGPF: Figs. 9.2, 12.1, 12.2, and 13.1; courtesy of the Helen Graham Park Foundation.

NAA: Papers of William Duncan Strong. Fig. 2.3 (Box 70 scrapbook p.16); courtesy of National Anthropological Archives, Smithsonian Institution, Suitland, MD.

PAHM: Theos Bernard Collection. Figs. 7.1 (15-28087), 7.2 (15-26194), 7.3 (15-28187), 8.1 (15-26424), 8.2 (15-26781), 8.3 (15-27154), 8.4 (15-27145), 8.5 (15-27324), 8.6 (15-28897), 8.7 (15-28907), 8.8 (15-28919), 8.9 (15-28908), 8.10 (15-28878), 8.11 (15-28920), 8.12 (15-28875), 8.13 (15-28896), 8.14 (15-28895), 8.15 (15-28850); courtesy of the Phoebe A. Hearst Museum of Anthropology and the Regents of the University of California.

Abbreviations

HGPF Archive: Park, Helen Graham, "Helen Graham Park Archive." Helen Graham Park Foundation, Miami Shores, FL.

TCB Diary: Bernard, Theos, "Tibet Diaries." 3 vols. (1937). Theos Bernard Papers, Bancroft Library; also VWB Archive #s 376.2, 376.3, 376.4.

Theos Bernard Papers: Bernard, Theos, "Theos Bernard Papers." BANC MSS 2005/161 c. The Bancroft Library, University of California, Berkeley.

VWB Archive: Bernard, Viola W., "Papers, 1918–2000." Columbia Health Sciences Library, Archives and Special Collections, Acc.#2000.10.13.

Works by Theos Bernard

Haṭha yoga; the report of a personal experience. Ph.D. diss., Columbia University, 1944. Reprinted as *Haṭha Yoga*. New York: Rider, 1950; London: Rider, 1950; New York: Samuel Wiser, 1967.
French translation: *Tout le Hatha Yoga*. Trans. and adapted by Roland Nagare and Antoine-Emile Fayon. Paris: Amiot Dumont, 1954.
German translation: *Hatha Yoga: ein Erfahrungsbericht aus Indien und Tibet*. Trans. Kurt Lamerdin. Stuttgart : Hans E. Günther Verlag, 1955.
Spanish translation: *Hatha yoga: una técnica de liberación*. Editorial Central, 1961; reprint, Buenos Aires: Siglo Veinte, 1966.
Heaven Lies Within Us. New York: Charles Scribner's Sons, 1939.
Spanish translation: *El Camino Practico del Yoga: El Cielo esta en Nosotros*. Trans. Aníbal Leal. Editorial Dedalo, 1955; reprint, Buenos Aires: Editorial La Pleyade, 1972.
Penthouse of the Gods. New York: Charles Scribner's Sons, 1939.
Land of a Thousand Buddhas. London: Rider, 1940.
Philosophical Foundations of India. London: Rider, 1945. Reprinted as *Hindu Philosophy*. New York: Philosophical Library, 1947.
A Simplified Grammar of the Literary Tibetan Language. Santa Barbara, CA: Tibetan Text Society, 1946.
"An American in Lhasa." *ASIA: Journal of the American Asiatic Association* (Mar. 1939): 139–147.
"An American in Lhasa, Part II." *ASIA: Journal of the American Asiatic Association* (Apr. 1939): 206–211.
"I Become a Lama." *ASIA: Journal of the American Asiatic Association* (Apr. 1939): 206–211.
"The Peril of Tibet." *ASIA: Journal of the American Asiatic Association* (Sept. 1939): 500–504.
"The Tibetan 'Wheel of Life.'" *Review of Religion* (May 1939): 400–401.
"Introduction to Tantrik Ritual." Master's thesis, Columbia University, 1936.
"Penthouse of the Gods." Lecture notes. Theos Bernard Papers, Bancroft Library.
"Tantric Yoga." Ph.D. diss. (rejected), Columbia University, 1938.
"Tantrik Yoga: A Clinical Report." Ph.D. diss. (draft), Columbia University, 1943.
"Tibet Diaries." 3 vols. (1937). Theos Bernard Papers, Bancroft Library; VWB Archive #376.
"Tibetan Saga." Theos Bernard Papers, Bancroft Library.

Archives

Bell, Charles. "Charles Bell Papers." Eur. Mss. Eur F-80. Oriental and India Office Collection, British Library.

Bernard, Theos. "Theos Bernard Papers." BANC MSS 2005/161 c. The Bancroft Library, University of California, Berkeley.

Bernard, Viola W. "Papers, 1918–2000." Columbia Health Sciences Library, Archives and Special Collections, Acc.#2000.10.13.

British Intelligence on China in Tibet, 1903–1950. OIOC, British Library. CIT-5 microfiche.

Evans-Wentz Papers. Collection M0278. Department of Special Collections, Green Library, Stanford University.

Gergan Dorje Tharchin Papers. Starr East Asian Library, Special Collections, Columbia University.

Pacific Geographic Society Records. Collection M0166. Department of Special Collections, Green Library, Stanford University.

Park, Helen Graham. "Helen Graham Park Archive." Helen Graham Park Foundation, Miami Shores, FL.

Records of the Bureau of Indian Affairs. RG-75. National Archives and Records Administration, Washington, DC.

Records of the Foreign Service Posts of the Department of State. RG 84. National Archives and Records Administration, College Park, MD.

Records of the Immigration and Naturalization Service, 1891–1957. RG-85. National Archives and Records Administration, Washington, DC.

Records of the U.S. Customs Service. RG-36. National Archives and Records Administration, Washington, DC.

Strong, William Duncan. "The Papers of William Duncan Strong." National Anthropological Archives, Smithsonian Institution, Suitland, MD.

Younghusband Papers. Mss. Eur 197. Oriental and India Office Collection, British Library.

Tibetan Language Sources

"'jig rten bde ba gzhan bde 'dod las byung, 'jig rten sdug bsngal rang bde 'dod las byung." *Mirror* 18, no. 8 (July 1, 1950), 8.

——. "a mi ri ka'i sa heb." *Mirror* 8, no. 12 (Mar. 13, 1937), 4 col. 2.

——. "a mi ri ka'i sbar ne de sa heb." *Mirror* 9, no. 7 (Jan. 2, 1938), 12.

——. "a mi ri ka'i sbar na te sa heb." *Mirror* 15 no. 2, (Dec. 1, 1946) 1.

——. "dar mdo rin po che." *Mirror* 15, no. 4/5 (Feb./Mar. 1947), 4 col. 2.

——. "dge ba'i bshes gnyen shes rab rgya mtsho." *Mirror* 8, no. 12 (Mar. 13, 1937), 7 col. 3.

——. "gsar 'gyu do dam pa'i sger zhu." *Mirror* 9, no. 1 (May 11, 1937), 6 col. 3.

——. "mi snyan pa'i gnas tshul." *Mirror* 27, no. 8/9 (May–June 1961), 5–6.

——. "sa zla'i dus bzang." *Mirror* 9, no. 2 (June 9, 1937), 3 col. 2.

——. "shin tu nas skyo ba'i gnas tshul." *Mirror* 26, no. 1 (June 1959), 5, col. 3.

——. "sngags chen bdar ba ho thog thu blo bzang bstan 'dzin 'jigs med dbang phyug gi rnam thar rags bsdus." *bod kyi lo rgyus rig gnas dpyad gzhi'i rgyu cha bdams bsgrigs* 4 (1991).

——. "so so'i gnas tshul [Miscellaneous events]." *Mirror* 9, no. 6 (Oct. 5, 1937), 4.

——. *udānavarga; ched du brjod pa'i tshoms.* Toh. 326. Sde-dge Bka'-'gyur, MDO vol. SA fol. 209a1–253a7.

Ding-ja Tse-ring-dor-je (*sding bya tshe ring rdo rje*). "nye rabs kyi bod dmag dang bod ljongs dmag spyi khang gi skor sogs 'brel yod 'ga' zhig." In *bod kyi lo rgyus rig gnas dpyad gzhi'i rgyu cha bdams bsgrigs,* vol. 8 (spyi'i 'don thengs 17 pa). Sichuan: People's Publishing House (*mi rigs dpe skrun khang*), 1994, 149–180.

Gedun Chöpel (*dge 'dun chos 'phel*). *Bod chen po'i srid lugs dang 'brel ba'i rgyal rabs deb ther dkar po.* Dharamsala: Sherig Parkhang, 1993.

——. "'jig rten ril mo 'am zlum po." *Mirror* 10, no. 1 (June 28, 1938), 11.

Jang-lung Ārya Paṇḍita Nga-wang-lo-sang-ten-pay-gyel-tsen (*lcang lung ārya paṇḍi ta ngag dbang blo bzang bstan pa'i rgyal mtshan, 1770–1845*). *rgya dkar nag rgya ser ka smi ra bal bod hor gyi yi ge dang dpe ris rnam grangs mang ba* [Assorted scripts and diagrams from India, China, Russia, Kashmir, Nepal, Tibet, and Mongolia]. University of Washington, xylograph 66–5 (29 fol.); also, *The Collected Works of Lcaṅ-luṅ Paṇḍi-ta Ṅag-dbaṅ-blo-bzaṅ-bstan-pa'i-rgyal-mtshan.* Delhi: Mongolian Lama Gurudeva (1975–1985), 4:fol. 555–612; also, Berlin ms. Tib. Bl. 151. DSB Berlin.

Ka-shö Chö-gyel-nyi-ma (*ka shod chos rgyal nyi ma*). "lha sdod dbyin ji ri car san gyi bod kyi nang srid la the jus ngan skul byas te bzos pa'i don rkyen zhig dang ngos bka' blon gnas dbyung btang skor." In *Bod kyi lo rgyus rig gnas dpyad gzhi'i rgyu cha bdams bsgrigs,* vol. 8 (spyi'i 'don thengs 17 pa). Sichuan: People's Publishing House (*mi rigs dpe skrun khang*), 1994, 232–238.

Sek-shing Lo-sang-don-drup (*sreg shing blo bzang don grub*). "de snga'i bod dmag ka dang sku srung dmag sgar gyi sgrig srol dang, rang nyid sku srung ru dpon byed mus su 1949 lo'i zing 'khrug langs pa'i 'brel yod gnad don 'ga' zhig." In *bod kyi lo rgyus rig gnas dpyad gzhi'i rgyu cha bdams bsgrigs,* vol. 8 (spyi'i 'don thengs 17 pa). Sichuan: People's Publishing House (*mi rigs dpe skrun khang*), 1994, 250–271.

English Language Sources

Abhedananda, Swami. *Journey into Kashmir and Tibet.* Calcutta: Ramakrishna Vedanta Math, 1967. (English translation of *Kasmira, Amaranatha, o Tibhata bhramana* [Calcutta: N.p., 1929].)

[Advertisement]. *San Francisco Chronicle,* Oct. 1, 1922, C-1.

Alter, Joseph. *Yoga in Modern India: The Body Between Science and Philosophy.* Princeton: Princeton University Press, 2004.

———. "Yoga at the Fin de Siècle: Muscular Christianity with a 'Hindu' Twist," *International Journal of the History of Sport* 23, no. 5 (2006): 759–776.

"American Became Only White Lama of Tibet." *Evening Standard* (UK), May 11, 1940.

Amiruddin, Begum Sultan Mir. "World Congress of Faiths." *Star of India* (Calcutta), Mar. 8, 1937, 4 col. 4.

"Arizona Statehood Post Offices & Postmasters, 1912–1979, Part XIII," *The Heliograph* 6, no. 3 (Summer 1992): 27–30.

Arnold, Elliot. "Nazis and Fascists are Filtering Into Tibet As a Key in World Drive, Expert Reports." *New York World-Telegraph*, Apr. 5, 1939.

Asian relations, being report of the proceedings and documentation of the First Asian Relations Conference, New Delhi, March–April, 1947. New Delhi: Asian Relations Organization, 1948.

Aśvaghoṣa. *Handsome Nanda.* Trans. Linda Covill. New York: New York University Press, 2007.

"Autonomy for Inner Mongolia." *Star of India* (Calcutta), Oct. 29, 1937, 1 col. 4.

Avalon, Arthur. *Principles of Tantra.* London: Luzac, 1914.

Avalon, Arthur, ed. *Sāradā-tilaka.* Tantrik Texts Series vols. 16–17. Calcutta: Agamanusandhana Samiti/Sanskrit Press Depository, 1933.

Bacot, Jacques, ed. *Dictionnaire tibétan-sanscrit.* Paris: P. Geuthner, 1930.

Bacot, Jacques, trans. *Une grammaire tibétaine du tibétain classique: Les slokas grammaticaux de Thonmi Sambhota, avec leurs commentaires.* Paris: P. Guenther, 1928.

Balmer, Randall. *Blessed Assurance.* Boston: Beacon, 1999.

"Bara Lama." *Star of India* (Calcutta), Feb. 26, 1937, 3 col. 5.

Barker, Ralph. *One Man's Jungle: A Biography of F. Spencer Chapman DSO.* London: Chatto & Windus, 1975.

Baudrillard, Jean. *America.* London: Verso, 1996.

Bell, Charles. "Pious Tibet Searches for a Little Child," *New York Times Magazine,* May 23, 1937, 12–13, 28.

Benedict, Ruth. *Patterns of Culture.* Boston: Houghton Mifflin, 1934.

Berg, A. Scott. *Lindbergh.* New York: Putnam, 1998.

Bernard, Glen. "The Art of Yoga." Unpublished ms. Theos Bernard Papers, Bancroft Library.

———. "The Rationale of Sex." Unpublished ms. Theos Bernard Papers, Bancroft Library.

Bernard, Pierre Arnold. *Vira Sadhana: A Theory and Practice of Veda.* New York: American Book Import Co., 1919.

"Bernstorff Active in Irish Plots Here." *New York Times,* Jan. 10, 1921, 3.

Bessac, Frank. "This Was the Trek to Tragedy." *Life,* Nov. 13, 1950, 130–141.

Bhattacharyya, Benoytosh. *An Introduction to Buddhist Esoterism.* Oxford: Oxford University Press, 1932.

Bhattacharyya, Benoytosh, ed. *Sādhanamālā.* 2 vols. Baroda: Oriental Institute, 1928.

Bogin, B. and H. Decleer. "Who was "this evil friend" ("the dog", "the fool", "the tyrant") in Gedun Chopel's Sad Song?" *The Tibet Journal* 22, no. 3 (1997): 67–78.

Boorman, Howard L. and Richard C. Howard. *Biographical Dictionary of Republican China.* New York: Columbia University Press, 1970.

Bowles, Gordon T. *The People of Asia.* New York: Scribner, 1977.

Brahmachary, Syamānanda. *Truth Revealed.* Benares: N.p., 1926.

The British Invasion of Tibet: Colonel Younghusband, 1904. London: The Stationery Office, 1999.

Bruce, Charles. *Assault on Mt. Everest.* London: Longmans, Green, 1922.

"'Buddhist Monk' Sued by Singer." *Tucson Citizen,* July 9, 1946.

Candler, Edmund. *The Unveiling of Lhasa.* London: E. Arnold, 1905.

Collier, John. "Office of Indian Affairs." In *Annual Report of the Department of the Interior.* Washington, DC: Government Printing Office, 1936.

"Colonel Lindbergh." *Star of India,* Feb. 27, 1937, 4.

Cosulich, Bernice. "Bernard Would Trade Tibet's Yak Meat for Yankee Hot Dog." *Arizona Daily Star,* Sept. 27, 1937.

Cotlow, Lewis N. "Farewell and Luck to You." *The Log of the Circumnavigator's Club* 38, no. 3 (Fall 1950): 8.

Crawford, Sharon. *Ganna Walska Lotusland: The Garden and Its Creators.* Santa Barbara, CA: Companion Press, 1996.

Crowley, Aleister. *Eight Lectures on Yoga.* London: Ordo Templi Orientis, 1939.

"Cycles of Psychism." *Theosophy* 31, no. 10 (Aug. 1943): 442–447.

Daniels, George. *American Science in the Age of Jackson.* Tuscaloosa: University of Alabama Press, 1968.

Darjeeling District Gazetteer. Calcutta: Bengal Secretariat Book Depot, 1907.

Das, Sarat Chandra. *Journey to Lhasa and Central Tibet.* London: John Murray, 1902.

Das, Sarat Chandra. *Narrative of a Journey to Lhasa in 1881–82.* Calcutta: Bengal Secretariat Press, 1885.

——. *Narrative of a Journey Round Lake Yamdo (Palti) and in Lhoka, Yarlung, and Sakya in 1882.* Calcutta: Bengal Secretariat Press, 1887.

——. *Tibetan-English Dictionary: With Sanskrit Synonyms.* Calcutta: Bengal Secretariat Book Depot, 1902.

Dasgupta, Sailendra Bejoy. *Kriya Yoga.* Calcutta: n.p., 1979.

David-Neel, Alexandra. *Secret Oral Teachings.* San Francisco: City Lights, 1988.

Dowling, Levi H. *The Aquarian Gospel of Jesus the Christ; The Philosophic and Practical Basis of the Religion of the Aquarian Age of the World and of the Church Universal; Transcribed from the Book of God's Remembrances, Known as the Akashic Records.* London: L. N. Fowler, 1911.

"Edna Bryner Schwab, Tibetan Scholar and Yale Benefactor." *Yale University Library Gazette* 44, no. 1 (July 1969): 21–29.

"Eight Months in Tibet." *Calcutta Statesman,* Oct. 28, 1937, 21.

Eimer, Helmut. *Die Xerokopie des Lhasa-Kanjur/The Xerox Copy of the Lhasa Kanjur.* Tokyo: The Reiyukai Library, 1977.

Evans-Wentz, W. Y. (Walter Yeeling). *Tibetan Yoga and Secret Doctrines.* London: Oxford University Press, 1935.

"Evolution." *Fortune,* July 1933, 4.

Fields, Rick. *How the Swans Came to the Lake*. Boston: Shambhala, 1992.

Forman, Harrison. "I See the King of Hell." *Harper's* 170 (Dec.1934–May 1935): 14–25.

——. *Through Forbidden Tibet: An Adventure Into the Unknown*. New York: Longmans, Green, 1935.

Francke, A. F. *Antiquities of Indian Tibet*. 1926; reprint, New Delhi: Asian Educational Services, 1992.

"Gandhi Disciple Rejuvenated; Mahatma Himself May Follow; '172-Year-Old' Yogi Claims Ancient Lore, Exercised in Bricked-up Chamber, Has Grown New Set of Teeth for Patient." *The Washington Post*, Feb. 27, 1938, 6.

"Ganna Walska Fights Mate's Support Suit." *Los Angeles Times,* July 9, 1946, A-1.

"Ganna Walska Is Freed." *New York Times,* July 14, 1946, 31.

Gedun Choephel and Samten Norboo, trans. *The White Annals*. Dharamsala: LTWA, 1978.

Ginsberg, Allen. *Indian Journals: Notebooks, Diary, Blank Pages, Writings*. San Francisco: City Lights, 1970.

Goldenweiser, Alexander. *History, Psychology, and Culture*. New York: Knopf, 1935.

Goldstein, Melvin. *History of Modern Tibet*. Vol. 1. Berkeley: University of California Press, 1989.

Gould, Basil. *The Jewel in the Lotus: Recollections of an Indian Political*. London: Chatto and Windus, 1957.

Gould, Basil and Hugh Richardson. *Tibetan Word Book*. London: Oxford University Press, 1943.

Hackett, Paul G. "Barbarian Lands: Theos Bernard, Tibet, and the American Religious Life." Ph.D. diss., Columbia University, 2008.

——. "Looking for a Lost Gita." *Nāma-rūpa* 7 (Fall 2007): 41–45.

Hall, Manly P. *The Secret Destiny of America*. Los Angeles: Philosophical Research Society, 1944.

A Handbook for Travelers in India Burma & Ceylon. London: J. Murray, 1910.

Harrer, Heinrich. "Flight of the Dalai Lama." *Life*, April 23, 1951.

——. *Seven Years in Tibet*. New York: E. P. Dutton, 1954.

Havnevik, Hanna. "The Life of Jetsun Lochen Rinpoche (1865–1951)." Ph.D. diss., University of Oslo, 1999.

"He Can't Work But He Stands on His Head For 3 Hours." *Gettysburg Times* (PA), July 13, 1946.

Hilton, James. *Lost Horizon*. New York: William Morrow, 1933.

Hopkins, Jeffrey, et al. "Tibetan-English Dictionary." Unpublished ms., 1993.

[Hopper, Hedda]. "Hedda Hopper's Hollywood." *Los Angeles Times,* Nov. 23, 1942, 14.

Hopper, Hedda. "Looking at Hollywood." *Chicago Daily Tribune*, Nov. 23, 1942, 20.

"The Hotels." *The Rangoon Gazette*, Sept. 10, 1936, 7.

Hughes, A. Daniel. *Tombstone Story: The Biography of an Arizona Pioneer*. Hicksville, NY: Exposition Press, 1979.

Illion, Theodore [Theodor Burang]. *Darkness Over Tibet*. London: Rider, 1937.

——. *In Secret Tibet*. London: Rider, 1937.

Illson, Murray. "Ex-Ivy Leaguers Aim to Be Monks: Three Studying at Buddhist Monastery in Jersey." *New York Times*, Dec. 15, 1963, 71 col.1.

"Indian Melodies Charm Denizens of the Jungle." *San Francisco Examiner*, May 25, 1914, 19.

International Congress of Free Christians and Other Religious Liberals. *New Pilgrimages of the Spirit. Proceedings and Papers of the Pilgrim Tercentenary Meeting of the International Congress of Free Christian and Other Religious Liberals, held at Boston and Plymouth, U.S.A., October 3-7, 1920.* Boston: Beacon Press, 1921.

Jackson, David. *A Saint in Seattle.* Boston: Wisdom, 2003.

"Jacob Wertheim Estate: Tobacco Manufacturer Leaves $6,038,284 Net to 38 Beneficiaries." *New York Times*, Dec. 24, 1921, 8.

Jacobsen v. United States, 7th Circuit Court of Appeals, 272 F. 399.

Jung, Carl. "The Dreamlike World of India." In *Civilization in Transition.* Princeton: Princeton University Press, 1964.

——. "The Kundalini Yoga: Notes on the Seminar By Prof. Dr. J. R. Hauer with Psychological Commentary by Dr. C. G. Jung." Ed. Mary Foote. Unpublished ms. Zürich, Autumn 1932.

——. *Memories, Dreams, Reflections.* New York: Vintage, 1989.

——. "Psychological Commentary on *The Tibetan Book of the Great Liberation*." In *Psychology and Religion: West and East.* Collected Works, v. 11. Princeton: Princeton University Press, 1969, 500.

Kimura, Hisao. *Japanese Agent in Tibet.* London: Serindia, 1990.

Kipling, Rudyard. *Kim.* New York: Doubleday, 1901.

Knight, George. *Intimate Glipses of Mysterious Tibet and Neighboring Countries.* London: Golden Vista Press, 1930.

von Koerber, Hans Nordewin. *Morphology of the Tibetan Language.* Los Angeles: Sutton Press, 1935.

Kuvalayananda, Swami. *Asanas.* Lonavala: Kaivalyadhama, 1924.

Laird, Thomas. *Into Tibet.* New York: Grove Press, 2002.

"Lama Geshe Chompell." *Journal of the Mahabodhi Society* 49, no. 8 (Aug. 1941): 3.

Landau, Rom. *God Is My Adventure—A Book on Modern Mystics, Masters, and Teachers.* London: Faber & Faber, 1935.

Landon, Kenneth P. ["K.P.L."]. "Review: Hatha Yoga. The Report of a Personal Experience by Theos Bernard." *Journal of Philosophy* 41, no. 19 (Sept. 1944): 530.

Landon, Perceval. *The Opening of Tibet.* New York: Doubleday, 1905.

Lapierre, Dominique and Larry Collins. *Freedom at Midnight.* New Delhi: Vikas Publishing House, 2005.

"Lily Pons Is Star of Opening Opera." *New York Times*, Nov. 12, 1946, 35.

"Lindbergh's Movements." *Star of India*, Feb. 25, 1937, 1.

"Lindberghs at Calcutta." *New York Times*, Mar. 1, 1937, 9.

"Lindberghs Still Missing." *Star of India*, Feb. 24, 1937, 1.

Lopez, Donald S. *Prisoners of Shangri-La.* Chicago: University of Chicago Press, 2000.

Love, Robert. *The Great Oom.* New York: Viking, 2010.

Macdonald, David. *Touring in Sikkim and Tibet.* Kalimpong: n.p., 1930.

——. *Twenty Years in Tibet.* London: Seeley, Service, 1932.

Macdonald-Bayne, M. *Yoga of the Christ.* London: L. N. Fowler, n.d.

Manuel, D. G. *A Gladdening River: Twenty-Five Years' Guild Influence Among the Himalayas.* London/Edinburgh: A. & C. Black, 1914.

Mao Tse-tung. *The Collected Works of Mao Tse-tung.* Peking: Foreign Language Press, 1977.

Marshall, P. J. *The British Discovery of Hinduism in the Eighteenth Century.* Cambridge: Cambridge University Press, 1970.

Maugham, Sumerset. *The Razor's Edge.* Garden City, NY: Doubleday, Doran & Co., 1944.

McGovern, William. *To Lhasa in Disguise.* New York: The Century Co., 1934.

McKay, Alex. *Tibet and the British Raj.* London: Curzon Press, 1997.

Meinheit, Susan. "The Rockhill Tibetan Collection at the Library of Congress." Paper presented at the XIth International Association for Tibetan Studies (IATS) Conference (Königswinter, Germany), 2006.

Melville, Herman. *Moby Dick.* New York: Bantam, 1981.

Mengele, Irmgard. *dGe-'dun-chos-'phel, A Biography of the 20th-century Scholar.* Dharamsala: LTWA, 1999.

Misra, Pankaj. "The Train to Tibet." *The New Yorker,* Apr. 16, 2007.

"Miss Wertheim Wed at Country Home." *New York Times,* May 31, 1929, 26.

"Mme. Walska Fights Her Yogi Husband's Suit." *Chicago Daily Tribune,* July 9, 1946, 6.

Morgan, William Stanley. *Amchi Sahib: A British Doctor in Tibet 1936–37.* Charlestown, MA: Acme Bookbinding, 2007.

Mullin, Glenn. *Path of the Bodhisattva Warrior.* Ithaca, NY: Snow Lion, 1988.

Mundy, Talbot. "Mystic India Speaks." *True Mystic Science* 1, no. 2 (Dec. 1938): 15–16, 63.

"New Autonomous Mongolian State." *Star of India* (Calcutta), Oct. 30, 1937, 1 col. 7.

"No Dalai Lama May Be Found." Ca. Jan.–Feb. 1938 [unidentified newspaper clipping].

"On the Aisle: Audience More Fun Than Opera at Met's Opening." *Chicago Daily Tribune,* Nov. 14, 1946, 29.

"'172-Year-Old Yogi' Turns Back the Years, He Reports, for Aging Follower of Gandhi." *New York Times,* Feb. 27, 1938, 35.

"Only a Hindoo Monk: Vive Kananda Believes Not in the Tricks of the Yogis." *Washington Post* Oct. 29, 1894, 6.

"Only White Lama of Tibet Finishing Book in Southland: Former American Lawyer Tells How He Came to Take Up Philosophy of Land of Shangri-La." *Los Angeles Times,* Aug. 13, 1939.

Pallis, Marco. *Peaks and Lamas.* New York: Knopf, 1949.

Petech, Luciano. *Aristocracy and Government in Tibet: 1728–1959.* Rome: IsMEO, 1973.

Phillips, Sandra S. "Adams and Stieglitz: A Friendship." *Art in America* (Jan. 2005).

"Political Associate of Gandhi, 77, Made 'Youthful' by Indian Yogi, 172." *The Atlanta Constitution,* Feb. 27, 1938, 1A.

Potter, Karl H. [Untitled book review]. *Philosophy East and West* 7, no. 3/4 (Oct. 1957–Jan. 1958): 146–149.

Prothero, Stephen. *The White Buddhist: The Asian Odyssey of Henry Steel Olcott.* Bloomington: Indiana University Press, 1996.

"Radio Listeners in Panic, Taking War Drama as Fact/Many Flee Homes to Escape 'Gas Raid From Mars'—Phone Calls Swamp Police at Broadcast of Welles Fantasy." *New York Times,* Oct. 31, 1938, 1.

Religions of the World. 2 vols. Calcutta: Ramakrishna Mission Institute of Culture, 1938.

"Religious Wealth In Tibet's Wilderness Seen By Bernard." *Arizona Daily Star,* Nov. 4, 1937.

Rhodes, Nicholas and Deki Rhodes. *S. W. Laden La: A Man of the Frontier.* Kolkata: Library of Numismatic Studies, 2006.

Richardson, Hugh. "Foreigners in Tibet." In Hugh Richardson, *High Peaks, Pure Earth.* London: Serindia, 1998, 409–419.

Richardus, Peter. *The Dutch Orientalist Johan van Manen: His Life and Work.* Leiden: Kern Institute, 1989.

R.M. "The Magic of Oxford." *The New Age: An Independent Socialist Review of Politics, Literature, and Art* 676 (New Series. Vol. I. No. 17) (Aug. 22, 1907): 260–261.

Robb, Inez. "The Old Met 'Opry' House 'Ain't What It Used to Be.'" *Washington Post,* Nov. 20, 1942, B-13.

Robbins, Mildred Brown. "From Where I Sit." *San Francisco Chronicle,* Aug. 11, 1946.

Robertson, Stewart. "The White Lama on Yoga." *Family Circle* 15, no. 8 (Aug. 25, 1939): 14–15, 18, 21.

Rockhill, William Woodville. *The Land of the Lamas: Notes of a Journey Through China, Mongolia and Tibet.* New York: Century Co., 1891.

"Rocklanders Get New Year Greeting from Rocky Tibet." *Rockland County Herald,* Feb. 26, 1938, 1, 4.

Rodrigues, Santan. *The Householder Yogi: Life of Shri Yogendra.* Bombay: Yoga Institute, 1982.

Roerich, Nicholas. "Remains." *The Mahabodhi Journal* 50, no. 2 (Feb. 1942): 60–63.

——. *Shambhala.* N.p., 1930.

Sambuddhananda, Swami. *The Message of the Himalayas.* Bombay: Saxon Press, 1953.

Sāṅkṛtyāyana, Tripiṭakâcharya Rāhula. "Sanskrit Palm-Leaf Mss. In Tibet." *Journal of the Bihar and Orissa Research Society* 20, no. 3/4 (1934): 21–43.

Satyananda Giri, Swami. *Yoganand Sanga.* N.p., n.d.

Schary, Edwin G. *In Search of the Mahatmas of Tibet.* London: Seeley, Service, 1937.

Scherrer-Schaub, C. A. and E. Steinkellner, eds. *Tabo studies II: manuscripts, texts, inscriptions, and the arts.* Rome: Istituto italiano per l'Africa e l'Oriente, 1999.

Schlagintweit, Emil. *Buddhism in Tibet.* London: Trübner, 1863.

Schneider, Herbert W. *Philosophy Will Never Be A Science.* Torino: Edizioni di «Filosofia», 1963.

Schurmacher, Emile C. "They Try to Come Back Alive." *Los Angeles Times,* June 5, 1949, F-14–15, 27.

Schwartzberg, Joseph E. *A Historical Atlas of South Asia.* Minneapolis: University of Minnesota Press, 1978.

"Secret Rites I Saw in Darkest Tibet, I Was a Lama." *Daily Mail* (UK), Nov. 13, 1937, 13, 16.

"Secrets of Tibet Were Revealed to Author." [Review of *Land of a Thousand Buddhas.*] *Psychic News* (UK), June 8, 1940.

Sennwald, Andre. "The Old-Fashioned Way." *New York Times*, July 14, 1934, 16, col. 5.

Sinh, Pancham. *Haṭha yoga Pradīpikā.* 2nd ed. Allahabad: Lalit Mohan Basu, The Panini Office, 1932.

Snelling, John. *Buddhism in Russia.* Shaftesbury, Dorset: Element, 1993.

"Still Modest." *New York Times*, Mar. 5, 1937, 20.

Stoddard, Heather. *Le Mendiant de l'Amdo.* Paris: Société d'Ethnolographie, 1985.

"Suit Discloses Fifth Ganna Walska Marriage." *Los Angeles Times,* May 26, 1946, A3.

T. Bernard v. A. Bernard. Complaint for Separate Maintenance. Superior Court of California, County of Santa Barbara, case no. 38378.

"Tales of Tibetan Trip Told by Member Of Clarkstown Country Club on Return From Six Months Tour of Exploration." *The Journal-News* [Nyack, NY], Nov. 27, 1937.

Tappan, Cora L.V. *Discourses Through the Mediumship of Cora L. V. Tappan; The New Science: Spiritual Ethics.* London: J. Burns, 1875.

Taring, Rinchen Dolma. *Daughter of Tibet.* Boston: Wisdom, 1986.

Taves, Brian. *Talbot Mundy, Philosopher of Adventure.* Jefferson, NC: McFarlane, 2006.

Taylor, Kathleen. "Arthur Avalon: The Creation of a Legendary Orientalist." In *Myth and Mythmaking: Continuous Evolution in Indian Tradition,* ed. Julia Leslie. Surrey, London: Routledge Curzon, 1996.

——. *Sir John Woodroffe, Tantra and Bengal.* London: Curzon, 2001.

Teichman, Eric. *Travels of a Consular Officer in Eastern Tibet.* Cambridge: Cambridge University Press, 1922.

"Theos Bernard: 'Penthouse of the Gods.'" *Reno Evening Gazette*, Mar. 18, 1939.

"Third Danish Expedition of Central Asia." *Explorer Journal* 28, no. 3 (Summer 1950).

Thomas, Lowell with Lowell Thomas Jr. "Out of This World: A Journey to Lhasa." *Collier's* 125, no. 6 (Feb. 11, 1950): 13–17, 70.

Thomas, Lowell Jr. *Out of This World: To Forbidden Tibet.* New York: Avon, 1950.

Thomas, Wendall. *Hinduism Invades America.* Boston: Beacon, 1930.

"Tibetan Books from a 'Peak Secretary.'" *Yale University Library Gazette* 35, no. 3 (Jan 1961): 126–133.

"The Tibetan Collection at Yale." *Yale University Library Gazette* 34, no. 3 (Jan 1960): 127–133.

"Tibetan New Year Greetings Here." *New York Sun,* Feb. 17, 1938.

Todd, Jesse T. "Imagining the Future of American Religion at the New York World's Fair, 1939–40." Ph.D. diss., Columbia University, 1996.

"Tragedy in China." *New York Times*, July 1, 1936, 24.

Tsarong, Dundul Namgyal. *In the Service of His Country.* Ithaca, NY: Snow Lion, 2000.

Tucci, Giuseppe. *Gyantse and Its Monasteries.* Indo Tibetica Part IV. vols. 1–3. Rome: Reale Academia d'Italia, 1941.

"$20,000 Yearly for Girls." *New York Times,* June 16, 1922, 13.

"U.A. Student to Study Primitive Indian Folk." *Arizona Daily Star*, July 10, 1936, 3.

[Unidentified]. *Johannesburg Star*, June 12, 1939.

U.S. Bureau of the Census. 1930.

U.S. Patent Office. *Official Gazette of the United States Patent Office*. Vol. 131. Washington, DC: Government Printing Office, 1907.

Vidyabhusana, Satis Chandra. *Bilingual index of Nyāya-bindu*. Calcutta: Asiatic Society, 1917.

Walska, Ganna. *Always Room at the Top*. New York: Richard R. Smith, 1943.

Wangyal, (Geshe) Ngawang. *The Door of Liberation*. Boston: Wisdom, 1995.

Wayman, Alex. "The Concept of Poison in Buddhism." *Oriens* 10, no. 1 (1957): 107–109.

"Wealthy Mrs. Donovan (Now in the Asylum) and Her Yogi Teacher." *American Weekly* supplement, May 4, 1941, 3.

"Wertheim Estate Put at $9,324,243; Accounting Covers Trusts Set Up by Investment House Head." *New York Times*, May 24, 1938, 16.

Who's Who in Tibet. Calcutta: Government of India Press, 1938.

Williams, T. Walter. "M. M. Mizzle Quits His Lamasery, Pursued by Sable Amazon on Yak." *New York Times*, Feb. 14, 1937, 41.

Williamson, Margret. *Memoirs of a Political Officer's Wife*. London: Wisdom, 1987.

"Wins Hawthornden Prize." *New York Times*, June 13, 1934, 21, col. 5.

W. N. "Yoga Studied First Hand." *Los Angeles Times*, Oct. 29, 1939, C-6.

Woodroffe, John. *Garland of Letters*. Madras: Ganesh & Co., 1922.

Woodroffe, John. *Shakti and Shâkta*. 1920; 2nd ed., London: Luzac, 1920.

——. *The World As Power: Power As Life*. Madras: Ganesh & Co., 1922.

——. *The World As Power: Reality*. Madras: Ganesh & Co., 1921.

Woodroffe, John and P. N. Mukhyopādhyāya. *The World As Power: Causality and Continuity*. Madras: Ganesh & Co., 1923.

——. *The World As Power: Power As Matter*. Madras: Ganesh & Co., 1923.

Yang, Twan. *Houseboy in India*. New York: John Day, 1943.

Yogananda, Paramahansa. *Whispers from Eternity*. Los Angeles: Self-Realization Fellowship, 1935.

——. *Autobiography of a Yogi*. Los Angeles: Self-Realization Fellowship, 1946.

"Yogi Magic Rejuvenates Elderly Follower of Gandhi." *Los Angeles Times*, Feb. 27, 1938, 1.

"Yogi Turns Back Years For Aged Indian Pandit." *Chicago Daily Tribune*, Feb. 27, 1938, 3.

"Yogi 'Turns Back Years' For Follower of Gandhi." *New York Herald Tribune*, Feb. 27, 1938.

Younghusband, Francis. *Life in the Stars*. New York: Dutton, 1928.

——. "An Explorer's Religion." *Atlantic Monthly* (Dec. 1936): 651–655.

INDEX

Bernard, Theos: Academy of Tibetan Literature, 319–320, 331, 355, 394; adopting Tibetan dress, 234–235, 242, 253, 457n84; American Institute of Yoga, 304; and Gedun Chöpel (*see* Gedun Chöpel); and Geshe Wangyal (*see* Wangyal, [Geshe] Ngawang); and his father, Glen, 7, 9, 63; and illustrated yoga manuscript, 124, 444n53; and Pur-bu-jok's *Collected Topics*, 356–357; and study of yoga, 9–10; approach to research, 33–34, 164; as a Buddhist, 283; as Padmasambhava, xii, 109, 145–146, 162, 183, 187, 245, 278, 293, 309, 343, 451n33; as reincarnate lama, 227, 249–250, 335; as Theos Gordon, 13; as Tibetan Lama, 174, 187, 200, 244, 252, 259, 283, 293, 309; as "White Lama," xi, 275, 290, 298, 306–307, 309, 343, 383, 405, 462n25, 464n10; *ASIA* (magazine) articles, 292–296; at the World Congress of Faiths (Calcutta), 137; attempt to bring Tibetans to America, 284; attempt to visit Lhasa (1947), 354, 357; attempts to attend Oxford, 263, 275, 279; attitude toward British, 151, 197, 246, 296, 462n31; Buddhism, study and knowledge of, 94, 148, 196, 352–356; claims of yogic powers, 342–344; college illness, 6, 21, 24, 281; critics of, 326–327, 392–393, 462n25, 470n23; death foretold, 127, 260, 381; disappearance—rumors and stories, 369–371, 375–376, 378, 381–384, 388–389, 401–402, 405–406, 427; early life, 2–3, 5, 284, 432n17; final activities, 423–426; Gtum-mo empowerment, 258–259; Hamati (namesake) (*see* Hamati, Sylvais); *Haṭha Yoga* dissertation, xiv, 328–329, 332, 461n23; *Heaven Lies Within Us*, 284, 286–288, 309, 326, 380, 392–393, 430n8, 461n21; in Kulu, 360–365;

influence on 1960s counterculture, 393; ingesting mercury, 123, 444n50; *Land of a Thousand Buddhas*, 292, 332, 462n28; last will, 467n3; lawsuit (1940–41), 306–310; lecture tour (1938–39), 159, 282–283; legal experience, 7; New York yoga studio and lectures, 299, 304–306, 312, 325; officially declared dead, 389; opinion of other visitors to Tibet, 168, 191, 227, 451n35, 456n66; opinion of the Tibetans, 226, 241, 467n4; opinion of Western culture, 166–167, 232, 247, 255–256, 321; opinions of academia, 20, 24, 31, 37, 38, 125, 280; *Penthouse of the Gods*, 281; Penthouse of the Gods (Santa Barbara, CA), 315; *Philosophical Foundations of India*, 331–332, 340, 392; project to translate the Tibetan Buddhist canon, 248, 319, 337; reckless behavior, 6, 24, 28, 203, 432n17, 434n11; reincarnations of, 403, 408–409, 471n36; relationship with Blanche DeVries, 201, 281; relationship with Ganna Walska (*see* Walska, [Madame] Ganna); relationship with Helen Park (*see* Park, Helen Graham); relationship with Viola Wertheim, 16, 19, 21, 28, 125–126, 150, 200, 244, 277–278, 329, 335, 383; religious experiences, 141–143, 189, 232, 241, 270, 430–31n8; religious views, 29, 247, 249–250, 253–255, 294; return to Kalimpong (1946), 350; second attempt for Ph.D., 324–326; *Simplified Grammar of the Literary Tibetan Language*, 337, 340, 357; *Tantric Yoga* dissertation (failed), 279–280; *Tantric Yoga* M.A. thesis, 37, 40–42, 44, 79, 306; Tibet diaries, 159, 202, 232, 449; Tibetan language study and proficiency, 124, 127, 136, 145–146, 152, 186, 190, 204, 216–218, 228, 263, 265, 352, 355–357, 463n35; Tibetan materials, xiii, 394; Tibetan materials, acquisitions by Harvard, Yale, and State Library of West Berlin, 394; Tibetan materials, acquisitions by U. C. Berkeley, 403–404; Tibetan Text Society of Santa Barbara, 337; Tibetland (Santa Barbara, CA), 315–319, 323–324, 339–341, 344, 383; *Twentieth Century India*, 347; understanding of religious truth, 40–41, 125, 163, 190; unpublished works, 331; work for Bureau of Indian Affairs, 20–21, 24, 26, 28–29, 33–35, 382; yoga practice, 9, 147, 277; yoga retreat (alleged), 107

Bernard, Viola Wertheim: censorship of personal papers, 440n20, 455n57; early life, 13–15, 432n2; later life, 402; opinion of Theos Bernard, 383, 430–31n8; opinions of religious practice, 30; relationship with Theos Bernard, 17, 21, 264, 277, 280, 282

Bhattacharyya, Benoytosh, 42–43, 45, 435n13

Bidyanidhi, Kaviraj Narendranath, 59, 74

Bonshö (Shapé/Cabinet Minister), 223

Bowles, Gordon T., 111, 227, 441n10

breath control (*prāṇāyāma*) practices, 51, 58, 102, 106, 123, 140, 302, 438n4, 441n3

British: attitude toward Tibet, 175, 191, 227, 384, 442n23; bureaucracy, 192, 194, 199; opinion of Theos Bernard, 296–298, 354, 377, 448n3

British Mission (Lhasa), 245–247

Cable, (Captain) Gordon, 168, 171–173, 179–180, 182, 188, 191–194, 260, 449n18, 450n28

Calcutta Statesman (newspaper), 227, 274, 460n3

Caraka Saṃhita, 51, 59, 262

Carpenter, Henry Albert, 94, 440n17

Categorical Sayings (udānavarga), 399–400

Chaksam Ferry, 158, 203, 208, 413

Chao Erh-feng, 206, 208, 440n8

Chapman, Frederick (Freddy) Spencer, 141, 144, 150, 159, 165, 167, 192, 289, 448n84, 449n16, 458n91

Chatterji, Sukumar, 49–53, 67, 71, 75–76, 81, 94, 306

Chhophel, Geshe. *See* Gedun Chöpel

China: attitude toward Tibet and Tibetans, 240, 472n10, 472n14; spies in Tibetan monasteries, 229, 231

Chödrak, Geshe, 121, 232

Chokte (Dorje Wangyal), 174, 176–179, 183–184, 186–187, 398–399, 450n31

Chomolhari, 164–165, 167, 192

Clarkstown Country Club. *See* Bernard, Pierre (Perry, P.A.), and Clarkstown Country Club

Columbia University, xiii, 10, 13, 15–16, 18, 20, 22, 24, 27–28, 32, 37–40, 83–84, 113, 279–280, 284, 309, 324–325, 327, 329, 361, 390–391, 402, 408, 430n8, 464n7, 466n23

Crable, Aura, 3, 8, 19, 431–432

Crowley, Aleister, 298

Cutting, Suydam, 141, 144, 159, 182, 237, 264, 266, 429n3, 459n95

Daily Mail (U.K.), xi, 275

Dalai Lama, Fifth, 213, 222–223

Dalai Lama, Fourteenth, 131, 200, 231, 239, 385–386, 395–396, 398, 407, 416

Dalai Lama, Thirteenth, 88, 111, 118, 121, 127, 130–131, 134, 139, 206, 208–214, 218–220, 222, 265, 386, 395, 439n8, 443n30, 451n37, 452n42; arrival in India, 453n44; as Avalokiteśvara, 454n45; modernization initiative, 210–211; prophecy, 212

Dardo Rinpoche, 356

Taring, Rinchen Dolma (Mary) and Jigme, 174–176, 195, 450n22

Tashi Lama. *See* Panchen Lama (Ninth)

Tashilhunpo Monastery, 130–131, 137–138, 211, 234, 266, 414, 417

Tengyur. *See* Tibetan Buddhist canon

Tethong (Shapé/Cabinet Minister), 223, 225, 266, 317

Tharchin, (Gergan) Dorje: activities in Lhasa, 203; and Buddhism, 262; British opinons of, 117; early life, 115–116; espionage for the British, 230–231, 239, 457n78; *Mirror (see Mirror* [newspaper]); relations with Kalimpong missionaries, 261; Tibet, early visits, 116–118, 386, 442n22, 442n26, 443n27, 443n30

Theosophical Society, 36, 49, 104, 108, 326

Tibet: academic study of, 407; and popular American culture, 406; aristocracy and monastic regional houses, 232; army, 117, 181, 213, 231, 446n68, 455n52, 472n14; British invasion (1904), 206, 445n67; British policies toward, 181; Chinese invasion (1950), 384, 445n59; Chinese occupation (1909–12), 130, 206; CIA activities in, 385, 391, 394; cultural similarity with Native Americans, 166, 226; currency exchange problems, 455n50, 456n73; first official contact with U.S. government, 452n41; modernization attempts, 130, 210; mythic image of, xiv; phonograph records from Lhasa, 440n19; political tumoil (1930s), 130, 181, 211, 213; postal system, 182, 261, 450n27; private schools in Lhasa, 206, 452n39; under Chinese governance, 410–416; Unification Party, 214; uprising against Chinese (1959), 395–396

Tibetan Buddhist canon, 42, 223, 241, 248, 414, 445n62; Bernard's copies of, 113–114, 138–139, 148, 217–218, 220, 234, 241, 260, 394; Bernard's

wish to translate, 137, 149, 319–320, 337; copy at Drepung, 249; editing by Sherap Gyatso, 121, 129, 131, 248

Tibetan Cabinet. *See* Kashag

Tibetan Wheel of Life, 94, 145, 305, 353, 464n7, 470n25

Tombstone, AZ, xi–xii, 3–8, 16, 84–85, 329, 381, 430n6, 431n15

Trekang (Shapé/Cabinet Minister), Kalön Lama, 120, 221–222, 266

Trimön (Shapé/Cabinet Minister), 243, 245

Trisam Bridge, 204, 217, 410

Trivikram Swami, 73–74, 82, 91, 107, 461n22

Tsarong, (Lord/Dzasak) Dasang Damdul: and escape of the Fourteenth Dalai Lama, 395–396; and Theos Bernard, 198, 214–215, 217, 228, 233, 235, 241–243, 251, 259, 263, 267, 279, 292, 356; early life, 206–210, 451n37, 452n39, 452n40, 454n48; governmental activities, 249, 396, 455n52; Lhasa estate, 204–206, 215, 216, 232, 249, 413, 451n37; modernization efforts, 210; obituary of, 396–398; photographic pursuits, 235, 262; removal from government, 175, 211; routing of Chinese occupation, 209

Tsarong, Kalön Wangchuk Gyalpo, 209

Tsarong, Lady (Lhacham), 133, 147, 153, 174, 195, 198, 204, 217, 226, 237, 267, 450n30

Tsiang, S. H. William (Chinese envoy to Tibet), 228–229, 266, 458n89

Tucci, Giuseppe, 227, 260, 264, 362, 456n66, 459n94, 462n28

Tucson, AZ, 5–7, 9–10, 84, 274, 282, 284, 310, 329, 344, 381, 402, 408

uḍḍiyāna bandha, 76, 125, 328

University of Arizona, xi, 4–6, 9, 16, 84, 282, 408, 431n10

University of Southern California, 64